INTERNATIONAL REVIEW OF CHILD NEUROLOGY SERIES

HEAD INJURY IN CHILDREN AND ADOLESCENTS

Edited by

Daune L MacGregor

Abhaya V Kulkarni

Peter B Dirks

Peter Rumney

© 2007 Mac Keith Press
30 Furnival Street, London EC4A 1JQ

Editor: Hilary M Hart
Managing Editor: Michael Pountney
Project Manager: Sarah Pearsall

The authors would like to thank Barbara Zimnowodzki for
her assistance with manuscript preparation

First published in this edition 2007

British Library Cataloguing-in-Publication data
A catalogue record for this book is available from the British Library

ISBN: 978 1 898683 50 6

Typeset by Keystroke, 28 High Street, Tettenhall, Wolverhampton

Printed by The Lavenham Press Ltd, Water Street, Lavenham, Suffolk
Mac Keith Press is supported by Scope

INTERNATIONAL REVIEW OF CHILD NEUROLOGY SERIES

HEAD INJURY IN CHILDREN AND ADOLESCENTS

Edited by

DAUNE L MACGREGOR

University of Toronto; Hospital for Sick Children, Toronto, Canada

ABHAYA V KULKARNI

University of Toronto; Hospital for Sick Children, Toronto, Canada

PETER B DIRKS

University of Toronto; Hospital for Sick Children, Toronto, Canada

PETER RUMNEY

University of Toronto; Bloorview Kids Rehab, Toronto, Canada

2007
MAC KEITH PRESS
for the
INTERNATIONAL CHILD NEUROLOGY ASSOCIATION

INTERNATIONAL REVIEW OF CHILD NEUROLOGY SERIES

CONTENTS

AUTHORS' APPOINTMENTS

Kim Bradley	Assistant Professor, University of Toronto, Canada; Speech, Language Pathologist
Helen M Branson	Fellow, Department of Diagnostic Imaging, Hospital for Sick Children, Toronto, Canada
Peter B Dirks	Associate Professor, University of Toronto; Staff Neurosurgeon, Hospital for Sick Children, Toronto, Canada
Trish Geisler	Instructor, Department of Occupational Therapy, University of Toronto; Occupational Therapist, Bloorview Kids Rehab, Toronto, Canada
Anne-Marie Guerguerian	Assistant Professor of Paediatrics and Critical Care Medicine, University of Toronto; Staff, Critical Care Medicine, Hospital for Sick Children, Toronto, Canada
Nicola Hunt	Researcher, Acquired Brain Injury Clinic, Toronto Western Hospital, University Health Network, Toronto, Canada
Jamie Hutchison	Associate Professor of Paediatrics and Critical Care Medicine, University of Toronto; Staff, Critical Care Medicine, Hospital for Sick Children, Toronto, Canada
Babita Kara	Researcher, Acquired Brain Injury Clinic, Toronto Western Hospital, University Health Network, Toronto, Canada
Abhaya V Kulkarni	Assistant Professor of Neurosurgery, University of Toronto; Staff Neurosurgeon, Hospital for Sick Children, Toronto, Canada
Daune L MacGregor	Professor of Paediatrics (Neurology), University of Toronto; Associate Paediatrician-in-Chief, Staff Neurologist, Hospital for Sick Children, Toronto, Canada
Charles Matouk	Research Fellow, Neurosurgery, University of Toronto, Toronto, Canada
Shay Menascu	Consultant in Pediatric Neurology, Edmond and Liliy Safra Children's Hospital, Tel-Aviv, Israel

Erin M Picard   Neuropsychologist, Bloorview Kids Rehab, Toronto, Canada

Rajesh RamachandranNair   Assistant Professor of Paediatrics (Neurology), McMaster University, McMaster Children's Hospital, Ontario, Canada

Maya Kishida Rattray   Speech-Language Pathologist

Peter Rumney   Assistant Professor of Paediatrics, University of Toronto; Staff Paediatrician, Bloorview Kids Rehab, Toronto, Canada

Chanth Seyone   Associate Professor of Psychiatry, University of Toronto; Director, Acquired Brain Injury Clinic, Toronto Western Hospital, University Health Network, Toronto, Canada

Manohar Shroff   Assistant Professor of Radiology, University of Toronto; Staff Neuroradiologist, Department of Diagnostic Imaging, Hospital for Sick Children, Toronto, Canada

Pamela Speed   Special Education Consultant, Toronto District School Board, Toronto, Canada

Mary L Stewart   Psychologist, Child Development Program, Bloorview Kids Rehab, Toronto, Canada

Shelly K Weiss   Assistant Professor of Paediatrics, University of Toronto; Staff Neurologist, Hospital for Sick Children, Toronto, Canada

Janet Woodhouse   Instructor, Department of Occupational Therapy, University of Toronto; Occupational Therapist, Bloorview Kids Rehab, Toronto, Canada

PREFACE

Traumatic brain injury in children and adolescents is a significant epidemiological and health problem in all countries of the world. Severe brain injury forever alters the lives of affected children and their families. What has become clear is that there is also a 'silent epidemic' of mild head injury and that many children – for what is now recognized as the result of individual genetic differences and vulnerabilities or injury characteristics – are at risk for significant long-term cognitive and behavioural disabilities of varying severity. The future will hold promise for children who have had traumatic brain injury – neuroprotective strategies, advanced treatment in neurointensive settings and new rehabilitation approaches will all play a role in reducing disability. Preventive measures – with the regulatory and legislative strength of governments – hold the key to reduction in the incidence of traumatic brain injury.

The authors dedicate this book to all children who have suffered traumatic brain injury. We trust that bringing together the work of the many experts who have contributed to the volume will provide a comprehensive framework for the care needed by children and their families after a traumatic brain injury has occurred.

Daune L MacGregor

1
ACUTE BRAIN INJURY

Charles Matouk and Abhaya V Kulkarni

EPIDEMIOLOGY OF CHILDHOOD BRAIN INJURY

Traumatic injury is the leading cause of death and long-term disability in children of all ages. In Western countries, more children die as the result of trauma than from all childhood diseases combined. Head trauma, in particular, is responsible for as much as 80% of all pediatric trauma-related deaths (Ommaya et al. 2002). A recent report from the National Center for Injury Prevention and Control (2000) estimates that deaths from traumatic brain injury in the pediatric population in the USA are 6, 20 and 38 times greater than those from HIV/AIDS, asthma and cystic fibrosis, respectively. In all, the numbers are staggering: in the USA, more than 3000 deaths, 29,000 hospitalizations and 400,000 emergency department visits each year (National Center for Injury Prevention and Control 2000).

Few population-based studies have sought to define specific incidence, mortality and case-fatality rates of traumatic brain injury in a pediatric population (Reid et al. 2001). Incidence rates of hospital admissions for pediatric traumatic brain injury range from 73.5 to 300 per 100,000 person-years (Kraus et al. 1986, 1987, National Center for Injury Prevention and Control 2000, Reid et al. 2001). Overwhelmingly, these cases comprise concussive syndromes and mild brain injuries. Severe traumatic brain injury in children almost exclusively results from falls and motor vehicle accidents (National Center for Injury Prevention and Control, 2000, Reid et al. 2001). In infants and young children, non-accidental traumatic brain injury ranks second to falls, and is the leading cause of traumatic death (Duhaime et al. 1998). Overall, mortality rates are approximately 10 per 100,000 person-years with the few reported case-fatality rates under 5% (Kraus et al. 1990, Reid et al. 2001). Mortality rates have fallen slightly over the last 20 years, and are not associated with an increased proportion of patients in a persistent vegetative state (Berney et al. 1995, Sosin et al. 1995, Levi et al. 1998). The reasons for improved survival are likely to be multi-factorial and include: (1) improvements in the design of motor vehicles and roadways; (2) increased usage of child safety seats and seat belts for infants and young children, respectively; (3) decreased rates of driving-under-the-influence; (4) better pre-hospital medical care and triage; and (5) technical innovations in critical care medicine (Sosin et al. 1995, Levi et al. 1998, Reid et al. 2001, Pfenninger and Santi 2002, Muszynski et al. 2005). Despite the considerable burden of pediatric trauma-related disability, no population-based outcome studies have been reported (National Center for Injury Prevention and Control 2000).

The epidemiology of pediatric traumatic brain injury differs substantively with age and sex. Numerous reports consistently demonstrate frequency peaks among adolescents and young children (Kraus et al. 1990, National Center for Injury Prevention and Control 2000, Reid et al. 2001). It is interesting that these age strata are generally characterized as developmental periods when physical abilities exceed the experience of the person. Mechanisms of injury and overall outcomes differ between age groups as well (National Center for Injury Prevention and Control 2000, Ommaya et al. 2002). In one large series of pediatric head trauma, Berney and colleagues (1995) concluded that infants and young children sustain more low-energy impacts (for example, falls from a low height), skull fractures and less neurological morbidity than older children. Children over the age of 9 years and adolescents behave in a similar way to adults, suffering more high-impact injuries (for example, motor vehicle accidents and higher falls) and correspondingly more severe traumatic brain injuries (Berney et al. 1994a, 1994b). Poor admission Glasgow Coma Scale (GCS) scores and younger age are poor prognostic factors in moderate and severe pediatric closed head injury (Benz et al. 1999, Morrison et al. 2004). Males are consistently found to be at higher risk for traumatic brain injury, a discrepancy accentuated with the increasing age of the child (Barancik et al. 1986, Kraus et al. 1987, Kraus et al. 1990, National Center for Injury Prevention and Control 2000, Gaines et al. 2004). This may reflect a predilection for risky behaviours, especially among adolescent males.

DIFFUSE AXONAL INJURY

First described nearly 50 years ago, the most important pathological correlate of severe accidental traumatic brain injury is diffuse axonal injury (DAI) (Strich 1956). Unlike the damage incurred by an intracranial space-occupying lesion, the damage in DAI is microscopic, often radiographically occult and widespread, affecting large regions of the cerebral hemispheres, brain stem and cerebellum (Meythaler et al. 2001). DAI is documented in over 20% of children who die from traumatic brain injury (Adams et al. 1989a, 1989b, Graham et al. 1989a). In survivors, the physical, medical, neurobehavioural and emotional sequelae can be devastating and lifelong. Currently, no specific therapies exist for the treatment of DAI, and results from recent clinical trials have been uniformly disappointing (Bullock et al. 1999). The success of childhood injury prevention initiatives and management of severe traumatic brain injury is in large part dependent on a better understanding of this complex pathophysiological condition. This section reviews the epidemiology, clinico-radiological characteristics and pathophysiological underpinnings of pediatric DAI. Non-accidental severe traumatic brain injury in infants and young children, the so-called 'shaken-baby syndrome', represents a distinct clinicopathological syndrome and is discussed separately at the end of this chapter.

EPIDEMIOLOGY OF DIFFUSE AXONAL INJURY

A minority (less than 1%) of all pediatric head trauma is considered severe (Levi et al. 1998, National Center for Injury Prevention and Control 2000). It is this relatively small proportion of cases that results in the most disability and nearly all mortality associated with pediatric traumatic brain injury. All cases result from violent forces and, in the pediatric population, are almost exclusively associated with motor vehicle accidents and falls (National Center for Injury Prevention and Control 2000, Ommaya et al. 2002). Violent collisions during sporting activities account for a small number of cases. Despite improvements in overall mortality from severe traumatic brain injury, the number of children referred to hospitals for acute management is increasing. Often, these children are more severely ill, require prolonged hospitalizations and present with a greater incidence of concomitant serious injuries, especially to the chest and face (Levi et al. 1998).

CLINICORADIOLOGICAL CHARACTERISTICS OF DIFFUSE AXONAL INJURY

DAI is a pathological diagnosis that can only be established at autopsy (Adams et al. 1989b). Nevertheless, it is often associated with a stereotypical clinicoradiological syndrome. Most frequently, patients with DAI present with coma of immediate onset after a motor vehicle accident, fall from significant height or, less commonly, violent collision during sporting activities (Meythaler et al. 2001). The clinical association of immediate loss of consciousness without an intervening lucid interval and appropriate mechanism of injury should immediately alert the clinician to the diagnosis. Early neuroimaging is essential to exclude neurosurgically accessible intracranial hematomas. Normal or near-normal initial neuroimaging all but confirms the diagnosis of DAI. In approximately 10% of patients with severe traumatic brain injury, CT and MR imaging demonstrate classical punctate, hemorrhagic lesions in the corpus callosum, grey–white matter interface of the cerebral hemispheres and ponto-mesencephalic junction (Meythaler et al. 2001). It is important to note that the degree of cortical contusion is not well correlated with outcome (Chiaretti et al. 1998, Tong et al. 2003, 2004). Admission Glasgow Coma Scale score is the most consistently reported predictor of poor outcome in pediatric DAI and is likely to reflect damage to the rostral brain stem, reticular activating system and other critical midline structures including the thalamus (Chiaretti et al. 1998, Meythaler et al. 2001, Campbell et al. 2004).

PATHOPHYSIOLOGY OF DIFFUSE AXONAL INJURY

The biomechanical forces required to produce DAI are well understood (Ommaya et al. 2002). Dynamic, impulsive forces result in acceleration–deceleration momentums with the brain moving relative to the skull. More important, perhaps, is the rotational (angular) component of acceleration producing differential displacements of adjacent brain layers and the characteristic shearing injuries of DAI. A great amount of force is required to reproduce these injury patterns in an experimental setting.

The term DAI is a misnomer. While the microscopic histopathological changes are certainly widespread, they do not occur randomly throughout the brain, but rather have a predilection for discrete anatomical sites. These include the corpus callosum, grey–white interface of the cerebral hemispheres, basal ganglia, rostral brain stem and superior cerebellar peduncles (Adams et al. 1989a, 1989b, Graham et al. 1989b, Meythaler et al. 2001). The multifocal (in contradistinction to diffuse) nature of the injuries is reflected in the increased use of the term *traumatic axonal injury* as a more appropriate descriptor (Meythaler et al. 2001).

The histopathology is characterized by Wallerian-type axonal degeneration which results from disruption of neurofilament subunits of the axonal cytoskeleton, damage to internal organelles and loss of membrane integrity. In severe traumatic brain injury, especially injuries resulting from high-speed traffic accidents, multiple mechanisms contribute to the brain pathology in addition to DAI, including cerebral contusion, vascular dissection, compromised cerebrovascular autoregulation and hypoxia-ischemia (Graham et al. 1989b, Meythaler et al. 2001). Their relative contribution to malignant cerebral edema of childhood and overall patient outcome is currently unclear. Two additional points deserve special mention. First, patterns of DAI that result from motor vehicle accidents and falls are similar in children and adults (Adams et al. 1989a, 1989b, Graham et al. 1989b). Second, the forces and injuries incurred as part of the 'shaken-baby syndrome' are markedly different, and constitute a distinct clinicopathological syndrome (Duhaime et al. 1998, Geddes et al. 2001b).

TRAUMATIC HEMATOMAS
Post-traumatic Hematoma
In contradistinction to head injury in adults, post-traumatic intracranial hematomas are decidedly uncommon in the pediatric population. Notwithstanding, they may be incurred after relatively trivial impacts and result in severe secondary cerebral injury if left untreated (Nelson et al. 1984). The pattern of post-traumatic hematomas varies significantly with the age of the pediatric patient. As a general rule, extra-axial hematomas are much more common than post-traumatic intracerebral hemorrhages. In neonates and young infants, acute subdural hematomas predominate. In toddlers and young children, extradural hematomas comprise the majority of post-traumatic hematomas. In older children and teenagers, the pattern of post-traumatic hematomas more closely reflects that seen in young adults with a higher proportion of intracerebral hematomas (Berney et al. 1994a, 1994b). This section reviews the clinical presentation and pathophysiology of the most common pediatric post-traumatic (accidental) hematomas: epidural, subdural and intracerebral.

Extradural Hematoma
Extradural hematomas complicate a small minority of pediatric head injuries (2 to 3%), but represent the major post-traumatic intracranial hematoma in toddlers

and young children (Nelson et al. 1984, Weber 1984, Moore and Persaud 1998, Sinnatamby 1999). They are rarely encountered in infants and neonates, in whom child abuse must be strongly suspected. An overlying linear skull fracture and sub-galeal hematoma are frequent accompaniments of pediatric extradural hematomas, but their presence is not invariable. Most frequently located in temporo-parietal regions, epidural hematomas result from a stripping away of the dura after a skull impact. Blood accumulates in the epidural space as a result of torn branches of the middle meningeal artery, disruption of osseous emissary veins or multiple dural bleeders (Nelson et al. 1984). Rarely, in posterior fossa extradural hematomas resulting from an occipital blow, violation of a venous sinus is the source of extra-dural hemorrhage. These latter lesions may result in precipitous and catastrophic neurological decline, and always warrant strong consideration for urgent surgical evacuation (Weber 1985, 1987).

On CT imaging, the classical lentiform shape of extradural hematomas reflects the confinement of hemorrhage by firm attachment of the dura at bony sutures. Clinically, a 'lucid interval' after a brief loss of consciousness followed by irritability, vomiting and increasing lethargy is often cited in pediatric patients with epidural hematomas. Notwithstanding, the clinical presentation is highly variable, and often non-specific. Definitive CT imaging must always be performed in a child who has sustained even a relatively minor head injury who does not continue to improve over the first 24 to 48 hours (Nelson et al. 1984). Because extradural hematomas often result from low-velocity skull impacts, underlying focal or diffuse parenchymal brain injury is typically not severe at presentation. With appropriate neurosurgical management, patients enjoy excellent neurological outcomes.

POST-TRAUMATIC (ACCIDENTAL) ACUTE SUBDURAL HEMATOMA

Acute subdural hematomas are the most common post-traumatic hematoma in neonates and young infants (Nelson et al. 1984, Berney et al. 1994a, 1994b). Especially in this age group, the treating clinician must always consider the possibility of child abuse. These cases represent a distinct clinicoradiological syn-drome, and will be discussed separately at the end of this chapter. In all pediatric age groups, accidental acute subdural hematomas result from violent forces, and often present in dramatic fashion with seizures, focal neurological deficits and a decreasing level of consciousness. Emergency surgical evacuation is mandatory for lesions with significant mass effect. Unfortunately, good neurological recovery is uncertain. Acute subdural hematomas result from disruption of convexity bridging veins, most commonly in parieto-occipital regions, with accumulation of blood in the subdural space (Berney et al. 1994a, 1994b). Even when subdural hematomas are very small in size and unlikely to cause significant mass effect, they are indicators of a severe cerebral injury and an attendant poor neurological prognosis.

POST-TRAUMATIC INTRACEREBRAL HEMATOMA

Intracerebral hematomas are the least common post-traumatic hematoma in the pediatric population (Nelson et al. 1984, Berney et al. 1994a, 1994b). They are most frequently observed in older children and teenagers as the result of violent forces, for example, motor vehicle accidents and falls from a great height. Often, the clinical picture of a severe closed head injury, i.e. diffuse axonal injury, dominates the child's presentation, and the presence of a substantive intracerebral hematoma is an unexpected finding on CT imaging. Frontal and temporal lobes are the predominant sites of intracerebral hemorrhage, and likely reflect local trauma to the brain against the uneven anterior cranial fossa floor and sphenoid ridge, respectively (Nelson et al. 1984).

Two general patterns of intracerebral hematoma may be discerned. Multiple, superficial cortical contusions result from rotational and shearing forces on the brain. These hemorrhagic foci may coalesce over hours and days to form the classical 'gliding contusions' characteristic of diffuse axonal injury. A local skull impact, alternatively, may result in a more focal, discrete intracerebral hematoma. These latter lesions are often associated with depressed skull fractures and penetrating injuries. Rarely, deep hemorrhagic lesions are observed in severe closed head injury, and likely result from disruption of penetrating vessels by severe transmitted forces through the substance of the brain (Nelson et al. 1984). The neurological recovery from traumatic intracerebral hematoma is frequently dependent on the overall severity of the concomitant diffuse axonal injury.

SKULL FRACTURES

Skull fractures frequently accompany both mild and severe traumatic brain injury in infants and children of all ages. A large, population-based study in Olmsted County, Minnesota, revealed that approximately 30% of head trauma is associated with skull fracture and an overall incidence rate of 44.3 per 100,000 person-years (Nelson et al. 1984). In infants and young children, the age-specific incidence is even higher (Nelson et al. 1984, National Center for Injury Prevention and Control 2000). The majority of skull fractures are simple linear fractures that heal spontaneously without neurological sequelae (Berney et al. 1994a, 1994b). Importantly, however, they serve as clinicoradiological indicators that confirm the diagnosis of head trauma and suggest the potential for more sinister intracranial pathology. Other less common fracture types occur almost exclusively in the pediatric population, and mandate urgent neurosurgical intervention to prevent severe neurological morbidity. This section will review distinguishing features of the pediatric skull and classification of pediatric skull fractures.

THE PEDIATRIC SKULL – WORK IN PROGRESS

The pediatric skull is substantively different from its adult counterpart. These special characteristics are important to keep in mind during the evaluation and management of skull fractures in children, especially the very young. Unlike the adult cranial vault, the bones of the pediatric skull do not interdigitate in sutures, but rather are attached by fibrous tissue. At their corners, these fibrous unions are known as fontanelles (Sinnatamby 1999). This discontinuity of the cranial vault, important in moulding of the fetal skull during birth and accommodation of the rapidly growing postnatal brain, limits its capacity to disperse an impact force, thereby increasing the probability of focal deformation and fracture (Moore and Persaud 1998, Ommaya et al. 2002). This anatomical circumstance is exacerbated by the much thinner calvarium of infants and young children. Indeed, the skull increases modestly in size between the ages of 16 and 20 years as the result of bone thickening prior to assuming its adult configuration (Moore and Persaud 1998). Biomechanical studies confirm that skull failure stress (the point at which the skull fails mechanically under external pressure) in the adult may be as much as eleven times greater than in the neonate (Ommaya et al. 2002). The clinical correlate of these anatomical and biomechanical characteristics is that linear skull fractures do occur in infants with low-energy impacts such as falls off a table or from a caregiver's arms (Weber 1984, 1985, 1987). This observation does not imply that significant intracranial pathology cannot ensue in the absence of skull fracture. The much greater elasticity of the pediatric skull permits deformation and the propagation of substantial impact forces to the brain (Ommaya et al. 2002).

CLASSIFICATION AND PATHOGENESIS OF PEDIATRIC SKULL FRACTURES

Pediatric skull fractures are classified as linear, basilar, depressed, growing and compound. Each of these pediatric skull fracture patterns is briefly reviewed.

Linear skull fractures are simple fractures that extend through the entire thickness of bone – cortex to cortex. Linear skull fractures are generally of little clinical significance other than that they confirm the diagnosis of head trauma. Sometimes asymptomatic, they are associated with the entire spectrum of traumatic brain injury from mild to severe. Clinical circumstances and anatomical location dictate the probability of potential complications. For example, infants and young children with simple linear skull fractures and an associated cephalhematoma may become anemic from extensive blood loss. Fractures extending through vascular channels in the skull may cause an underlying epidural hematoma. Traumatic venous sinus thrombosis in association with an overlying linear fracture has rarely been reported in the literature. Splayed sutures have the same clinical significance as linear skull fractures in infants and young children (Nelson et al. 1984).

Basilar skull fractures are linear fractures involving the bones at the base of the skull. These fractures are further subdivided by anatomical location: anterior skull base, temporal bone and occipital condyle. Fractures of this type require large impact forces and confirm suspicions of a serious blow to the head. Often associated with dural tears, the treating clinician must remain alert to the possibility of a cerebrospinal fluid (CSF) leak and its complications – meningitis and cerebral abscess formation. Multiple cranial nerve palsies are also well documented (Yildirim et al. 2005). Temporal bone fractures may be associated with disruption of the contents of the middle ear resulting in vertigo and hearing loss. Bruising over the mastoids (Battle's sign) and hemotypanum are often present (Lee et al. 1998). Occipital condylar fractures, especially those resulting from forced rotation and lateral bending, may be associated with occipito-cervical instability (Tuli et al. 1997, Neeman and Bloom 2003).

Depressed skull fractures result from focal, high-energy impacts to the skull. By definition, the outer table of at least one of the fracture edges must lie below the level of the inner table of the surrounding intact skull (Ersahin et al. 2000). In neonates and young infants, a special type of depressed skull fracture is observed: the 'ping-pong' fracture. It results from a focal indentation of skull bone, typically in the frontal and parietal regions, without a definite break in the bony cortex. Ping-pong fractures are the equivalent to orthopedic 'green stick' fractures and most commonly result from deformation of the soft neonatal skull against the mother's sacral promontory during uterine contractions or the application of forceps during delivery (Dupuis et al. 2005).

Growing skull fractures are a rare but well recognized complication of head trauma in the pediatric population. Variably called post-traumatic leptomeningeal cyst, meningocele spuria, traumatic ventricular cyst and craniocerebral erosion, growing skull fractures are characterized by progressive diastatic enlargement of the fracture line (Ersahin and Gulmen 1998, Ersahin et al. 2000). Without treatment, they are responsible for significant neurological morbidity including paralysis, seizures and headache. Three elements are required for the development of a growing skull fracture: a widely diastatic linear fracture (> 4 mm), underlying dural tear and intracranial expansive force (most commonly, the rapidly growing brain of a young child) (Lende and Erickson 1961, Lende 1974). Growth of the skull fracture over time is likely related primarily to bony erosion of the skull fracture edges by the constant pulsations of the underlying brain. Indeed, the diastatic fracture often behaves as a 'neosuture' resulting in asymmetrical expansion of the pediatric skull (Drapkin 2006). An underlying porencephalic cyst and/or cystic encephalomalacia are often observed and also likely result from misdirection of cerebral pulsations onto the surface of the brain. In extreme cases, the pathology is sometimes referred to as a *cranial burst fracture* and implies extracranial extrusion of brain tissue underneath an intact scalp (Ellis et al. 2000). These injuries require prompt recognition and neurosurgical intervention to prevent increased neurological morbidity.

Any of these fracture types may be associated with an overlying scalp defect. These *compound skull fractures* constitute a neurosurgical emergency to minimize the risk of intracranial infections.

CONCUSSION IN SPORT

The potential for concussion to adversely impact on the normal cognitive, behavioural and social development of children is generating increased concern among parents, sporting associations and the medical community. This is reflected by a sharp increase in the number of medical publications citing 'sports' and 'concussion' over the last ten years. Despite recent consensus guidelines for the management of sport-related concussion in adults (Quality Standards Committee 1997, Aubry et al. 2002, McCrory et al. 2004), few pragmatic guidelines exist to alert clinicians to important differences in the management of childhood concussion (Committee on Quality Improvement 1999, Davis and McCrory 2005). In this section, the definition, classification and pathophysiology of sport-related concussion are reviewed. When appropriate, features particular to childhood concussion are highlighted.

EPIDEMIOLOGY OF CONCUSSION IN CHILDREN

Data from well controlled studies are lacking to estimate the incidence, age-specific frequencies and outcome of sport-related concussion in children (McCrory et al. 2004). Mild brain injuries comprise the majority (approximately 85%) of pediatric traumatic brain injuries, many of which are incurred during amateur or recreational sporting activities (Yeates et al. 1999, McCrory et al. 2004). In one large secondary analysis of emergency department visits in the National Hospital Ambulatory Medical Care Survey (NHAMCS) for the years 1998–2000, bicycle and sports accidents together comprised the largest cause (26.4%) of mild traumatic brain injury in children aged 5 to 14 years (Bazarian et al. 2005). These results are particularly concerning given that a large percentage of student athletes underreport concussion for a myriad of reasons, including underestimating the seriousness of the injury, fear of suspension from competition and general lack of awareness of probable concussion (McCrea et al. 2004).

THE VIENNA STATEMENT (2001) – A REVISED DEFINITION OF CONCUSSION

The definition of concussion remains contentious (Johnston et al. 2001). The first modern description of concussion is attributed to the great Arabic physician, Rhazes, in the tenth century, who postulated a perturbed physiological state rather than structural brain injury as most characteristic of the concussed state (McCrory and Berkovic 2001). This understanding is reflected in the consensus definition proposed by the Committee of Head Injury Nomenclature of the Congress of Neurological Surgeons (CNS) in 1966 (CNS 1966). Although this definition was an important step forward, it failed to account for many of the common symptoms of concussion (Aubry et al. 2002, McCrory et al. 2005). More recently, increased confusion has arisen from the colloquial usage of the term 'concussion' and euphemisms like 'ding' to refer to almost any brain injury incurred during sport. The popularity of the Glasgow Coma Scale (GCS) in the prognostication of severe traumatic brain injury

TABLE 1.1
The Vienna Statement

Definition: Sports concussion is defined as a complex pathophysiological process affecting the brain, induced by traumatic biomechanical forces.

Shared clinical, pathological and biomechanical injury characteristics help define the concussive head injury:

1 Concussion may be caused by a direct blow to the head, face, neck or elsewhere on the body with "impulsive" force transmitted to the head.
2 Concussion typically results in the rapid onset of short-lived impairment of neurological function that resolves spontaneously.
3 Concussion may result in neuropathological changes, but the acute clinical symptoms largely reflect a functional disturbance rather than structural injury.
4 Concussion results in a graded set of clinical syndromes that may or may not involve loss of consciousness. Resolution of the clinical and cognitive symptoms typically follows a sequential course.
5 Concussion is typically associated with grossly normal structural neuroimaging studies.
6 Post-concussive symptoms may be prolonged or persistent.

---

has introduced the term 'mild brain injury' into the general medical lexicon, further obscuring the definition of concussion (Jennett and Bond 1975, Johnston et al. 2001). To address these concerns, a revised definition of concussion was proposed at the first International Conference on Concussion in Sport (Vienna, 2001). It defines sports concussion as 'a complex pathophysiological process affecting the brain, induced by traumatic biomechanical forces'. Several common clinical, pathological and biomechanical injury characteristics help define concussive head injury, and are summarized in Table 1.1 (Aubry et al. 2002). Although specific consideration of childhood concussion is lacking, the revised definition of concussion in the Vienna Statement enjoys widespread support (Aubry et al. 2002, McCrory et al. 2004, 2005).

THE PRAGUE STATEMENT (2004) – A SIMPLIFIED CLASSIFICATION OF CONCUSSION IN SPORT

A major development of the Vienna Group was the recommendation to abandon the more than 25 published injury-grading scales in the assessment of the concussed athlete (Aubry et al. 2002, Bazarian et al. 2005). This philosophical shift reflects the emerging consensus that concussion severity is a determination that can only be made in retrospect after complete resolution of neurological sequelae (McCrory et al. 2005). In their place, the Prague Group proposed a simplified, binary classification of concussion in sport, emphasizing its utility in the management of injured athletes (McCrory et al. 2005). A 'simple concussion' gradually resolves over a period of 7 to 10 days without untoward or persistent neurological consequences. A 'complex concussion' is characterized by persistent symptoms, prolonged loss of consciousness (more than one minute), convulsive or motor phenomena, or a history of multiple concussions over time (McCrory et al. 2005). Athletes with simple concussion do not need to be aggressively investigated, and generally return to play after symptom resolution. In this majority subset of injured children, the risk of clinically significant intracranial pathology is exceedingly low (approximately 0.02%) (Committee on Quality Improvement 1999, Davis and McCrory 2005). Athletes with complex concussion, however, warrant neuroimaging and formal neuropsychological testing to exclude serious intracranial pathology and guide return-to-play decisions (McCrory et al. 2005).

The general applicability of this classification schema in the management of pediatric concussion has not been verified, and there remains significant heterogeneity, even amongst experts, in the diagnosis and management of childhood sport-related concussion (Davis and McCrory 2005). The Prague Group classification of concussion in sport fails to account for important biomechanical and pathophysiological features that distinguish pediatric and adult concussion (McCrory et al. 2004).

PATHOPHYSIOLOGY OF CONCUSSION – CHILDREN ARE NOT LITTLE ADULTS

Although its pathophysiological substrate is incompletely understood, concussion is generally thought to reflect a transient or functional perturbation in neuronal function (McCrory and Berkovic 2001). In experimental models, this is accompanied by alterations in metabolic, neurotransmitter and ionic neuronal parameters (McCrory et al. 2001). Whether a concomitant structural injury accompanies these physiological perturbations is a longstanding controversy that remains unresolved. The increased availability and usage of more sensitive neuroimaging modalities (diffusion-weighted and functional MR imaging) and comprehensive neuropsychological assessments in the evaluation of the concussed athlete may provide novel insights (Kushner 2002, Jantzen et al. 2004).

Regardless of its precise pathophysiological basis, concussion in sport results from the application of acceleration–deceleration forces to the moving brain (McCrory et al. 2001). The effects of rotational acceleration are likely to be particularly deleterious as they result in shearing forces and distortion of neural structures (McCrory et al. 2001, Ommaya et al. 2002). This mechanism is likely to be responsible for concussion in sport across all age groups.

The adage, 'Children are not little adults', has received increased attention in concussion management and guideline development (McCrory et al. 2004, 2005). Despite similar concussive symptomatology and neurocognitive sequelae, important developmental and biomechanical characteristics distinguish pediatric concussive head injuries and must be considered in their management (McCrory et al. 2004). First, the repercussions of even a single, simple concussion on the developing brain are currently not known, but have the potential to adversely impact a child's scholastic, social and behavioural development with longstanding consequences. Second, poor neuropsychological outcomes from pediatric concussive head injury may be masked by the continued cognitive growth of the child. This often confounds meaningful interpretation of serial neuropsychological evaluations (McCrory et al. 2004). Third, it is now well appreciated that a substantively greater force is required to produce similar concussive symptoms in an injured child compared with an adult, and this should alert the treating clinician to a potentially more serious injury (Holbourn 1943, Ommaya et al. 2002, McCrory et al. 2004). Fourth, a rare but potentially disastrous clinical syndrome of impaired cerebral autoregulation, diffuse cerebral swelling and subsequent brain stem herniation and death has been described almost exclusively in children and adolescents. Because this injury pattern was traditionally associated with repeated mild head injuries over a short period of time, it is often referred to as the 'second impact syndrome'. Whether repetitive mild head injuries predispose to this condition is currently contested, but it more likely represents an idiosyncratic reaction to a head injury of any severity (McCrory and Berkovic 1998, McCrory et al. 2004). Support for this view comes from recent genetic studies implicating the *CACNA1A* calcium channel subunit gene in delayed cerebral edema after mild brain injury (Kors et al. 2001). Finally, to date, no pragmatic consensus guidelines have been developed for the management of childhood sport-related concussion (McCrory et al. 2004, 2005). Until such time, a conservative management strategy is warranted to minimize the risk of potentially catastrophic neurological outcomes.

NON-ACCIDENTAL TRAUMATIC BRAIN INJURY IN INFANTS – THE SHAKING-IMPACT SYNDROME

An unfortunate peculiarity in the evaluation of pediatric head trauma is the high frequency of non-accidental or inflicted traumatic brain injury in infants and young children. All those involved in the evaluation of pediatric trauma must be aware of the shaking-impact syndrome and its potentially dire consequences. This section will review its epidemiology, clinicoradiological definition and pathophysiology.

EPIDEMIOLOGY OF NON-ACCIDENTAL TRAUMATIC BRAIN INJURY

Non-accidental head injury is the single leading cause of traumatic death in infancy (Billmire and Myers 1985, Overpeck et al. 1998). In young children, it is the leading cause of serious head injury (Duhaime et al. 1998). In one early series, approximately 80% of head trauma-related deaths in infants and young children (less than 2 years old) resulted from child abuse (Bruce and Zimmerman 1989). Even among survivors, developmental and neurologic morbidity is severe (Duhaime et al. 1996, Barlow et al. 2004). The adverse emotional, economic and societal costs cannot be overstated (Duhaime et al. 1998, Ettaro et al. 2004).

A recent population-based study in infants and young children in North Carolina revealed an incidence of inflicted traumatic brain injury of 17.0 per 100,000 person-years. Incidence rates of 29.7 and 3.8 per 100,000 person-years were reported for infants and children older than 12 months, respectively (Keenan et al. 2003), consistent with previous reports documenting the most at risk as the very young (Duhaime et al. 1987, Hadley et al. 1989, Overpeck et al. 1998, Barlow and Minns 2000). Specific risk factors for infant homicide have been reported and include early age at childbearing (17 to 19 years old), fewer years of completed education, lack of prenatal care, and preterm birth or disability of the newborn (Klein and Stern 1971, Duhaime et al. 1998, Overpeck et al. 1998). Male perpetrators (fathers, step-fathers and mother's boyfriends) are responsible for approximately 60% of all cases of inflicted traumatic brain injury. Female babysitters and mothers account for a disturbing number of cases (17.3 and 12.6%, respectively) (Starling et al. 1995).

A COMPLEX CLINICORADIOLOGICAL DIAGNOSIS MANDATES A MULTI-DISCIPLINARY APPROACH

Although no single feature is pathognomonic, the constellation of clinical and radio-logical signs is unique to the shaking-impact syndrome of inflicted traumatic brain injury in infancy. A clinical history that is vague, changes over time or is inconsistent with the developmental stage of the infant must immediately alert the clinician to the diagnosis (Duhaime et al. 1998). Neurological examination of the abused infant typically demonstrates the tell-tale signs of raised intracranial pressure: lethargy, irritability, vomiting, poor feeding, breathing abnormalities, a full fontanelle, splayed sutures, opisthotonus, sixth nerve palsy and seizures. Approximately half of all patients will have severe neurological impairment and are unresponsive or moribund at the time of first evaluation (Hahn et al. 1983, Duhaime et al. 1998, King et al. 2003).

CT imaging of the brain is the cornerstone in the diagnosis of inflicted trau-matic brain injury in infants and young children (Duhaime et al. 1998). In nearly all cases, subdural hemorrhage (acute, chronic or acute-on-chronic) is documented over the cerebral convexities. Rarely massive, these subdural collections are, however, extensive and often bilateral. A predilection for subdural blood to collect in the posterior interhemispheric fissure and along the tentorium is well documented (Merten et al. 1984). Although brain contusions are sometimes observed, much more common is the association of subdural hemorrhage with unilateral or bilateral cerebral hypodensity and profound loss of grey–white differentiation (Han et al. 1989, Duhaime et al. 1998). These neuroimaging features may only be evident a few days after injury in severely compromised children, and portend a poor neuro-logical outcome (Han et al. 1990). The presence of subarachnoid blood frequently accompanies overlying calvarial fractures most commonly observed in occipital and parieto-occipital regions. Epidural hemorrhage is exceedingly rare in this patient population, and may be related to the lack of large arteries in these regions and the firm adherence of the dura to the infant skull (Geddes et al. 2001a, 2001b).

The utility of other neuroimaging modalities in the evaluation of traumatic inflicted brain injury is less certain. Skull x-rays may be more sensitive than CT scans in the detection of skull fractures (Duhaime et al. 1998). MR imaging is useful in equivocal cases of suspected abuse for the characterization of small, posterior fossa subdural hemorrhages, the residua of previous bleeds and shear parenchymal hemorrhages (gliding contusions) (Petitti and Williams 1998, Demaerel et al. 2002).

In addition to a dedicated clinical and radiological evaluation of the child's central nervous system, a detailed examination of the infant by a multi-disciplinary team is essential for the accurate and timely diagnosis of the shaking-impact syndrome. A systematic search for past or present evidence of soft tissue and musculoskeletal injuries is mandatory. This includes a complete skeletal survey and may include a radionuclide bone scan. Multiple posterior or lateral rib fractures and metaphyseal fractures are particularly suggestive of the diagnosis. Extracranial abnormalities are documented in 30 to 70% of all cases (Merten et al. 1984, Duhaime et al. 1998). A dilated fundoscopic examination by an ophthalmologist reveals posterior segment (retinal) hemorrhages in as many as 65 to 95% of abused infants (Duhaime et al. 1998, Becker and Gupta 1999). Early involvement of pediatricians and pediatric intensivists is important to exclude bleeding diatheses and rare metabolic syndromes (osteogenesis imperfecta, Menkes kinky hair syndrome, glutaric aciduria type I) that may mimic inflicted traumatic brain injury, as well as to treat concomitant cardiorespiratory, biochemical and hematological abnormalities (Hartley et al. 2001, Ganesh et al. 2004). At the Hospital for Sick Children in Toronto, a multi-disciplinary SCAN (Suspected Child Abuse and Neglect) program is activated when child abuse is suspected and serves as an important liaison with the Children's Aid Society and legal authorities.

THE PATHOPHYSIOLOGY OF NON-ACCIDENTAL TRAUMATIC BRAIN INJURY – 'SHAKEN-BABY SYNDROME' OR 'SHAKING-IMPACT SYNDROME'

Since the initial description of the 'whiplash shaken-baby syndrome' by Caffey (1974), controversy has surrounded the type and magnitude of biomechanical forces required to cause such extensive damage to the infant brain (Caffey 1974, Duhaime et al. 1998). Most experts agree that shearing rotational forces (in contradistinction to translational forces) are required to produce the constellation of severe intracranial pathology observed in infants and young children with inflicted traumatic brain injury. This solitary observation has profound medico-legal implications as it underscores the improbability of incurring such a catastrophic injury from simple falls in the home or at play (Duhaime et al. 1998, Ommaya et al. 2002). These latter types of injuries, characterized by predominantly translational forces, are usually trivial. More controversial is whether the magnitude of rotational forces generated by shaking alone is sufficient to account for the severe intracranial injuries. In the vast majority of cases, evidence of blunt head trauma is documented, and likely to be required, to produce the so-called 'shaken-baby syndrome' (Duhaime at al. 1987, 1998, Geddes et al. 2001a, 2001b). This clinical observation is supported by several biomechanical studies in rats (Smith et al. 1998), rhesus monkeys (Ommaya et al. 2002) and an anthropomorphic surrogate infant 'dummy' model (Duhaime et al. 1987). These experiments clearly demonstrate the greatly increased magnitude of angular deceleration and relative ease of subdural hemorrhaging when the head suddenly stops on impact with a solid surface. Whether some cases of inflicted traumatic brain injury result from shaking alone remains controversial, but these are likely to represent a minority of cases and require extremely violent, repetitive shaking. Accordingly, some authors have proposed the term 'shaking-impact syndrome' to more accurately reflect the biomechanical forces most responsible for the condition (Bruce and Zimmerman 1989, Duhaime et al. 1998).

To date, very few studies have specifically investigated the neuropathological findings in severe inflicted traumatic brain injury (Vowles et al. 1987, Hadley et al. 1989, Gleckman et al. 1999). In a recent series, Geddes and colleagues made the following two important observations (Geddes et al. 2001a, 2001b). First, microscopic evidence of global neuronal hypoxia-ischemia accompanied by macroscopic swelling of the brain and clinical stigmata of raised intracranial pressure represents the typical clinicopathological condition of infants and young children who die from inflicted traumatic brain injury. Second, histopathological criteria of diffuse axonal injury are lacking in the overwhelming majority of cases. These findings underscore the contribution of prolonged hypoxia as a fundamental determinant of injury severity. This view is consistent with frequent reports of apnea in cases of inflicted traumatic brain injury that may result from a stretching of the neuraxis and damage to the lower brain stem and upper cervical cord (Johnson et al. 1995, Dumaine et al. 1998). Future studies are required to determine the relative contributions of reactive hyperemia, vascular occlusion, seizure activity and mechanical trauma in the pathogenesis of this unfortunate and complex clinical entity (Duhaime et al. 1998).

REFERENCES

Adams JH, Doyle D, Ford I, Graham DI, McGee M, McLellan DR (1989a) Brain damage in fatal non-missile head injury in relation to age and type of injury. *Scott Med J* 34: 399–401.

Adams JH, Doyle D, Ford I, Gennarelli TA, Graham DI, McLellan DR (1989b) Diffuse axonal injury in head injury: definition, diagnosis and grading. *Histopathology* 15: 49–59.

Aubry M, Cantu R, Dvorak J, Graf-Baumann T, Johnston K, Kelly J, Lovell M, McCrory P, Meeuwisse W, Schamasch P (2002) Summary and agreement statement of the First International Conference on Concussion in Sport, Vienna 2001. Recommendations for the improvement of safety and health of athletes who may suffer concussive injuries. *Br J Sports Med* 36: 6–10.

Barancik JI, Chatterjee BF, Greene-Cradden YC, Michenzi EM, Kramer CF, Thode HC Jr, Fife D (1986) Motor vehicle trauma in northeastern Ohio. I: Incidence and outcome by age, sex, and road-use category. *Am J Epidemiol* 123: 846–861.

Barlow KM, Minns RA (2000) Annual incidence of shaken impact syndrome in young children. *Lancet* 356: 1571–1572.

Barlow K, Thompson E, Johnson D, Minns RA (2004) The neurological outcome of non-accidental head injury. *Pediatr Rehabil* 7: 195–203.

Bazarian JJ, McClung J, Shah MN, Cheng YT, Flesher W, Kraus J (2005) Mild traumatic brain injury in the United States, 1998–2000. *Brain Inj* 19: 85–91.

Becker H, Gupta BK (1999) Recognizing abusive head trauma in children. *JAMA* 282: 1421. (Author reply: 1422.)

Benz B, Ritz A, Kiesow S (1999) Influence of age-related factors on long-term outcome after traumatic brain injury (TBI) in children: a review of recent literature and some preliminary findings. *Restor Neurol Neurosci* 14: 135–141.

Berney J, Favier J, Froidevaux AC (1994a) Paediatric head trauma: influence of age and sex. I. Epidemiology. *Childs Nerv Syst* 10: 509–516.

Berney J, Froidevaux AC, Favier J (1994b) Paediatric head trauma: influence of age and sex. II. Biomechanical and anatomo-clinical correlations. *Childs Nerv Syst* 10: 517–523.

Berney J, Favier J, Rilliet B (1995) Head injuries in children: a chronicle of a quarter of a century. *Childs Nerv Syst* 11: 256–264.

Billmire ME, Myers PA (1985) Serious head injury in infants: accident or abuse? *Pediatrics* 75: 340–342.

Bruce DA, Zimmerman RA (1989) Shaken impact syndrome. *Pediatr Ann* 18: 482–484, 486–489, 492–494.

Bullock MR, Lyeth BG, Muizelaar JP (1999) Current status of neuroprotection trials for traumatic brain injury: lessons from animal models and clinical studies. *Neurosurgery* 45: 207–217; discussion 217–220.

Caffey J (1974) The whiplash shaken infant syndrome: manual shaking by the extremities with whiplash-induced intracranial and intraocular bleedings, linked with residual permanent brain damage and mental retardation. *Pediatrics* 54: 396–403.

Campbell CG, Kuehn SM, Richards PM, Ventureyra E, Hutchison JS (2004) Medical and cognitive outcome in children with traumatic brain injury. *Can J Neurol Sci* 31: 213–219.

Chiaretti A, Visocchi M, Viola L, De Benedictis R, Langer A, Tortorolo L, Piastra M, Polidori G (1998) [Diffuse axonal lesions in childhood]. *Pediatr Med Chir* 20: 393–397.

Committee on Quality Improvement, American Academy of Pediatrics. Commission on Clinical Policies and Research, American Academy of Family Physicians (1999) The management of minor closed head injury in children. *Pediatrics* 104: 1407–1415.

Congress of Neurological Surgeons (1966) Committee of Head Injury Nomenclature: glossary of head injury. *Clin Neurosurg* 12: 386–394.

Davis G, McCrory P (2005) Paediatric sport related concussion pilot study. *Br J Sports Med* 39: 47.

Demaerel P, Casteels I, Wilms G (2002) Cranial imaging in child abuse. *Eur Radiol* 12: 849–857.

Drapkin AJ (2006) Growing skull fracture: a posttraumatic neosuture. *Childs Nerv Syst* 22: 394–397.

Duhaime AC et al. (1987) The shaken baby syndrome. A clinical, pathological, and biomechanical study. *J Neurosurg* 66: 409–415.

Duhaime AC, Christian C, Moss E, Seidl T (1996) Long-term outcome in infants with the shaking-impact syndrome. *Pediatr Neurosurg* 24: 292–298.

Duhaime AC, Christian CW, Rorke LB, Zimmerman RA (1998) Nonaccidental head injury in infants – the 'shaken-baby syndrome'. *N Engl J Med* 338: 1822–1829.

Dupuis O et al. (2005) Comparison of 'instrument-associated' and 'spontaneous' obstetric depressed skull fractures in a cohort of 68 neonates. *Am J Obstet Gynecol* 192: 165–170.

Ellis TS, Vezina LG, Donahue DJ (2000) Acute identification of cranial burst fracture: comparison between CT and MR imaging findings. *Am J Neuroradiol* 21: 795–801.

Ersahin Y, Gulmen V (1998) Growing skull fractures: a clinical study of 41 patients. *Acta Neurochir (Wien)* 140: 519.

Ersahin Y, Mutluer S, Mirzai H, Palali I (1996) Pediatric depressed skull fractures: analysis of 530 cases. *Childs Nerv Syst* 12: 323–331.

Ersahin Y, Gulmen V, Palali I, Mutluer S (2000) Growing skull fractures (craniocerebral erosion). *Neurosurg Rev* 23: 139–144.

Ettaro L, Berger RP, Songer T (2004) Abusive head trauma in young children: characteristics and medical charges in a hospitalized population. *Child Abuse Negl* 28: 1099–1111.

Gaines BA, Shultz BL, Ford HR (2004) Nonmotorized scooters: a source of significant morbidity in children. *J Trauma* 57: 111–113.

Ganesh A, Jenny C, Geyer J, Shouldice M, Levin AV (2004) Retinal hemorrhages in type I osteogenesis imperfecta after minor trauma. *Ophthalmology* 111: 1428–1431.

Geddes JF, Hackshaw AK, Vowles GH, Nickols CD, Whitwell HL (2001a) Neuropathology of inflicted head injury in children. I. Patterns of brain damage. *Brain* 124: 1290–1298.

Geddes JF, Hackshaw AK, Vowles GH et al. (2001b) Neuropathology of inflicted head injury in children. II. Microscopic brain injury in infants. *Brain* 124: 1299–1306.

Gleckman AM, Bell MD, Evans RJ, Smith TW (1999) Diffuse axonal injury in infants with nonaccidental craniocerebral trauma: enhanced detection by beta-amyloid precursor protein immunohistochemical staining. *Arch Pathol Lab Med* 123: 146–151.

Graham DI et al. (1989a) Fatal head injury in children. *J Clin Pathol* 42: 18–22.

Graham DI et al. (1989b) Ischaemic brain damage is still common in fatal non-missile head injury. *J Neurol Neurosurg Psychiatry* 52: 346–350.

Hadley MN, Sonntag VK, Rekate HL, Murphy A (1989) The infant whiplash–shake injury syndrome: a clinical and pathological study. *Neurosurgery* 24: 536–540.

Hahn YS, Raimondi AJ, McLone DG, Yamanouchi Y (1983) Traumatic mechanisms of head injury in child abuse. *Childs Brain* 10: 229–241.

Han BK, Towbin RB, De Courten-Myers G, McLaurin RL, Ball WS Jr (1989) Reversal sign on CT: effect of anoxic/ischemic cerebral injury in children. *Am J Neuroradiol* 10: 1191–1198.

Han BK, Towbin RB, De Courten-Myers G, McLaurin RL, Ball WS Jr (1990) Reversal sign on CT: effect of anoxic/ischemic cerebral injury in children. *Am J Roentgenol* 154: 361–368.

Hartley LM, Khwaja OS, Verity CM (2001) Glutaric aciduria type 1 and nonaccidental head injury. *Pediatrics* 107: 174–175.

Holbourn AHS (1943) Mechanics of head injury. *Lancet* 4: 438.

Jantzen KJ, Anderson B, Steinberg FL, Kelso JA (2004) A prospective functional MR imaging study of mild traumatic brain injury in college football players. *Am J Neuroradiol* 25: 738–745.

Jennett B, Bond M (1975) Assessment of outcome after severe brain damage. *Lancet* 1: 480–484.

Johnson DL, Boal D, Baule R (1995) Role of apnea in nonaccidental head injury. *Pediatr Neurosurg* 23: 305–310.

Johnston KM, McCrory P, Mohtadi NG, Meeuwisse W (2001) Evidence-based review of sport-related concussion: clinical science. *Clin J Sport Med* 11: 150–159.

Keenan HT et al. (2003) A population-based study of inflicted traumatic brain injury in young children. *JAMA* 290: 621–626.

King WJ, MacKay M, Sirnick A (2003) Shaken baby syndrome in Canada: clinical characteristics and outcomes of hospital cases. *CMAJ* 168: 155–159.

Klein M, Stern L (1971) Low birth weight and the battered child syndrome. *Am J Dis Child* 122: 15–18.

Kors EE et al. (2001) Delayed cerebral edema and fatal coma after minor head trauma: role of the CACNA1A calcium channel subunit gene and relationship with familial hemiplegic migraine. *Ann Neurol* 49: 753–760.

Kraus JF, Fife D, Cox P, Ramstein K, Conroy C (1986) Incidence, severity, and external causes of pediatric brain injury. *Am J Dis Child* 140: 687–693.

Kraus JF, Fife D, Conroy C (1987) Pediatric brain injuries: the nature, clinical course, and early outcomes in a defined United States population. *Pediatrics* 79: 501–507.

Kraus JF, Rock A, Hemyari P (1990) Brain injuries among infants, children, adolescents, and young adults. *Am J Dis Child* 144: 684–691.

Kushner D (2002) Toward an evidence-based approach in the management of concussion: the role of neuroimaging. *Am J Neuroradiol* 23: 1442–1444.

Lee D, Honrado C, Har-El G, Goldsmith A (1998) Pediatric temporal bone fractures. *Laryngoscope* 108: 816–821.

Lende RA (1974) Enlarging skull fractures of childhood. *Neuroradiology* 7: 119–124.

Lende RA, Erickson TC (1961) Growing skull fractures of childhood. *J Neurosurg* 18: 479–489.

Levi L et al. (1998) Severe head injury in children – analyzing the better outcome over a decade and the role of major improvements in intensive care. *Childs Nerv Syst* 14: 195–202.

McCrea M, Hammeke T, Olsen G, Leo P, Guskiewicz K (2004) Unreported concussion in high school football players: implications for prevention. *Clin J Sport Med* 14: 13–17.

McCrory PR, Berkovic SF (1998) Second impact syndrome. *Neurology* 50: 677–683.

McCrory PR, Berkovic SF (2001) Concussion: the history of clinical and pathophysiological concepts and misconceptions. *Neurology* 57: 2283–2289.

McCrory P, Johnston KM, Mohtadi NG, Meeuwisse W (2001) Evidence-based review of sport-related concussion: basic science. *Clin J Sport Med* 11: 160–165.

McCrory P, Collie A, Anderson V, Davis G (2004) Can we manage sport related concussion in children the same as in adults? *Br J Sports Med* 38: 516–519.

McCrory P et al. (2005) Summary and agreement statement of the 2nd International Conference on Concussion in Sport, Prague 2004. *Br J Sports Med* 39: 196–204.

Merten DF, Osborne DR, Radkowski MA, Leonidas JC (1984) Craniocerebral trauma in the child abuse syndrome: radiological observations. *Pediatr Radiol* 14: 272–277.

Meythaler JM, Peduzzi JD, Eleftheriou E, Novack TA (2001) Current concepts: diffuse axonal injury-associated traumatic brain injury. *Arch Phys Med Rehabil* 82: 1461–1471.

Moore KL, Persaud TVN (1998) *The Developing Human: Clinically Oriented Embryology.* Philadelphia: WB Saunders.

Morrison WE, Arbelaez JJ, Fackler JC, De Maio A, Paidas CN (2004) Gender and age effects on outcome after pediatric traumatic brain injury. *Pediatr Crit Care Med* 5: 145–151.

Muszynski CA, Yoganandan N, Pintar FA, Gennarelli TA (2005) Risk of pediatric head injury after motor vehicle accidents. *J Neurosurg* 102: 374–379.

Nassogne MC et al. (2002) Massive subdural haematomas in Menkes disease mimicking shaken baby syndrome. *Childs Nerv Syst* 18: 729–731.

National Center for Injury Prevention and Control (2000) Traumatic brain injury in the United States: assessing outcomes in children. Summary and recommendations from the Expert Working Group. Atlanta, GA, October 26–27. JA Langlois (ed). Division of Acute Care, Rehabilitation Research and Disability Prevention, National Center for Injury Prevention and

Control, Department of Health and Human Services, Centers for Disease Control and Prevention.

Neeman Z, Bloom AI (2003) Occipital condyle fractures in the pediatric population. *Radiographics* 23: 1699–1701. (Author reply: 1699–1701.)

Nelson EL, Melton LJ 3rd, Annegers JF, Laws ER, Offord KP (1984) Incidence of skull fractures in Olmsted County, Minnesota. *Neurosurgery* 15: 318–324.

Ommaya AK, Goldsmith W, Thibault L (2002) Biomechanics and neuropathology of adult and paediatric head injury. *Br J Neurosurg* 16: 220–242.

Overpeck MD, Brenner RA, Trumble AC, Trifiletti LB, Berendes HW (1998) Risk factors for infant homicide in the United States. *N Engl J Med* 339: 1211–1216.

Paterson CR, Burns J, McAllion SJ (1993) Osteogenesis imperfecta: the distinction from child abuse and the recognition of a variant form. *Am J Med Genet* 45: 187–192.

Petitti N, Williams DW 3rd (1998) CT and MR imaging of nonaccidental pediatric head trauma. *Acad Radiol* 5: 215–223.

Pfenninger J, Santi A (2002) Severe traumatic brain injury in children – are the results improving? *Swiss Med Wkly* 132: 116–120.

Quality Standards Subcommittee (1997) Practice parameter: the management of concussion in sports (summary statement). Report of the Quality Standards Subcommittee. *Neurology* 48: 581–585.

Reid SR, Roesler JS, Gaichas AM, Tsai AK (2001) The epidemiology of pediatric traumatic brain injury in Minnesota. *Arch Pediatr Adolesc Med* 155: 784–789.

Sinnatamby CS (1999) *Last's Anatomy: Regional and Applied, 10th edn.* New York: Churchill Livingstone.

Smith SL, Andrus PK, Gleason DD, Hall ED (1998) Infant rat model of the shaken baby syndrome: preliminary characterization and evidence for the role of free radicals in cortical hemorrhaging and progressive neuronal degeneration. *J Neurotrauma* 15: 693–705.

Sosin DM, Sniezek JE, Waxweiler RJ (1995) Trends in death associated with traumatic brain injury, 1979 through 1992. Success and failure. *JAMA* 273: 1778–1780.

Starling SP, Holden JR, Jenny C (1995) Abusive head trauma: the relationship of perpetrators to their victims. *Pediatrics* 95: 259–262.

Strich SJ (1956) Diffuse degeneration of the cerebral white matter in severe dementia following head injury. *J Neurochem* 19: 163–185.

Tong KA et al. (2003) Hemorrhagic shearing lesions in children and adolescents with posttraumatic diffuse axonal injury: improved detection and initial results. *Radiology* 227: 332–339.

Tong KA et al. (2004) Diffuse axonal injury in children: clinical correlation with hemorrhagic lesions. *Ann Neurol* 56: 36–50.

Tuli S, Tator CH, Fehlings MG, Mackay M (1997) Occipital condyle fractures. *Neurosurgery* 41: 368–376. (Discussion: 376–377.)

Vowles GH, Scholtz CL, Cameron JM (1987) Diffuse axonal injury in early infancy. *J Clin Pathol* 40: 185–189.

Weber W (1984) [Experimental studies of skull fractures in infants]. *Z Rechtsmed* 92: 87–94.

Weber W (1985) [Biomechanical fragility of the infant skull]. *Z Rechtsmed* 94: 93–101.

Weber W (1987) [Predilection sites of infantile skull fractures following blunt force]. *Z Rechtsmed* 98: 81–93.

Yeates KO et al. (1999) Postconcussive symptoms in children with mild closed head injuries. *J Head Trauma Rehabil* 14: 337–350.

Yildirim A, Gurelik M, Gumus C, Kunt T (2005) Fracture of skull base with delayed multiple cranial nerve palsies. *Pediatr Emerg Care* 21: 440–442.

2

DIAGNOSTIC IMAGING

Helen M Branson and Manohar Shroff

INTRODUCTION

Pediatric head injury accounts for almost half of all new cases of traumatic brain injury. Pediatric trauma can be divided into three groups: (1) birth trauma (trauma occurring as a result of the birth process); (2) accidental trauma (this usually occurs in adolescent and teenage children and results in pathology and radiology similar to adults); and (3) non-accidental trauma. In this chapter, we will discuss accidental trauma and non-accidental trauma.

CANADIAN HEAD CT GUIDELINES

The CT head rule was developed for *adults* with minor head injury. Minor head injury is defined as witnessed loss of consciousness, definite amnesia, or witnessed disorientation in a patient with a GCS score of 13–15 (Stiell et al. 2001). Routine use of CT in every instance of minor head injury is not cost-effective as 96% of these scans do not contribute to management of the patient. Though this rule has not been validated in children, one could presumably use similar criteria in older verbal children and teenagers. Using this rule, head CT is indicated for patients with minor head injury and one of the following:

- High risk (for neurological intervention):
  - GCS score < 15 two hours after injury
  - suspected open or depressed skull fracture
  - any sign of basal skull fracture (hemotympanum, raccoon eyes (periorbital hematoma), cerebrospinal fluid otorrhea or rhinorrhea and Battle's sign (postauricular bruising))
  - vomiting - two or more episodes
- Medium risk (for brain injury on CT):
  - amnesia before impact > 30 minutes
  - dangerous mechanism (pedestrian struck by motor vehicle, occupant ejected from motor vehicle, fall from height > 3 feet (1 m) or five stairs)

IMAGING MODALITIES

CT and MRI are the best imaging modalities. CT is the accepted first-line investigation. However, MRI is more sensitive for post-traumatic brain injury except for fractures and subarachnoid hemorrhage (Besenski 2002). Skull x-rays are no longer considered accurate because there is poor correlation between brain injury and the presence of skull fractures (Parizel at al. 2005). CT in the majority of large centres is now multi-detector, often with 16 or more detector rows which provide isotropic data sets and allow for multiplanar and 3D reconstructions (Parizel et al. 2005). Thin section images can then be reconstructed from the data set to assess, for example, tiny fractures in the petrous temporal bone and base of skull without the need to rescan the patient. Images in trauma should be viewed at three window width and level settings:

1 Brain window (54 W, 35 L) for parenchymal and large extra-axial hemorrhage
2 Bone algorithm (2500 W, 500 L) for fractures
3 Intermediate setting or abdomen window (350 W, 40 L) for subtle small extra-axial hemorrhage

PRACTICALITIES OF IMAGING

In the ideal environment all children would remain still for imaging. In the setting of head injury, neurological status can be extremely varied, from wide awake and playful, with a skull fracture diagnosed after an uncomplicated fall, to comatose, intubated and ventilated patients.

The aim of imaging, however, is the same: to obtain diagnostic quality images, as quickly as possible. Comatose patients are intubated and ventilated and usually the only degradation to imaging is from the spinal board which can produce a streak artifact. Most developmentally normal children over the age of 6 will otherwise remain still for an unenhanced scan of the brain. There are techniques for settling small babies, including feed and sleep, although most post-trauma patients are fasted which has implications for this technique. Distractors include a 'disco-ball' (Fig. 2.1) strung from the ceiling and soothers. Then there is the group of patients that require sedation or general anaesthesia, which carries its inherent risks.

RADIATION ISSUES

The advent of helical CT has led to a dramatic increase in the use of CT. The estimated annual number of CT examinations in the United States rose from 2.8 million in 1981 to 20 million in 1995. CT examinations contribute dispro-portionately to the collective radiation dose to the population. In Britain, though the number of CT examinations is 4%, the contribution of CT radiation to the collective dose is 40%. It is well accepted that lifetime radiation risk estimation for excess probability of fatal cancer is larger for children than for adults. In addition to this factor, it is also well established that the effective radiation dose is higher in children due to their smaller mass, and the effective doses are highest in newborns. Effective doses range from 1.5 to 6 mSv in head CT examinations and 3.1 to 5.3 mSv in abdomen CT examinations (Huda et al. 1997). Data from atom bomb

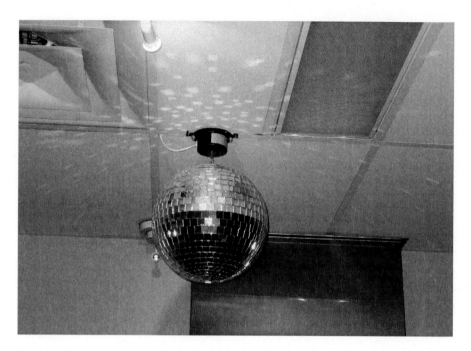

Fig. 2.1. This disco ball is ideal for settling infants, usually up to 10–12 months. With the room lights dimmed it can be mesmerizing to the patient, avoiding the need for sedation.

survivors have shown that individuals exposed 50 years ago to doses comparable to those associated with helical CT show a small but significant excess incidence of cancer (Hall 2002). The risk to the individual child is small, but the benefit gained from the scan needs to outweigh the risk. When individual risks are multiplied by the number of CT scans performed worldwide annually, it becomes a public health issue (Brenner et al. 2001). The aim of this discussion is to emphasize that CT should be done only when indicated, and when done should be performed by skilled personnel who will make all efforts to reduce radiation by making an appropriate choice of peak kilovoltage and milliampere-second settings.

THE SCOUT VIEW

The scout view is invaluable. It is good to generally assess for soft tissue swelling and fractures sometimes not visible in the transaxial plane. The scout view should also be used to look at the upper cervical spine for any gross misalignment or pre-vertebral soft tissue swelling.

EXTRA IMAGING

Consideration should be given to post-contrast imaging in a number of circumstances. If a fracture or hematoma crosses a venous sinus then a CT venogram

(CTV) should be performed to assess venous sinus integrity (Figs 2.2 and 2.3). If a fracture crosses a major vascular canal, specifically the carotid canal, then a CT angiogram (CTA) can be performed to assess for vessel injury.

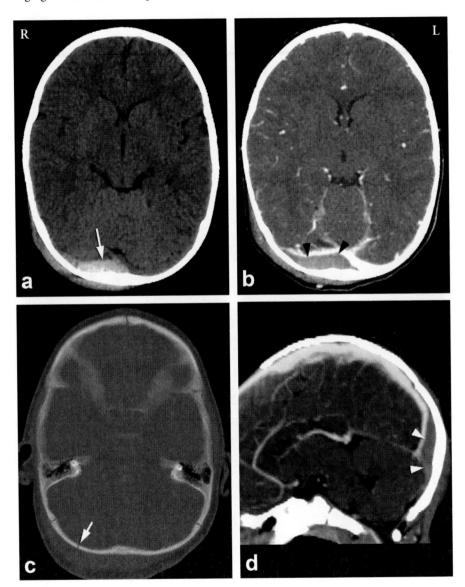

Fig. 2.2. Unenhanced CT (a) and CT venogram (CTV) (b and d) on a 10-month male patient who fell on a wooden floor demonstrates an acute right posterior fossa epidural hematoma (long arrow) with an undisplaced right occipital bone skull fracture (short arrow). CTV demonstrates anterior displacement and compression of the right transverse sinus (arrowheads).

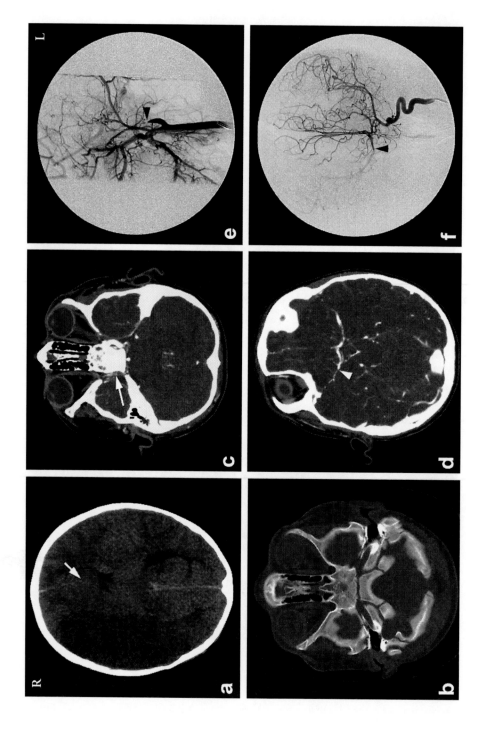

CLASSIFICATION
CLOSED HEAD INJURY
Closed head injury is defined as head injury where the dura remains intact (Besenski 2002), and accounts for approximately half of all new cases of traumatic brain injury in children (Khoshyomn and Tranmer 2004).

Classic imaging pattern

1   Plain film: This is now obsolete. The presence or absence of a fracture does not correlate with severity of brain injury (Besenski 2002).
2   CT: Intra-axial lesions consist of contusions and hematoma. Contusion and hematoma represent a spectrum based on size. If more than two-thirds of the lesion is blood then it is considered a hematoma (Khoshyomn and Tranmer 2004). Contusion may be underneath the point of impact, e.g. under a skull fracture –*coup* contusions; or at a remote location to the point of contact – *contrecoup* contusions (Khoshyomn and Tranmer 2004).

    There are four types of extra-axial lesions: extradural, subdural, subarachnoid and intraventricular hemorrhage (Figs 2.4 and 2.5). These are all readily demonstrated on CT. Herniation is also readily assessed (Fig. 2.6) and skull fractures are well seen on bone algorithm images and, if needed, 3D reconstructions (Figs 2.7 and 2.8).
3   MRI: MRI can demonstrate almost all of the above and gives more detail and often shows small contusions, subdural hematoma and ischemia not seen on CT. One of the limitations of MRI is the visualization of subarachnoid hemorrhage in the suprasellar region due to CSF flow artifacts on FLAIR T2 images.

Complications
One of the main complications to assess for is herniation. There are four types:

1   Subfalcine
2   Ascending and descending transtentorial
3   Tonsillar
4   Extracerebral

Fig. 2.3. (opposite) Unenhanced CT on a 2-year-old male demonstrates acute right middle cerebral artery territory infarction with early subfalcine herniation to the left with edema after head trauma (fig. a – small arrow). Images through the skull base demonstrate no fracture (fig. b). CT angiogram demonstrates non-enhancement of the right internal carotid artery (fig. c – large arrow) just after the carotid bifurcation extending to the right middle cerebral artery (fig. d – arrowhead) consistent with post-traumatic dissection. This was diagnosed on CT and confirmed on angiogram (black arrowheads).

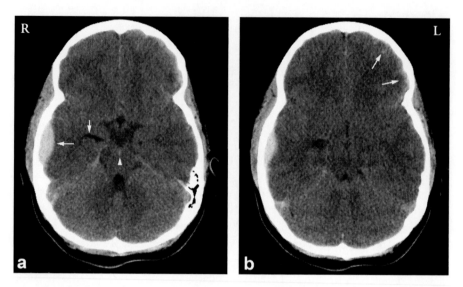

Fig. 2.4. This axial non-contrast CT on a 9-year-old boy demonstrates a right temporal extra-axial hematoma likely to be epidural (fig. a – long arrow) causing local mass effect and dilatation of the temporal horn of the right lateral ventricle (short arrow). There is also subarachnoid hemorrhage in the interpeduncular cistern (arrowhead). In fig. b, an axial scan, multiple tiny left frontal contusions (arrows) are seen and the right temporal extra-axial hematoma is again identified.

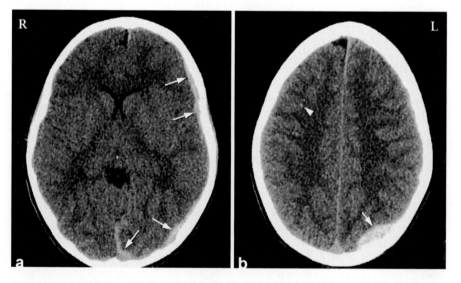

Fig. 2.5. This axial non-contrast CT demonstrates an acute left temporo-parietal subdural hematoma (long arrows in fig. a) with mild effacement of ipsilateral cerebral sulci. In the same child a tiny right frontal contusion is noted at the grey–white junction (arrowhead in fig. b) with a left parietal extra-axial hematoma (short arrow in fig. b).

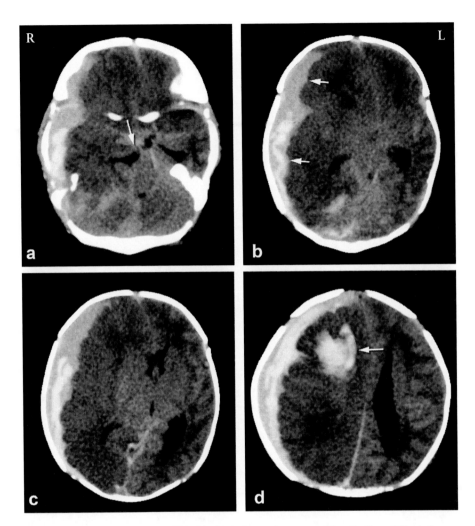

Fig. 2.6. This axial non-contrast CT of the brain in a male neonate (Day 0) after a difficult forceps extraction delivery demonstrates an acute large right cerebral subdural hematoma (fig. b – short arrows) with right cerebral infarction and right frontal intraparenchymal hematoma (fig. d – long arrow). Note the mass effect with subfalcine and right uncal herniation (fig. a – long arrow).

Late complications include cerebral and cerebellar atrophy with skull remodelling. The basal ganglia and brainstem can also atrophy with thalamic dystrophic calcification (Fig. 2.9).

PENETRATING HEAD INJURY

Penetrating head injury is defined as head injury where the dura is torn (Besenski 2002). It represents a small percentage of all head injury in children. In children, this

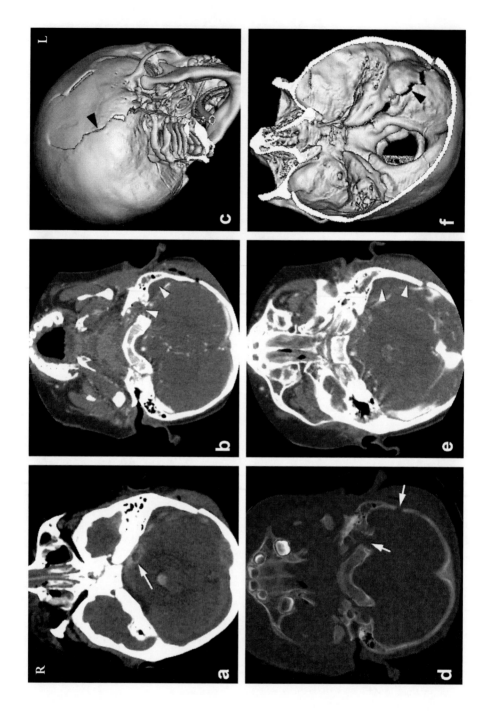

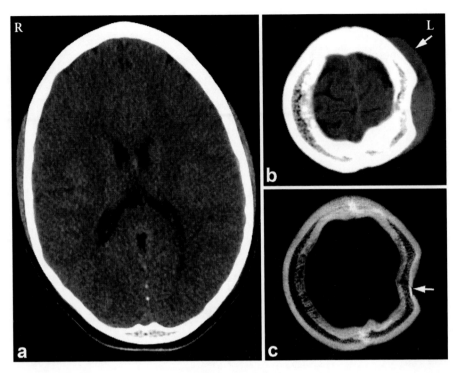

Fig. 2.8. In this 10-year-old girl, with blunt trauma to the left parietal region, no intracranial hematoma is detected (fig. a). Intermediate soft tissue windows (fig. b) and bone window (fig. c) images show a scalp hematoma and a depressed parietal bone fracture (arrows).

type of injury mainly involves household items such as scissors, television antennas and kitchen utensils (Koestler and Keshavarz 2001); in adults, penetrating injury more often results from gunshot wounds and stabbings. The orbits and paranasal sinuses, particularly the maxillary and ethmoid sinuses, are at risk of injury (Al-Sebeih et al. 2002).

Fig. 2.7. (opposite) This 2.5-year-old male pulled a television onto his head. There is a displaced fracture through the left parietal bone extending into the posterior fossa with diastasis of the jugular foramen (fig. d – small arrows), best demonstrated on the 3D reformat (figs c and f – black arrowhead). There is intraventricular hemorrhage with clot in the left cerebellopontine angle (fig. a – long arrow) and acute sinovenous thrombosis in the left internal jugular vein at the skull base and left sigmoid sinus (figs b and e – arrowheads).

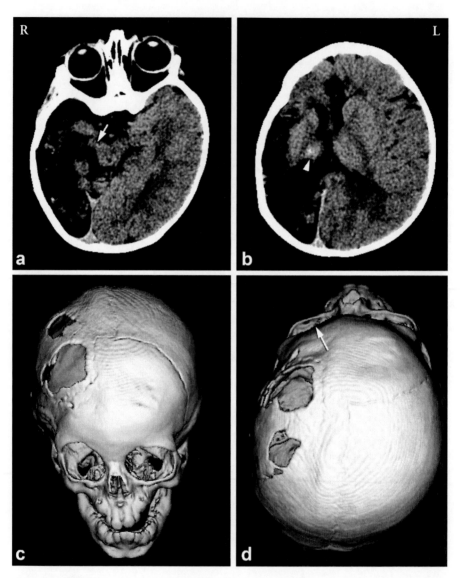

Fig. 2.9. Images obtained 17 months after head trauma demonstrate right cerebral cortical atrophy, atrophied right basal ganglia along with atrophied and calcified right thalamus (fig. b – arrowhead) with skull vault distortion. Note the atrophied right middle cerebral peduncle (fig. a – arrow). 3D CT reformats on the same child (figs c and d) show thinning and remodelling of the right cerebral skull vault with prior burr holes and elevation and recession of the right orbital roof due to volume loss.

Classic imaging pattern

1 Plain film: Skull x-rays may show a typical 'slot' fracture, a depressed fracture or retained foreign body (Domingo et al. 1994). Plain x-rays may also be normal if the foreign body is non-radioopaque. X-rays can show depth of penetration of metallic foreign bodies (Fig. 2.10).

2 CT: Penetrating objects may be metallic and their trajectory pathway can be well demonstrated on CT (Fig. 2.11) with tract hematoma (Domingo et al. 1994). Intracerebral hematoma may require surgical drainage. Intracerebral complications include intra- and extra-axial hematoma, pneumocephalus, herniation, cerebral edema and infarction (Deb et al. 2000).

3 MRI: Detection of early signs of ischemia is accomplished using diffusion weighted sequences. MRI is more sensitive to intracranial complications and useful in follow-up for late complications including abscess formation.

4 Angiography: Angiography may be indicated to assess vascular injury.

Complications
Intracranial infection is the most serious complication and may be devastating. Domingo et al. investigated 54 patients under the age of 14 who were admitted with penetrating injury and found the incidence of septic complications to be as high as 43%. Another delayed complication is growing skull fractures which result from a tear in the dura from a skull fracture (Makkat et al. 2001).

DIFFUSE AXONAL INJURY
Diffuse axonal injury is thought to be the result of widespread tearing of axons during acceleration, deceleration, and brain rotation (Parizel et al. 2005).

Classic imaging pattern

1 Plain film: There are usually no findings. There may be soft tissue swelling or a fracture.

2 CT: CT classically demonstrates eccentric hemorrhage in the corpus callosum, with or without hemorrhage in the brainstem, forniceal columns, grey–white junction and anterior commissure (Zimmerman et al. 1978). There are often also signs of cerebral edema. CT will classically underestimate these foci of hemorrhage (Parizel et al. 2005). CT can also be normal.

3 MRI: MRI is the modality of choice (Fig. 2.12). It can detect hemorrhagic and non-hemorrhagic lesions. Gradient echo T2* sequences are sensitive to susceptibility effects and very useful to assess for blood products. Diffusion weighted images are very sensitive for the detection of cytotoxic edema and areas of acute brain tissue injury.

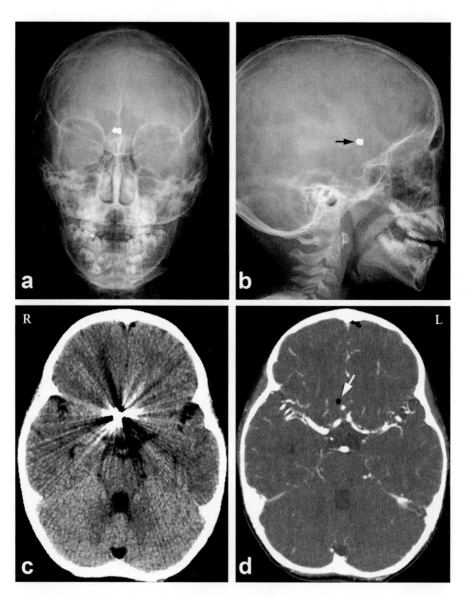

Fig. 2.10. Imaging on this 6-year-old male demonstrates a bullet centred on the anterior interhemispheric fissure, best seen on skull x-ray (figs a and b – black arrow). Unenhanced CT demonstrates metallic artifact making assessment of adjacent brain parenchyma inadequate (fig. c). CT angiogram demonstrates normal enhancement of the circle of Willis, in particular the anterior cerebral arteries. A small focus of pneumocephalus is demonstrated adjacent to the right anterior cerebral artery (fig. d – white arrow).

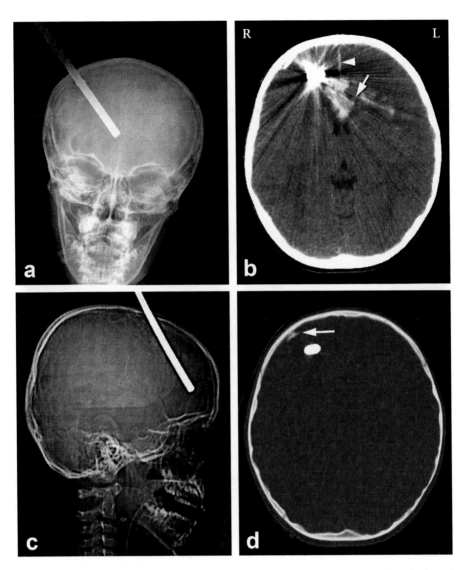

Fig. 2.11. This 6-year-old female was struck by an arrow. The arrow penetrated the right frontal bone and skull parenchyma with hemorrhage and contusion in both frontal lobes and the genu of the corpus callosum (fig. b – small arrow). There is a tiny amount of subdural blood in the anterior interhemispheric fissure (fig. b – arrowhead). Fig. d demonstrates a tiny displaced bone fragment (large arrow).

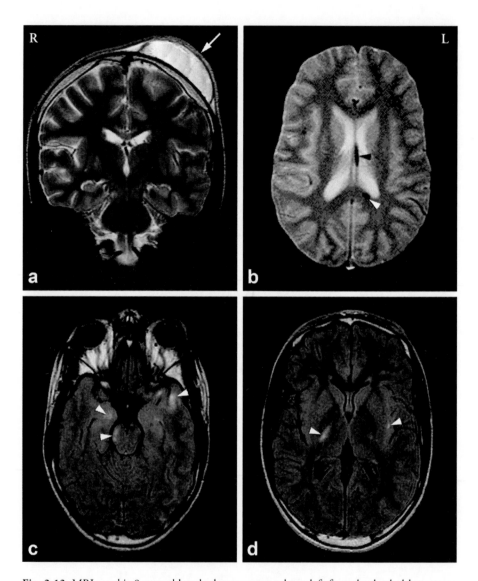

Fig. 2.12. MRI on this 8-year-old male demonstrates a large left frontal subgaleal hematoma (fig. a – long arrowhead) with hemorrhagic and non-hemorrhagic shear injuries in the body (fig. b - black arrowhead) and splenium of the corpus callosum (fig. b – white arrowhead), the temporal lobe and right posterior limb of the internal capsule (figs c and d – white arrowheads). The CT was normal.

Complications

1 Early: Cerebral edema and herniation.
2 Late: Within several weeks, there is ventricular enlargement due to atrophy with focal hypodensities in the cerebral white matter (Zimmerman et al. 1978). Late complications will include Wallerian degeneration, if there is significant tissue injury. Rarely Wallerian degeneration can occur in the acute phase.

SUSPECTED CHILD ABUSE/NON-ACCIDENTAL INJURY

Most inflicted head injuries occur in infants and toddlers. Most are of the rapid and dynamic type, which involves a stationary head being struck by a moving object or a moving head being struck by a stationary object, or both the head and object moving at the same time and colliding (Kleinman 1998). The more devastating injuries are the indirect injuries, which occur with sudden acceleration and deceleration of the head (Kleinman 1998).

Classic imaging pattern

The dynamic type of contact injury results in skull fracture, focal cortical injury and extra-axial hemorrhage (Kleinman 1998). Indirect injuries include subdural hematoma without skull fracture, and hypoxic-ischemic (Fig. 2.13a–d) edema, swelling often with herniation (Kleinman 1998). With the advent of multi-slice CT, a three-dimensional reformat can be provided to demonstrate these fractures.

1 Plain film: Skull x-rays may show scalp hematoma and swelling with or without skull fracture. Skull fractures secondary to non-accidental injury are often parieto-occipital or occipital (Kleinman 1998). Simple linear fractures and also complex comminuted fractures that cross sutures can both be found in cases of abuse (Kleinman 1998). Thus no pattern of skull injury is diagnostic of abuse. It was thought that all cases of suspected child abuse that have a head CT should also have a skull x-ray as fractures lying in the transaxial plane (even relatively large ones) can be missed on CT (Stoodley 2005).
2 CT: The most common finding is that of acute generalized cerebral edema (Zimmerman et al. 1978). CT classically demonstrates acute hyperdense subdural hematomas. Often these are small and they may be multi-compartmental, and they most often occur over the cerebral convexities (Stoodley 2005). Zimmerman et al. (1979a) were the first to describe the finding of parieto-occipital acute interhemispheric subdural hematomas occurring with more frequency in abuse. Often acute subdural hematomas occur in the high parietal convexities, and may be difficult to see on axial CT as they merge with the high-density skull. Thin-section axial CT can be performed with sagittal and coronal reformats, making these easier to detect.

If a skull fracture is in the transaxial plane, that is, parallel to the plane of CT, the fracture may not be detectable with CT. With multi-detector CT a 3D image may be produced, making detection of skull fractures easier. Cerebral infarction and edema with herniation may also be detectable (Fig. 2.13).

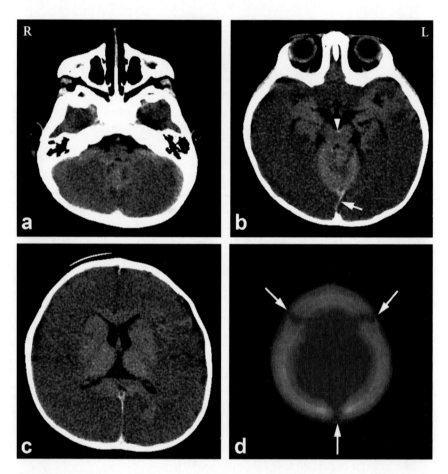

Fig. 2.13. This 10-month-old male presented with a history of uncontrolled seizures. Unenhanced CT of the brain demonstrates diffuse cerebellar and cerebral infarction with blood in the interpeduncular cistern (fig. b – arrowhead). There is a tiny amount of subdural blood adjacent to the tentorium (fig. b – small arrow). The basal ganglia are relatively spared. Bone algorithm demonstrates splitting of the sutures consistent with cerebral edema (arrowheads). Fundoscopy confirmed retinal hemorrhage. The patient died three days later.

3 MRI: CT is relatively insensitive for detection of non-hemorrhagic contusions and infarction and white matter shear injury (Suh et al. 2001). MRI is very sensitive to hemorrhage except for subarachnoid (Kleinman 1998), and, as bone does not

produce artifact, small subdural collections adjacent to the skull are easily imaged (Fig. 2.14). MRI can image the breakdown products of hemoglobin, allowing imaging of differing stages of blood which may give some information regarding injury timing (Kleinman 1998). The use of diffusion weighted imaging and fluid-attenuated inversion recovery (FLAIR) allows early detection of ischemia and shear injury. This is especially important in young infants with unmyelinated white matter where ischemia is difficult to detect on CT. Diffusion weighted imaging detects changes in the random motion of water and, along with an ADC (apparent diffusion coefficient) value or map, assigns a measure to this. It allows differentiation between cytotoxic and vasogenic edema (Suh et al. 2001).

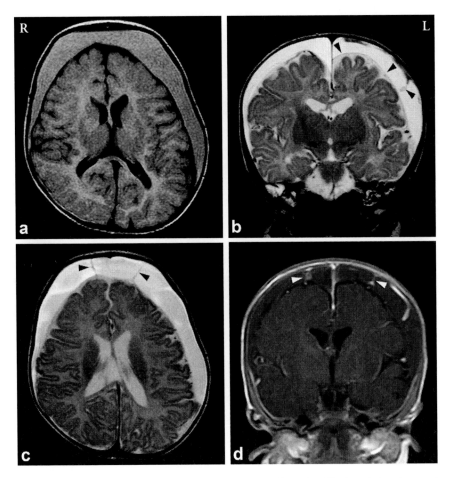

Fig. 2.14. MRI with axial FLAIR (fig. a), coronal and axial FSE T2 (figs b and c) and coronal post-gadolinium demonstrates chronic bicerebral subdural hematoma with membrane formation (arrowheads) which enhance.

Early MRI demonstrates multi-compartment subdural hematoma, with cerebral infarction and various types of herniation and mass effect. Suh et al. found some differences in distribution and pattern of diffusion weighted abnormalities in non-accidental versus accidental injury. Overall, in non-accidental injury the injuries appeared more diffuse and more likely to be posterior with sparing of the anterior temporal lobe and fronto-basal temporal lobes (Suh et al. 2001). Suh et al. also found a greater incidence of white matter shearing injury and intraparenchymal hematoma in accidental injury (Suh et al. 2001).

MRI is sensitive to blood products and allows differentiation of differing chemical forms of blood to enable and attempt injury/hemorrhage timing (see Table 2.1).

TABLE 2.1

Stage	Biochemical form	T1 MRI	T2 MRI
Hyperacute	Fe II oxyhb	Iso-low	High
Acute	Fe II deoxyhb	Iso-low	Low
Early subacute	Fe III methb	High	Low
Late subacute	Fe III methb	High	High
Early chronic	Fe III transferrin	High	High
Chronic	Fe III ferritin and hemosiderin	Iso-low	Low

Source: Modified from Kleinman 1998: 297.

Complications

Wallerian degeneration with a large cortical infarct may be demonstrated in the brainstem. This can be acute or chronic. Follow-up imaging may demonstrate cerebral atrophy, with calcification which may be cortical or in the basal ganglia. Chronic subdural hematoma may indicate chronic injury and requires further investigation.

Associated findings

Cervical spine injury should be assessed in all trauma cases. In a large majority of patients this can be assessed clinically and/or with plain film. In patients who undergo CT for cerebral scanning, there are certain markers on the head CT which may indicate spine injury. These include:

1 Soft tissue swelling/edema/hematoma: the inferior-most CT image on a brain scan should include an image of the cervical cord with a normal 'cup' of cerebrospinal fluid surrounding it (Fig. 2.15). The scans should be continued inferiorly until this is obtained.

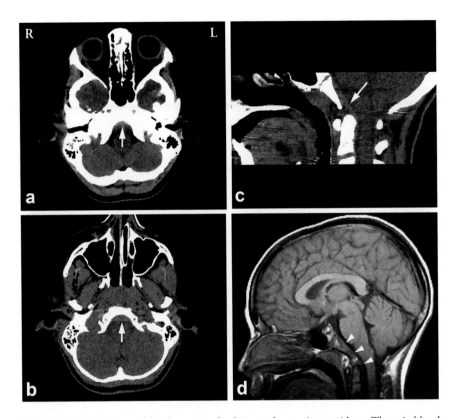

Fig. 2.15. This 10-year-old girl was involved in a tobogganing accident. There is blood posterior to the clivus, faintly seen on the routine 5 mm axial unenhanced CT (fig. a – small arrow), and clearly seen on the 1.25 mm axial reformatted images (fig. b – small arrow). Sagittal reformats demonstrate blood and air beneath the tectorial membrane which is lifted off the clivus (fig. c – long arrow), consistent with occipito-atlantal injury. Sagittal T1 MRI demonstrates blood along the clivus (fig. d – arrowheads).

2 Gross abnormalities/alignment of the upper cervical spine: on most scout views of the brain the upper cervical spine is included in the images. It is prudent to assess this image for gross malalignment for rare cases where plain film imaging of the spine has not been obtained. If an abnormality has been detected, CT imaging of the spine can be performed at the same time. Many pediatric centres advocate scans from the occiput to C3 in children with major trauma, as this is the major fulcrum of injury for young children up to 8 years of age.

REFERENCES

Al-Sebeih K, Karagiozov K, Jafar A (2002) Penetrating craniofacial injury in a pediatric patient. *J Craniofacial Surg* 13(2): 303–307.

Barr LL (1999) Neonatal cranial ultrasound. *Radiol Clin North Am* 37(6): 1127–1146.

Besenski N (2002) Traumatic injuries: imaging of head injuries. *Eur Radiol* 12: 1237–1252.

Brenner DJ, Elliston CD, Hall EJ, Berdon WE (2001) Estimated risks of radiation-induced cancer from pediatric CT. *Am J Roentgenol* 176: 289–296.

Deb S, Acosta J, Bridgeman A, Wang D, Kennedy S, Rhee P (2000) Stab wounds to the head with intracranial penetration. *J Trauma* 48(6): 1159–1162.

Domingo Z, Peter JC, de Villiers JC (1994) Low-velocity penetrating craniocerebral injury in childhood. *Pediatr Neurosurg* 21: 45–49.

Hall EJ (2002) Lessons we have learned from our children: cancer risks from diagnostic radiology. *Pediatr Radiol* 32(10): 700–706.

Huda W, Atherton JV, War DE, Cumming WA (1997) *Radiology* 203(2): 417–422.

Khoshyomn S, Tranmer BI (2004) Diagnosis and management of pediatric closed head injury. *Sem Ped Surg* 13(2): 80–86.

Kleinman P (1998) Head trauma. In: *Diagnostic Imaging of Child Abuse*. St Louis, MO: Mosby, ch. 15.

Koestler J, Keshavarz R (2001) Penetrating head injury in children: a case report and review of the literature. *J Emerg Med* 21(2): 145–150.

Makkat S, Vandevenne JE, Parizel PM, De Schepper AM (2001) Multiple growing fractures and cerebral venous anomaly after penetrating injuries: delayed diagnosis in a battered child. *Pediatr Radiol* 31(5): 381–383.

Ment LR, Bada HS, Barnes P, Grant PE, Hirtz D, Papile LA, Pinto-Martin J, Rivkin M, Slovis TL (2002) Practice parameter: Neuroimaging of the neonate: report of the quality standards subcommittee of the American Academy of Neurology and Practice Committee of the Child Neurology Society. *Neurology* 58(12): 1726–1738.

Parizel PM, Van Goethem JW, Oszarlak O, Maes M, Phillips CD (2005) New developments in neuroradiological diagnosis of craniocerebral trauma. *Eur Radiol* 15: 569–581.

Schutzman SA, Greenes DS (2001) Pediatric minor head trauma. *Ann Emerg Med* 37(1): 65–74.

Stiell IG, Wells GA, Vandemheen K, Clement C, Lesiuk H, Laupacis A, McKnight RD, Verbeek R, Brison R, Cass D, Eisenhauer MA, Greenberg GH, Worthington J (2001) The Canadian CT Head Rule for patients with minor head injury. *Lancet* 357: 1391–1396.

Stoodley N (2005) Neuroimaging in non-accidental head injury: if, when, why and how? *Clin Radiol* 60: 22–30.

Suh D, Davis P, Hopkins K, Fajman N, Mapstone T (2001) Non-accidental pediatric head injury: diffusion-weighted imaging findings. *Neurosurgery* 49: 309–320.

Tavani E, Zimmerman R, Clancy R, Licht D, Mable W (2003) Incidental intracranial hemorrhage after uncomplicated birth: MRI before and after neonatal heart surgery. *Neuroradiology* 45: 253–258.

Zimmerman RA, Bilaniuk LT, Bruce D, Dolinskas C, Obrist W, Kuhl D (1978) Computed tomography of pediatric head trauma: acute general cerebral swelling. *Radiology* 126: 403–408.

Zimmerman RA, Bilaniuk LT, Bruce D, Schut L, Uzzell B, Goldberg HI (1979a) Computed tomography of craniocerebral injury in the abused child. *Radiology* 130: 687–690.

Zimmerman RA, Bilaniuk L, Genneralli T (1979b) Computed tomography of shearing injuries of the cerebral white matter. *Radiology* 127: 393–396.

3
MILD CLOSED HEAD INJURY

Shay Menascu and Daune L MacGregor

INTRODUCTION

There is a high incidence of mild closed head injury in children but there was little research interest until studies in adult patients determined that even mild injury could significantly affect employability and other daily activities. The definition of mild closed head injury is most accurately based on functional outcome – not all children who have a mild head injury will have traumatic brain injury. Children with mild traumatic brain injury (MTBI) may appear unaffected until they return to school, where memory problems, impaired concentration and inefficient learning skills become evident. Other symptoms may include irritability and hyperactivity.

DEFINITIONS, INCIDENCE AND EPIDEMIOLOGY

The formal definition of mild closed head injury agreed upon by most clinicians correlates with a Glasgow Coma Scale score of 13–15, and is associated with temporary loss of consciousness, with symptoms of vomiting, lethargy, headache and rarely seizures – which occur immediately after the blow or impact (see Table 3.1).

The mechanisms of injury can vary from an acute direct blow to the head, to acceleration and deceleration injuries not necessarily associated with impact. Similarly, mild head injury may be the result of a severe whiplash injury which

TABLE 3.1
Signs and symptoms of mild/traumatic brain injury

Cognitive symptoms	Physical symptoms	Behavioural changes
Difficulties associated with: • Attention/concentration • Memory • Orientation • Decision making • Problem solving • New learning	• Headaches • Fatigue • Dizziness • Uneven gait • Nausea • Visual disturbances (e.g. blurring) • Seizures • Changes in sleep pattern • Changes in eating habits	• Depression • Anxiety • Irritability • Emotional/impulse control difficulties • Reduced initiative/ motivation

involves linear movement of the head (with acceleration and deceleration) and rotation of the head.

Concussion is defined as an instantaneous decrease or loss of consciousness associated with a head injury, with the duration of altered consciousness useful in estimating the severity of injury. Duration of post-traumatic amnesia (PTA) is felt to provide a reasonably accurate estimate of the end of altered consciousness (Satz et al. 1997). PTA is also called *anterograde amnesia* and is measured to the point when memory for life events becomes continuous once again after the injury. It is extremely difficult to determine the duration of PTA in children – in small children, non-specific signs such as crying, irritability and lethargy may be helpful.

It is difficult to obtain accurate statistics on the incidence and prevalence of mild closed head injuries in children. Using the Glasgow Coma Scale (Bullock 1997) as a measure of injury severity, the majority of closed head injuries are mild. About 85% of all head injuries requiring medical treatment are mild in nature, as documented in the United States National Coma Data Bank (Bijur et al. 1996).

It is recognized that many mild head injuries do not result in assessment by health care providers and thus the incidence is likely to be an underestimate. There is additional confusion in determining an accurate incidence depending on whether or not lacerations and abrasions of the face and scalp, with no defined impairment of consciousness, are included in the category of mild closed head injury.

Studies have shown that boys are at a higher risk for closed head injury than girls, with the ratio rising from approximately 1.5:1 in pre-school children, to 2:1 in school-aged children and adolescents (Semrud-Clikeman 2001). The incidence also varies with age and is relatively stable from birth to age 5, with documentation of MTBI in 160 per 100,000 children above age 5. There is a gradual increase in early adolescence, with the peak of 290 per 100,000 reported by the age of 18 years.

The incidence rate also varies in relation to family socioeconomic status. A study done in San Diego county in the USA (Silver and Oakland 2003) showed the incidence to be greater in children from families with median range income compared to children from higher family income groups. This relationship was not affected by the child's age or ethnic origin.

APOE GENOTYPE

Recent studies have demonstrated an interesting relationship of outcome after head trauma in relation to the apolipoprotein E (APOE) genotype. Previous studies have demonstrated that APOE has a correlation with an increased incidence of Alzheimer's disease. Head trauma in association with the presence of the APOE epsilon 4 allele has been found to be associated with earlier-onset Alzheimer's disease in older patients, possible poor outcome following head trauma in young patients, and increased severity of chronic traumatic brain injury in sports where there is repeated recurrent head trauma (boxing). Kutner et al. (2000) reported that professional

(American) football players heterozygous for the epsilon 4 allele showed decreased neurocognitive performance when compared with peers who did not possess the allele. This represents the first documentation of a genetic factor predisposing to poor outcome after head injury (Samson 2002).

AGE

In relation to sports-related head injury, it may be assumed that, because of a lower level of skill and playing experience, young athletes would be at higher risk for concussion. Proctor and Cantu (2000) reported that after age 12, adolescent head and neck injuries increased as a function of increasing age. This is more evident in contact sports (Gillis 2004). This finding is supported by other studies, such as that by Tysvaer and Storli (1989) in which abnormal electroencephalographic results were noted in 35% of active adult soccer players when compared to controls. Other studies have reported that number of years of playing soccer correlates with a greater degree of neurocognitive impairment (Webbe et al. 2003). Kutner et al. (2000) reported that the number of concussive and sub-concussive events increased with playing experience. There is some debate as to whether the mechanism of these findings relates to a history of concussion *per se* or cumulative sub-concussive incidents.

GENDER

There are few clinical studies observing differential outcome by gender after sports-related mild traumatic brain injury. It would seem likely that women would be at risk for more severe injury and post-concussion effects because of lower body mass and smaller neck size and supporting musculature. Mendelow and Crawford (1997), however, have reported that concussion-inducing collisions in women's sports are less severe because of overall lower body mass (entering into the force–mass relationship). A meta-analysis of gender differences in outcome determined that women had worse outcomes than men after head injury – primarily somatic symptoms (Putukian and Echemendia 2003).

BIOMECHANICS OF BRAIN PATHOLOGY

Trauma to the head and neck can produce brain injuries which may be focal or diffuse. There is, as well, disruption of brain function at the cellular level. Injuries are classified as either primary or secondary. Primary injury is the direct result of trauma and can include skull fractures, contusions and lacerations, as well as mechanical disruption of nerve fibres and blood vessels. Secondary injury is indirect from the trauma and related to edema, hypoxia, increased intracranial pressure and hemorrhage (McLean and Anderson 1997).

The mechanism of injury also relates to whether or not the head is in motion at the time of the impact, or in a stationary position. Head impact velocity is assumed to be greater if there is an association with high-speed movement (such as in motor vehicle accidents), although it is noted that this is not always a constant relationship. The nature of the brain injury strongly relates to the location of the impact on the head.

INJURY ADJACENT TO THE LOCATION OF THE IMPACT
Here there is local deformity of the skull at the point of impact with direct contact being produced between brain tissue and the bony skull. This is more evident in situations where there is a displaced skull fracture. In animal studies, Shatsky et al. (1986) found that impact to the occipital region does not lead to skull deformity and there were no underlying brain lesions observed. Impact in the temporal regions of the skull, however, did show transient deformity with involvement of the under-lying brain tissue and associated traumatic injury. Nahum et al. (1977) studied cadaver skulls and estimated that for a contact area of approximately 1 square inch (6.5 cm^2), the force required to produce a clinically significant skull fracture of the frontal bones was twice that required in the temporoparietal regions.

INJURY REMOTE FROM THE LOCATION OF THE IMPACT
Brain trauma may be found remote from the site of the original impact (Zhang et al. 2004). The term 'contrecoup' describes an injury to the brain which is opposite to the side of original impact. Contrecoup injuries are thought to be the result of rapid, localized pressure changes originating near the surface of the brain, with cavitation effects as the brain moves relative to the bony skull.

HEAD IMPACT AND BRAIN INJURY SEVERITY
Studies by Tomei et al. (1981) with primate models documented that a combination of linear and angular acceleration of the head results in a more serious injury than similar acceleration in only a sagittal plane. There is a relationship between impact in sagittal and coronal planes with more complex damage being produced than in each plane separately (Rees 2003).

PATHOPHYSIOLOGY
Mild traumatic brain injury results in a disturbance of function at the neuronal level. Brain function can be severely impaired with no observable pathophysiological evidence on standard neurodiagnostic testing. Changes may be observed only on autopsy studies, with degeneration of the neurons and axons in different areas of the brain (Baker and Dilip 2000).

If there is deformity of the skull, skull fractures and contusions can occur at the site of impact. Movement forces may also result in tearing or disruption of blood vessels with focal contusion and hemorrhage as well as shearing or straining of white matter nerve fibres. Shear and strain forces are responsible for diffuse axonal injury which then results in the process of Wallerian degeneration in distal axonal projections (de Kruijk et al. 2002b).

The frontal and temporal areas are particularly vulnerable to focal contusion because of proximity to the bony anterior and middle fossa of the skull. Shear and strain injuries are most common at the boundaries between white and grey matter (basal ganglia, periventricular regions, superior cerebellar peduncles, and other major fibre tracts) (Bullock 1997).

A number of neurochemical events also occur in head injury, with production of free radicals and excitatory amino acids with the disruption of normal calcium homeostasis. Cell membrane integrity is affected by excessive production of free radicals. Excessive neuro-excitation results from activation of N-methyl-D-aspartate (NMDA) and muscarinic cholinergic receptors. Traumatized brain tissue shows membrane depolarization and secondary release of neurotransmitters. Activation of NMDA receptors then results in excessive cellular calcium entry with activation of intracellular enzymes, thus producing a cascade of membrane depolarization and effect on function (Biegon et al. 2004). This excitotoxicity may account for severe effects of hypoxic-ischemic injury and traumatic brain injury on the hippocampus (the location of many glutamate receptors). These events are defined as one form of secondary injury which exacerbates the more direct physical traumatic brain injury (Bullock 1997).

PREDICTORS OF POST-TRAUMATIC COMPLICATIONS

Outcome prediction after traumatic brain injury is difficult – particularly with mild traumatic brain injury. An attempt to identify different serum and cerebrospinal fluid markers after head trauma has shown that S-100B and neuron-specific enolase (NSE) correlate with a Glasgow Coma Scale outcome score indicating severe brain injury. S-100 is an acidic calcium-binding protein with the isoform S-100B in high concentration in neurons and Schwann cells. It appears highly specific for lesions affecting the central nervous system (Pelinka 2004). The concentration of S-100B after severe and moderate brain injury shows a correlation with clinical predictors of poor outcome. S-100B also correlates with radiological abnormalities in moderate to severe head injury and has been associated with the severity of forgetfulness in patients with mild head injury. Savola et al. (2004) suggested that S-100B may be used as a marker in patients with mild to severe head injury as a predictor of outcome.

COGNITIVE AND PSYCHOLOGICAL SEQUELAE

The neuropsychological sequelae of mild closed head injury are variable, with deficits including decrease in intellectual function and language skills, problems with attention and memory as well as executive function, and reduced academic achievement with abnormal behaviour.

A high percentage of children after mild closed head injury can be found to have difficulties on linguistic skills testing (including object description and verbal fluency). These skills are highly important for school performance and deficits in these areas may contribute to the academic difficulties experienced on return to school after mild closed head injury (Levin et al. 2004). Severity of memory problems correlates with the severity of the injury and can be determined on a wide variety of verbal tests including word recognition and learning of word lists (Levin et al. 2004).

There is a spectrum of attentional problems which may be experienced after MTBI. The attention problems may include poorer response modulation, low ability to concentrate and a slower reaction time to various stimuli. A study by Max et al. (1999) demonstrated that in comparison to a matched group of children without preceding head injury, these difficulties are more evident in younger children with head injury than in older children with the same type of injury.

Post-traumatic behavioural changes may include irritability, poor anger control or different forms of attention deficit disorder. Levin et al. (2005) compared a group of children with mild head trauma to a matched group of children with orthopedic injuries but found there were no significant differences in the development of new psychiatric disorders. It had been reported, however, that the rate of new psychiatric disorders was markedly elevated in a group of children who suffered severe brain injury (Bloom et al. 2001).

INTERVENTION

It is important after a child has suffered a mild traumatic brain injury to be aware of possible symptomatology which may be easily misdiagnosed or ignored. It has been stated that mild head injury deserves the same attention, consideration and treatment resources as severe head injury. This is particularly important in younger children in whom there is difficulty in severity assessment (Barry et al. 1996).

Post-injury intervention may require assistance and support from a number of different sources. Return to school is important and a number of studies have shown that provision of a classroom program similar to the one the child was enrolled in pre-accident is key; and, if possible, the same classroom should be adapted to meet the special new needs of the child (Wade et al. 1998).

DIAGNOSTIC EVALUATION

The diagnosis is made if there is a history or any suspicion of head trauma in a conscious patient. The most important problem in assessment of a patient with mild head injury is evaluating the risk of acute intracranial bleeding or increased intra-cranial pressure. These considerations may arise if there are persisting behavioural or cognitive problems. Head CT is most sensitive in detection of intracranial hemor-rhage, although MRI is useful in detection of non-hemorrhagic lesions (Simon et al.

2001). Unfortunately, studies evaluating the need to screen (MRI) patients present-ing to emergency rooms with mild closed head injury have not been conclusive (Adams et al. 2001). Evaluation included status after a defined observation period, the presence or absence of skull fracture and overnight hospital admission.

PROGNOSIS AND PREDICTORS OF OUTCOME

Outcome in the first 24 hours after head injury is entirely dependent on the development of intracranial complications not observed during first assessment. Kashluba et al. (2004) reported that intracranial hematomas occur in approximately 1% of patients with mild traumatic brain injury – and 10% of these will result in death. Outcome is excellent if there is drainage of intracranial hematomas before clinical deterioration has occurred.

If there are no acute continuing complications, most children with mild closed head injury make a recovery within days or weeks (de Kruijk et al. 2002b). Rarely, neurobehavioural symptoms and other neuropsychological deficits will persist for months or years. In the future, assessment will involve anatomic and functional neuroimaging with neuropathological association to evaluate outcome.

OUTCOME AND RECOVERY

Ewing-Cobbs et al. (2004) indicated that there is a wide variability in the neuro-psychological difficulties seen in children after traumatic brain injury, and they thus recommended assessment regardless of the level of severity.

A study by de Kruijk et al. (2002a) evaluated the effect of bed rest after mild traumatic brain injury, and concluded that bed rest was no more effective than no bed rest at all. The authors felt that, at most, bed rest probably had some placebo effect within the first few weeks after injury.

Adams et al. (2001) studied the cost benefit of mandatory hospital admission after isolated mild closed head injury in children (with concussion and/or a brief loss of consciousness). These children were routinely admitted despite normal neuro-logical examination, negative findings on neuroimaging (head CT) and a Glasgow Coma Scale score of 15 at the time of presentation. The conclusion was that, in this selected population, mandatory admission was not necessary (Simon et al. 2001). Wade et al. (2003) evaluated the effectiveness of intervention following the acute phase, with treatment which included different psychotropic modulation, anti-convulsant medications, rehabilitation and educational programs with different parental education and support. The results indicated that these interventions seemed to aid recovery and assist in the process of getting the child to return to pre-injury status.

There is a need for more studies to evaluate the outcome for children and the implications of mild closed head injury. Areas to be evaluated include the overall quality of life, health care utilization, the influence of the family, and the effects on school and school performance after a child has had a closed head injury. It will be of particular interest to use advanced neuroimaging in order to improve understanding of the underlying neuropathology and neurophysiology of mild closed head injury and correlate these studies with neuropsychological and behavioural outcome. Prospective longitudinal studies will be helpful, with the overall aim being provision of improved treatment and adequate support for children recovering from a mild closed head injury.

REFERENCES

Adams J, Frumiento C, Shatney-Leach L et al. (2001) Mandatory admission after isolated mild closed head injury in children: is it necessary? *J Pediatr Surg* 36:119–121.

Baker RJ, Dilip R (2000) Sports related mild traumatic brain injury in adolescents. *Indian J Pediatr* 67(5): 317–321.

Barry CT, Taylor HG, Klein S et al. (1996) Validity of neuro-behavioral symptoms reported in children with traumatic brain injury. *Child Neuropsych* 2: 213–226.

Biegon A, Fry PA, Paden CM et al. (2004) Dynamic changes in *N*-methyl-D-aspartate receptors after closed head injury in mice: implications for treatment of neurological and cognitive deficits. *Proc Natl Acad Sci* 4: 5117–5122.

Bijur PE, Haslum M, Golding J (1996) Cognitive outcomes of multiple mild head injuries in children. *J Dev Behav Pediatr* 17: 143–147.

Bloom DR, Levin HS, Ewing-Cobbs L, Saunders AE, Song J, Fletcher JM, Kowatch RA (2001) Lifetime and novel psychiatric disorders after pediatric traumatic brain injury. *J Am Acad Child Adolesc Psychiatry* 40(5): 572–579.

Bullock R (1997) *Head Injury: Pathophysiology and Management of Severe Closed Injury.* London: Chapman and Hall.

de Kruijk JR, Leffers P, Meerhoff S et al. (2002a) Effectiveness of bed rest after mild traumatic brain injury: a randomised trial of no versus six days of bed rest. *J Neurol Neurosurg Psychiatry* 73: 167–172.

de Kruijk JR, Leffers P, Menheere CA et al. (2002b) Prediction of post-traumatic complaints after mild traumatic brain injury: early symptoms and biochemical markers. *J Neurol Neurosurg Psychiatry* 73: 727–732.

Ewing-Cobbs L, Barnes M, Fletcher JM, Levin HS (2004) Modeling of longitudinal academic achievement scores after pediatric traumatic brain injury. *Dev Neuropsychol* 25: 107–133.

Gillis D (2004) Concussion in football: when is it safe to return to the game? *Neurol Today* 2: 62–64.

Kashluba S, Paniak C, Blake T et al. (2004) A longitudinal, controlled study of patient complaints following treated mild traumatic brain injury. *Arch Clin Neuropsychol* 19: 805–816.

Kutner KC, Erlanger DM, Tsai J et al. (2000) Lower cognitive performance of older football players possessing apolipoprotein E epsilon4. *Neurosurgery* 47: 651–657.

Levin HS, Hanten G, Zhang L et al. (2004) Changes in working memory after traumatic brain injury in children. *Neuropsychology* 18(2): 240–247.

Levin HS, McCauley SR, Josic CP, Boake C, Brown SA (2005) Predicting depression following mild traumatic brain injury. *Arch Gen Psychiatry* 62: 523–528.

McLean AJ, Anderson RWG (1997) Biochemistry of closed head injury. *Head Inj* 2: 25–27.

Max JE, Koele SL, Smith WL et al. (1998) Psychiatric disorders in children and adolescents after severe traumatic brain injury: a controlled study. *J Am Acad Child Adolesc Psychiatry* 37(8): 832–840.

Max JE, Roberts MA, Koele SL et al. (1999) Cognitive outcome in children and adolescents following severe traumatic brain injury: influence of psychosocial, psychiatric, and injury-related variables. *J Int Neuropsychol Soc* 5: 58–68.

Mendelow AD, Crawford PJ (1997) Primary and secondary head injury. In: Reilly P, Bullock R (eds) *Head Injury*. London: Chapman and Hall, pp 71–77.

Nahum AM, Smith RW, Ward CC (1977) Intracranial pressure dynamics during head impact. *Proc 21st Stapp Car Crash Conference*, SAE No. 770922, pp 339–366.

Pelinka LE (2004) Serum markers of severe traumatic brain injury. *Indian J Crit Care Med* 8: 190–193.

Proctor MR, Cantu RC (2000) Head and neck injuries in young athletes. *Clin Sports Med* 19: 693–715.

Putukian M, Echemendia RJ (2003) Psychological aspects of serious head injury in the competitive athlete. *Clin Sports Med* 22: 617–630.

Rees PM (2003) Contemporary issues in mild traumatic brain injury. *Arch Phys Med Rehabil* 84(12): 1885–1894.

Samson K (2002) APOE (4) status may affect severity, recovery from milder brain trauma. *Neurol Today* 4: 35–36.

Satz P, Zaucha K, McCleary C et al. (1997) Mild head injury in children and adolescents: a review of studies (1970–1995). *Psychol Bull* 122: 107–131.

Savola O, Pyhtinen J, Leino T et al. (2004) Effects of head and extracranial injuries on serum protein S100B levels in trauma patients. *J Trauma* 56: 1229–1234.

Semrud-Clikeman M (2001) *Traumatic Brain Injury in Children and Adolescents: Assessment and Intervention*. New York: Guilford Press.

Shatsky SA, Ramirez A (1986) Recovery from acute subdural hematoma. *Am J Pediatr Hematol Oncol* 8(1): 18–27.

Silver CH, Oakland TD (2003) Helping students with mild traumatic brain injury: collaborative roles within schools. *Am Psychol* 58: 985–992.

Simon B, Letourneau P, Vitorino E et al. (2001) Pediatric minor head trauma: indications for computed tomographic scanning revisited. *J Trauma* 51: 231–238.

Tomei DI, Adams JH, Gennarelli TA (1981) Acceleration induced head injury in the monkey. II. Neuropathology. *Acta Neuropathol (Berl)* 7: 26.

Tysvaer AT, Storli OV (1989) Soccer injuries to the brain: a neurologic and encephalographic study of active football players. *Am J Sports Med* 17: 573–578.

Wade DT, King NS, Wenden FJ et al. (1998) Routine follow up after head injury: a second randomised controlled trial. *J Neurol Neurosurg Psychiatry* 65: 177–183.

Wade SL, Taylor HG, Yeats KO et al. (2003) Long-term parental and family adaptation following pediatric brain injury. *J Pediatr Psychol* 28: 251–263.

Webbe FM, Barth JT (2003) Short-term and long-term outcome of athletic closed head injuries. *Clin Sports Med* 22: 577–592.

Zhang L, Yang KH, King AI (2004) A proposed injury threshold for mild traumatic brain injury. *J Biomech Eng* 126(2): 226–236.

4

ACUTE AND EMERGENCY MANAGEMENT

Charles Matouk, Jamie Hutchison, Anne-Marie Guerguerian and Abhaya V Kulkarni

URGENT EVALUATION AND STABILIZATION

ROLE OF HEAD INJURY IN THE INITIAL EVALUATION OF THE TRAUMA PATIENT

It is imperative that pediatricians and adult traumatologists understand the urgent evaluation and stabilization of the pediatric neurotrauma patient in order to minimize secondary injury to the developing brain and prevent poor neurological outcomes. Although injury severity is the most important determinant of long-term neurological outcome, in general, pediatric head injury patients have better outcomes than their adult counterparts.

The pre-hospital management of pediatric head trauma is focused on the principles and standard practices established by the Pediatric Advanced Life Support System (PALS). In particular, attention to the ABCs (airway, breathing and circulation) is imperative to minimize secondary brain injury. A concerted effort must be made to prevent hypoxemia and to stabilize the patient's hemodynamic profile *en route* (Adelson et al. 2003a, 2003b). Importantly, full cervical spine immobilization is mandatory. In large metropolitan areas, transport to a dedicated pediatric trauma centre or level I adult trauma centre with added qualifications for pediatric treatment is preferable and correlated with better patient outcomes (Adelson et al. 2003c).

In the trauma room, a complete primary and secondary survey is rapidly performed. Appropriate review of the neurological system can be accomplished in a few minutes and dictates subsequent management decisions. Initial evaluation is focused on a determination of the patient's level of consciousness, pupillary reactions and best motor response. It is important to document the patient's admission Glasgow Coma Scale (GCS) score as a baseline for subsequent neurological examinations. A decreased level of consciousness, any neurological symptomatology or significant mechanism of injury mandates urgent CT. Early consultation with a pediatric neurosurgeon is warranted in the initial evaluation and resuscitation of the pediatric neurotrauma patient to make decisions regarding definitive surgical management and the need for intracranial pressure (ICP) monitoring (Adelson et al. 2003d). When confronted with a patient demonstrating clinical signs of brain herniation, mild hyperventilation and prompt administration of mannitol are recommended (Adelson et al. 2003e, 2003f). Although anti-seizure prophylaxis should not be routinely administered in severe traumatic brain injury and does not prevent the development of post-traumatic epilepsy, it has been demonstrated to reduce the frequency of early post-traumatic seizures and should be administered to children at particularly high risk (Adelson et al. 2003g).

INTENSIVE CARE MANAGEMENT OF SEVERE PEDIATRIC HEAD INJURY

Children presenting with severe traumatic brain injury require specialized, intensive care management involving pediatric intensivists working with the pediatric neuro-surgeons and traumatologists. This level of care requires an understanding of the basic physiology of intracranial pressure, cerebral perfusion, and cerebral blood flow.

INTRACRANIAL PHYSIOLOGY

The cranium is a semi-closed space filled with brain tissue, blood, and cerebral spinal fluid (CSF) with the foramen magnum as the outlet. The volume of one of these components can increase without causing increased intracranial pressure (ICP) by displacing other components (the Monroe-Kellie doctrine). When the volume of one of these three intracranial components expands beyond the displacement capacity of the other two components, a rise in ICP occurs (Fig. 4.1). Rapid and/or sustained elevations in ICP compromise cerebral blood flow, leading to cerebral ischemia, further injury, cerebral edema, and further rises in ICP, and, ultimately, herniation of the brain across the tentorium or through the foramen magnum can occur. For these reasons, limiting increases in ICP is one of the essential goals of management in severe traumatic brain injury (TBI).

Cerebral blood flow (CBF) is determined by cerebral perfusion pressure (CPP), cerebral oxygen (O_2) consumption, and arterial carbon dioxide ($PaCO_2$) and oxygen (PaO_2) tension. Maintaining adequate CBF and O_2 delivery is important in order to prevent secondary hypoxic-ischemic injury (Fig. 4.2). Cerebral perfusion pressure is expressed in terms of mean arterial pressure (MAP) and ICP as CPP = MAP – ICP; mean arterial blood pressure is the inflow pressure to the brain, and ICP is the outflow pressure to the brain. Under normal conditions, ICP is low (< 20 mmHg), CPP is primarily dependent on MAP, and cerebral vascular autoregulation maintains an adequate CBF over a wide range of CPP (50–150 mmHg). After injury, auto-regulation may become impaired; decreased CPP from increased ICP or hypotension can limit CBF.

MANAGEMENT

The management of children with severe traumatic brain injury (defined using a Glasgow Coma Scale score less than or equal to 8) recommended in this section was formulated using systematic reviews of the literature published in English before 2003 by the Canadian Critical Care Trials Group. Fourteen interventions related

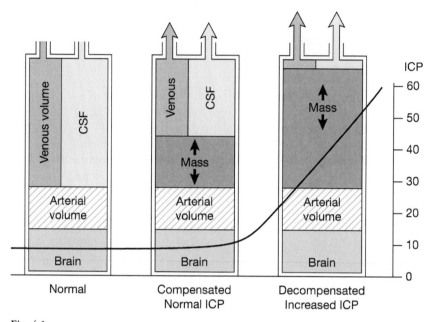

Fig. 4.1.

Source: MC Rogers (ed) (1996) *Textbook of Pediatric Intensive Care.* Baltimore, MD: Williams and Wilkins.

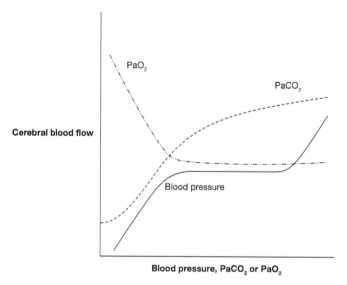

Fig. 4.2. Cerebral blood flow

to early resuscitation, monitoring, and the management of intracranial hypertension were evaluated in terms of their impact on outcomes related to death, neurological morbidity, physiologic outcomes and safety. Following literature reviews, summaries and discussions, consensus statements for management were developed using a modified Delphi technique (Hutchison et al. submitted).

It is recommended that the management of children with severe TBI include early endotracheal intubation using rapid sequence induction of anesthesia by experienced personnel (Sing et al. 1996, Stocchetti et al. 1996, Meyer et al. 2000, Cooper et al. 2001), with cervical spine precautions, early fluid resuscitation, and analgesia and sedation. In general, hypoxia, shock and hypotension should be prevented and treated rapidly with oxygen and intravenous fluids, and transfusion of blood products if necessary, during transport and in the emergency room, operating room and intensive care unit (Chesnut et al. 1993, Pigula et al. 1993, Kokoska et al. 1998). Children should be transported to a centre able to provide neurosurgical, trauma team and critical care evaluation, monitoring, and urgent surgical intervention if required.

The traumatic brain injury may be one of multiple injuries following trauma. Fractures and organ injuries may contribute to hypoxia, hemorrhage and hemorrhagic or cardiogenic shock (myocardial contusion, tamponade), which may contribute to secondary brain injury; all injuries should be evaluated and managed in consultation with the appropriate surgical and medical expertise. Patients should be administered intravenous normal saline at a maintenance rate and intravenous fluid should not be restricted below this rate. Blood pressure should be monitored invasively. ICP should be monitored in patients with an abnormal CT scan or who are judged to be at risk of intracranial hypertension (during an operative procedure while under anesthesia, because the level of consciousness cannot be assessed).

ICP greater than 20–25 mmHg should be treated (Bowers and Marshall 1980). The head of the bed should be kept at 30 degrees and the ICP transducer referenced to zero at the level of the tragus. The patient should be positioned with the head in the midline with the head slightly extended on the neck in a firm cervical spine collar. Reversible causes of ICP elevation include a constrictive c-spine collar, hypercarbia, hypoxia, hyperthermia (lower espophageal temp. >37.5°C), inadequate sedation/analgesia, suctioning and technical problems with the ICP monitor. These should be excluded or corrected before proceeding with further treatment. ICP elevation should then be treated with cerebrospinal fluid drainage (Mollman et al. 1988), mannitol (Kirkpatrick et al. 1996), and/or hypertonic saline (Simma et al. 1998). Normovolemia should be maintained during treatment with mannitol.

There are insufficient data in children to recommend a specific CPP management; however, hypotension should be prevented and treated aggressively. For refractory intracranial hypertension, we recommend mild to moderate hyperventilation followed by barbiturate therapy if necessary (Pittman et al. 1989). Sustained severe hyperventilation should not be used (Skippen et al. 1997). Neurosurgical intervention should be considered to remove a hematoma or an expanding contusion. Core temperature should be monitored and fever prevented (Natale et al. 2000) during the entire period of cerebral edema and ICP monitoring. Neuromuscular blocking agents should be used intermittently for intubation, to prevent procedure-induced ICP rise if unresponsive to analgesia/sedation, to facilitate ventilation in severe respiratory failure, and to prevent shivering during active cooling. Neuromuscular blocking agents should not be used continuously (Hsiang et al. 1994).

Until more information is available in children, recommendations cannot be made about the use of jugular venous oxygen saturation monitoring, induced hypothermia therapy, or de-compressive craniectomy in children with diffuse cerebral edema. Steroids have no role in the treatment of severe TBI in children (Roberts et al. 2004).

Severe elevations in ICP or herniation syndromes are an emergency and acute hyperventilation can be used to lower ICP while other therapies are being implemented. CT imaging and neurosurgical evaluation should be performed immediately.

Patients should be managed in an intensive care unit with attention to supportive care including nutrition and skin care. These patients are at particular risk for nosocomial infections such as ventilator-associated pneumonia and central line, external ventricular drain and urinary tract infections. In general, the principles of care used for patients with severe TBI can be used for the care of patients with moderate TBI; however, ICP monitoring is not required in most cases. Patients may evolve to neurological death and the Canadian Guidelines for care of the patient with neurological death can be used for these patients (Shemie et al. 2006).

SURGICAL MANAGEMENT OF PEDIATRIC HEAD TRAUMA

Decisions regarding surgical intervention persist even after the initial evaluation and resuscitation of the trauma patient and are typically heralded by an unexpected deterioration in level of consciousness or failure to improve in a timely fashion. This section reviews the surgical management principles of the most common and perilous pediatric traumatic head injuries.

SKULL FRACTURES

Skull fractures are frequent accompaniments of head trauma in adults, and even more prevalent in the pediatric population (Nelson et al. 1984, National Center for Injury Prevention and Control 2000). Special consideration must be given to infants presenting with overlying subgaleal hematomas as blood loss is often substantial and can precipitate anemia and cardiovascular failure (Raffel and Litofsky 1994). Hospitalization and close monitoring of hemodynamic indices are warranted in these cases.

Growing skull fractures (or post-traumatic leptomeningeal cysts) are a rare but serious complication of widely diastatic linear fractures (> 4 mm) and concomitant underlying dural tear in the pediatric population (Lende and Erickson 1961, Lende 1974). Most commonly, they occur in the parietal region. When associated with progressive neurological deficits and seizure disorders, surgical correction of growing fractures is recommended. The surgical principles include repair of the dural defect with a dural graft, reconstruction of the skull defect, and excision of excessive scalp tissue. Rarely, ventriculoperitoneal and cystoperitoneal shunting are required for the management of ventricular or leptomeningeal cyst enlargement, respectively (Raffel and Litofsky 1994).

The management of depressed skull fractures is dictated by their association with an overlying scalp defect, i.e. closed versus open fracture patterns. In closed depressed skull fractures, intracranial contamination is not a concern. Indications for surgical repair are limited to patients with neurological deficits and underlying parenchymal brain injury. The incidence of post-traumatic epilepsy is likely not changed by surgical intervention. Alternatively, open (or compound) depressed skull fractures represent a significant risk of intracranial infection, and warrant prompt neurosurgical action for satisfactory decontamination and repair of dural and skull defects (Raffel and Litofsky 1994, Ersahin et al. 1996). 'Ping-pong' fractures represent a special case of depressed skull fracture in neonates and young infants. The majority of defects resolve spontaneously, and few require surgical correction (either by an open procedure or application of external suction) (Dupuis et al. 2005).

EXTRADURAL HEMATOMAS

Extradural (or epidural) hematomas (EDH) are uncommon complications of pediatric traumatic head injury (2 to 3% of all pediatric head injury admissions). They constitute a majority of post-traumatic intracranial hematomas in children between 9 and 15 years old (Dhellemmes et al. 1985, Aronyk 1994). Treated appropriately, they afford an excellent neurological outcome. Typically the result of low-energy impacts associated with falls, EDH are frequently associated with an overlying simple linear skull fracture and subgaleal collection. In asymptomatic patients, these clinico-radiographic findings constitute important diagnostic clues. Urgent CT of the head is mandatory in all such patients to rule out EDH. It is important to remember that the pediatric skull is relatively 'elastic', and fractures are not invariably associated with the condition.

The majority of pediatric EDH are localized in the temporal and parietal regions with associated linear skull fractures extending across branches of the middle meningeal artery. In these most typical cases, the extradural collection results from accumulation of arterial blood from a torn branch of the middle meningeal artery. Alternatively, disruption of an osseous emissary venous channel or bleeding from multiple small foci on the dural surface are culprit lesions (Aronyk 1994).

Regardless of the precise source of bleeding, management principles are similar and straightforward. In a symptomatic child, urgent craniotomy, evacuation of the hematoma and obliteration of the epidural space by tacking the dura to the craniotomy flap are warranted. Occasionally, an EDH is identified in a neurologically intact child with no or minimal headache, often 24 to 48 hours after the time of injury. Non-surgical management of these children is optional, but should only be considered in specialized pediatric neurosurgical centres with 24-hour supervision by trained nursing personnel and access to prompt CT imaging. If the EDH is worrisome in any way (larger than 1.5 cm in maximal dimension, associated with an overlying fracture crossing a main branch of the middle meningeal artery, middle or posterior cranial fossa location, concomitant intraparenchymal injury, evidence of midline shift), prompt surgical intervention must be considered. Any change in the patient's neurological condition (even worsening headache) should provoke repeat imaging as EDH may accumulate in a delayed fashion. This is especially relevant in patients undergoing treatment for raised ICP or who have a CSF leak (Aronyk 1994). The surgical treatment of pediatric EDH is gratifying, with patients having excellent outcomes as long as the intervention is performed prior to neurological deterioration. Awaiting progressive neurological symptoms and signs prior to hematoma evacuation is inappropriate and results in a worse neurological outcome.

Posterior fossa extradural hematomas
Posterior fossa EDH are rare lesions, but occur more frequently in childhood than in the adult population. Associated with a potentially catastrophic clinical course, they deserve special consideration in the management of pediatric head injury. Typically the result of an occipital blow, posterior fossa EDH are associated with an overlying occipital skull fracture that crosses a venous sinus in approximately 80% of cases (Aronyk 1994). Consequently, unlike most temporo-parietal EDH, venous (not arterial) blood accumulates in the extradural space. Because blood may accumulate slowly, patients may present with headache, vomiting, irritability and unsteady gait several days after the time of injury. This delayed presentation may complicate accurate diagnosis because subacute blood appears isodense to brain on CT imaging. Deformation or effacement of the fourth ventricle is sometimes the only radiological clue. Neurological deterioration can be precipitous and catastrophic. Surgical evacuation of the hematoma should be seriously considered in all patients.

ACUTE SUBDURAL HEMATOMAS
Pediatric subdural hematomas (SDH) are, unfortunately, often a serious finding in the pediatric population. In many cases, non-accidental traumatic brain injury must be suspected and comprehensively investigated by a multi-disciplinary team (Duhaime et al. 1998). In these very young patients, the SDH and the patient's moribund condition all but confirm the severity of the underlying diffuse paren-

chymal injury. Infrequently, large acute SDH warrant surgical evacuation. However, in comatose infants and young children presenting with large bilateral SDH and underlying hemispheric hypodensities on CT imaging, the prognosis may be worse than in accidental injuries (Keenan et al. 2004, Barlow et al. 2005, Keenan et al. 2006). A neurosurgeon's role in these cases is typically limited to the insertion of an ICP monitor to facilitate medical management of intracranial hypertension.

Infants and older children may also sustain an acute SDH after accidental traumatic brain injury – for example, a fall from a great height or a motor vehicle accident. In general, urgent surgical evacuation of any sizeable subdural hematoma is mandatory. The child's prognosis is more reflective of the extent of underlying parenchymal injury and clinical condition at first presentation.

INTRACEREBRAL HEMATOMAS
Post-traumatic intracerebral hematomas are infrequent in children, and less common than extradural, subdural or subarachnoid hemorrages (Aronyk 1994). In most cases, they represent confluent cortical contusions in the setting of severe diffuse axonal injury after a motor vehicle accident or a fall from a considerable height (Statham and Todd 1990, Aronyk 1994). A minority of intracerebral hematomas are deep-seated and likely result from disruption of penetrating vessels. Overwhelmingly, the management of pediatric intracerebral hematoma is non-surgical, and most hematomas will resolve over two to three weeks. Efforts are directed at preventing secondary injury and include optimizing tissue oxygenation and aggressive control of raised ICP. Several common pitfalls must be avoided. First, isolated intracerebral hematomas are exceedingly rare in children of any age. A concerted search for evidence of a penetrating injury must be undertaken to gauge the risks of intracranial infection, CSF fistula and occult vascular injuries, including traumatic aneurysms and carotid-cavernous fistulas. Second, an atypical radiological appearance should suggest the possibility of an underlying vascular malformation. In these cases, cerebral angiography is warranted. Finally, massive intracerebral hematomas and those impinging on the ventricular system and disrupting the adequate flow of CSF may be considered for surgical evacuation as an adjunct to the medical management of raised ICP. In the case of the former, most pediatric surgical intracerebral hematomas are located in the orbito-frontal or temporal tip regions (Aronyk 1994).

PENETRATING HEAD INJURY
Penetrating head injuries constitute a minority of traumatic pediatric head injuries and, as in the adult population, are classified as non-missile penetrating injuries and missile injuries. Children are prone to non-missile penetrating injuries that result from falls or home and playground accidents. These injuries often involve nails, pencils and sharp sticks. Missile injuries are overwhelmingly comprised of gunshot wounds, although BB guns and air pellet rifles are capable of causing substantive

intracranial damage in children (Luerssen 1994). Each case is highly individualized, and requires assessment by an experienced neurosurgical team.

In the case of non-missile penetrating injuries, strong consideration should be given to pre-operative angiography in addition to prompt CT imaging if the object has damaged a region in proximity to large arteries or dural sinuses. The protruding foreign object should not be removed prior to adequate surgical exposure in the operating theatre. This includes a craniotomy performed around the object and dural opening to facilitate control of brain hemorrhage when the foreign body is extracted. Debridement of devitalized tissue, removal of easily accessible impacted bone fragments and a water-tight dural closure are mandatory to minimize the risk of intracranial infection. Antibiotic and seizure prophylaxis are appropriate.

In the case of gunshot wounds, the brain injury is generally much more severe. Patients who arrive in the trauma room comatose with a bullet trajectory that crosses the midline or passes through the geographic centre of the brain have a dismal prognosis, and are not surgical candidates. In salvageable patients, prompt identification of entry and exit wounds in the trauma room is important for forensic purposes and facilitates debridement of devitalized tissue and removal of easily accessible impacted bone and bullet fragments in the operating suite. Evacuation of superficial hematomas is also desirable to aid in the medical management of raised ICP. In general, deep-seated, remote bullet fragments should not be removed, and every effort should be made to confine debridement of brain parenchyma to the bullet tract so as not to damage surrounding functional brain tissue. Water-tight dural closure is mandatory to minimize the risk of CSF fistula and intracranial infection. Antibiotic and seizure prophylaxis are appropriate. Finally, strong consideration should be given to insertion of an ICP monitor, especially in patients whose poor neurological condition precludes informative serial neurological examinations.

REFERENCES

Adelson PD, Bratton SL, Carney NA et al. (2003a) Guidelines for the acute medical management of severe traumatic brain injury in infants, children, and adolescents. Chapter 2. Trauma systems, pediatric trauma centers, and the neurosurgeon. *Pediatr Crit Care Med* 4: S5–8.

Adelson PD, Bratton SL, Carney NA et al. (2003b) Guidelines for the acute medical management of severe traumatic brain injury in infants, children, and adolescents. Chapter 3. Prehospital airway management. *Pediatr Crit Care Med* 4: S9–S11.

Adelson PD, Bratton SL, Carney NA et al. (2003c) Guidelines for the acute medical management of severe traumatic brain injury in infants, children, and adolescents. Chapter 4. Resuscitation of blood pressure and oxygenation and prehospital brain-specific therapies for the severe pediatric traumatic brain injury patient. *Pediatr Crit Care Med* 4: S12–18.

Adelson PD, Bratton SL, Carney NA et al. (2003d) Guidelines for the acute medical management of severe traumatic brain injury in infants, children, and adolescents. Chapter 5. Indications for intracranial pressure monitoring in pediatric patients with severe traumatic brain injury. *Pediatr Crit Care Med* 4: S19–24.

Adelson PD, Bratton SL, Carney NA et al. (2003e) Guidelines for the acute medical management of severe traumatic brain injury in infants, children, and adolescents. Chapter 12. Use of hyperventilation in the acute management of severe pediatric traumatic brain injury. *Pediatr Crit Care Med* 4: S45–48.

Adelson PD, Bratton SL, Carney NA et al. (2003f) Guidelines for the acute medical management of severe traumatic brain injury in infants, children, and adolescents. Chapter 17. Critical pathway for the treatment of established intracranial hypertension in pediatric traumatic brain injury. *Pediatr Crit Care Med* 4: S65–67.

Adelson PD, Bratton SL, Carney NA et al. (2003g) Guidelines for the acute medical management of severe traumatic brain injury in infants, children, and adolescents. Chapter 19. The role of anti-seizure prophylaxis following severe pediatric traumatic brain injury. *Pediatr Crit Care Med* 4: S72–75.

Aronyk KE (1994) Post-traumatic hematomas. In: Cheek WR (ed) *Pediatric Neurosurgery: Surgery of the Developing Nervous System.* Philadelphia: WB Saunders.

Barlow KM, Thomson E, Johnson D, Minns RA (2005) Late neurologic and cognitive sequelae of inflicted traumatic brain injury in infancy. *Pediatrics* 116: 174–185.

Bowers SA, Marshall LF (1980) Outcome in 200 consecutive cases of severe head injury treated in San Diego County: a prospective analysis. *Neurosurgery* 6: 237–242.

Chesnut RM, Marshall SB, Piek J et al. (1993) Early and late systemic hypotension as a frequent and fundamental source of cerebral ischemia following severe brain injury in the Traumatic Coma Data Bank. *Acta Neurochir Suppl (Wien)* 59: 121–125.

Cooper A, DiScala C, Foltin G et al. (2001) Prehospital endotracheal intubation for severe head injury in children: a reappraisal. *Semin Pediatr Surg* 10: 3–6.

Dhellemmes P, Lejeune JP, Christiaens JL et al. (1985) Traumatic extradural hematomas in infancy and childhood. Experience with 144 cases. *J Neurosurg* 62: 861–864.

Duhaime AC, Christian CW, Rorke LB et al. (1998) Nonaccidental head injury in infants – the 'shaken-baby syndrome'. *N Engl J Med* 338: 1822–1829.

Dupuis O, Silveira R, Dupont C et al. (2005) Comparison of 'instrument-associated' and 'spontaneous' obstetric depressed skull fractures in a cohort of 68 neonates. *Am J Obstet Gynecol* 192: 165–170.

Ersahin Y, Mutluer S, Mirzai H et al. (1996) Pediatric depressed skull fractures: analysis of 530 cases. *Childs Nerv Syst* 12: 323–331.

Hsiang JK, Chesnut RM, Crisp CB et al. (1994) Early, routine paralysis for intracranial pressure control in severe head injury: is it necessary? *Crit Care Med* 22: 1471–1476.

Hutchison JS, Skippen P, Kirpalani H et al. (submitted) Guidelines for acute management of severe traumatic brain injury (TBI) in children and adolescents. *Can Med Assoc J.*

Keenan HT, Runyan DK, Marshall SW, Nocera MA, Merten DF (2004) A population-based comparison of clinical and outcome characteristics of young children with serious inflicted and noninflicted traumatic brain injury. *Pediatrics* 114: 633–639.

Keenan HT, Runyan DK, Nocera M (2006) Child outcomes and family characteristics 1 year after severe inflicted or noninflicted traumatic brain injury. *Pediatrics* 117: 317–324.

Kirkpatrick PJ, Smielewski P, Piechnik S et al. (1996) Early effects of mannitol in patients with head injuries assessed using bedside multimodality monitoring. *Neurosurgery* 39: 714–720. (Discussion: 720–711.)

Kokoska ER, Smith GS, Pittman T et al. (1998) Early hypotension worsens neurological outcome in pediatric patients with moderately severe head trauma. *J Pediatr Surg* 33: 333–338.

Lende RA (1974) Enlarging skull fractures of childhood. *Neuroradiology* 7: 119–124.

Lende RA, Erickson TC (1961) Growing skull fractures of childhood. *J Neurosurg* 18: 479–489.

Luerssen TG (1994) Acute traumatic cerebral injuries. In: Cheek WR (ed) *Pediatric Neurosurgery: Surgery of the Developing Nervous System.* Philadelphia: WB Saunders.

Meyer G, Orliaguet G, Blanot S et al. (2000) Complications of emergency tracheal intubation in severely head-injured children. *Paediatr Anaesth* 10: 253–260.

Mollman HD, Rockswold GL, Ford SE (1988) A clinical comparison of subarachnoid catheters to ventriculostomy and subarachnoid bolts: a prospective study. *J Neurosurg* 68: 737–741.

Natale JE, Joseph JG, Helfaer MA et al. (2000) Early hyperthermia after traumatic brain injury in children: risk factors, influence on length of stay, and effect on short-term neurologic status. *Crit Care Med* 28: 2608–2615.

National Center for Injury Prevention and Control (2000) Summary of recommendations from the Expert Working Group of the National Center for Injury Prevention and Control. Traumatic brain injury in the United States: assessing outcomes in children.

Nelson EL, Melton LJ 3rd, Annegers JF et al. (1984) Incidence of skull fractures in Olmsted County, Minnesota. *Neurosurgery* 15: 318–324.

Pigula FA, Wald SL, Shackford SR et al. (1993) The effect of hypotension and hypoxia on children with severe head injuries. *J Pediatr Surg* 28: 310–314. (Discussion: 315–316.)

Pittman T, Bucholz R, Williams D (1989) Efficacy of barbiturates in the treatment of resistant intracranial hypertension in severely head-injured children. *Pediatr Neurosci* 15: 13–17.

Raffel C, Litofsky NS (1994) Skull fractures. In: Cheek WR (ed) *Pediatric Neurosurgery: Surgery of the Developing Nervous System, 3rd edn.* Philadelphia: WB Saunders.

Roberts I, Yates D, Sandercock P et al. (2004) Effect of intravenous corticosteroids on death within 14 days in 10008 adults with clinically significant head injury (MRC CRASH trial): randomised placebo-controlled trial. *Lancet* 364: 1321–1328.

Shemie SD, Doig C, Dickens B et al. (2006) Severe brain injury to neurological determination of death: Canadian forum recommendations. *Can Med Assoc J* 174: 1–13.

Simma B, Burger R, Falk M et al. (1998) A prospective, randomized, and controlled study of fluid management in children with severe head injury: lactated Ringer's solution versus hypertonic saline. *Crit Care Med* 26: 1265–1270.

Sing RF, Reilly PM, Rotondo MF et al. (1996) Out-of-hospital rapid-sequence induction for intubation of the pediatric patient. *Acad Emerg Med* 3: 41–45.

Skippen P, Seear M, Poskitt K et al. (1997) Effect of hyperventilation on regional cerebral blood flow in head-injured children. *Crit Care Med* 25: 1402–1409.

Statham PF, Todd NV (1990) Intracerebral haematoma: aetiology and haematoma volume determine the amount and progression of brain oedema. *Acta Neurochir Suppl (Wien)* 51: 289–291.

Stocchetti N, Furlan A, Volta F (1996) Hypoxemia and arterial hypotension at the accident scene in head injury. *J Trauma* 40: 764–767.

5

COMPREHENSIVE MULTIDISCIPLINARY REHABILITATION

Peter Rumney

The literature on the rehabilitative process after traumatic brain injury in adults and children clearly shows that the earlier the intervention, the better for the speed and quality of recovery. In Ontario and the rest of Canada the network of primary care centres and tertiary care trauma centres is relatively well established and provides onsite stabilization, with supported transfer to appropriate trauma care centres, quite reliably. Multiple pediatric specialties are available to address the multisystem issues seen in polytrauma and ensure the minimization of the initial pathologic process whenever possible.

Once medical and surgical stabilization has been addressed, then the acute care thrust becomes one of secondary prevention of complications. Prolonged immobilization and ventilation often lead to pulmonary compromise with atelectasis and secondary pneumonia which may have an aspiration component as well. Preventing these complications hastens the recovery process and the transition to the acute rehabilitation phase. It has also been shown that the medical/infective setbacks that occur in acute care settings may have a long-term detrimental effect on functional outcome in the individual (Kalisky et al. 1985, McLean et al. 1995). Our own evaluation of severity indicators within the acquired brain injury (ABI) rehabilitation program has show that the best indicators of duration of stay in hospital for rehabilitation therapy relate to the initial duration of coma, duration of ventilation in the intensive care unit and the presence of pneumonia in the acute care environment (Hugh Macmillan Rehabilitation Centre 1994). With the effort to produce overall reduction of average lengths of stay in hospital, the prudent avoidance of complications is also clearly cost-effective (Sirios et al. 2004).

The initiation of rehabilitation care in acute care includes the provision of good nursing care to minimize secondary complications such as decubitus ulcers, joint contractures, deep venous thrombosis and atelectasis/pulmonary aspiration. The close medical monitoring of predictable sequelae of severe central nervous system trauma and early treatment is also required; such complications include SIADH (syndrome of inappropriate antidiuretic hormone), peptic ulcers (stress-induced), hypercalcemia, seizures, hypoglycemia, possible electrolyte imbalance, lower-extremity thromboses, and secondary infections through prolonged urinary catheterization, central lines, necessary foreign bodies (orthopedic fixators), gastrostomy and nasogastric feeding tubes and tracheostomy sites. With the increasing prevalence of multiple-resistant staphylococcus aureus, and vancomycin-resistant enterococci, the process of treatment of these infections has become increasingly challenging.

After the transfer from the intensive care setting, formal therapy assessment and treatment can be started. Referrals to the therapy team, including physiotherapy, occupational therapy, speech language pathology, and social work, can be made, beginning the assessment process and starting the long process of educating the family about the traumatic brain injury (TBI).

Practitioners in acute care and rehabilitation have regular exposure to the long-term consequences of TBI (Moscato et al. 1994), but families have very skewed and unrealistic perceptions about the recoverability of central nervous system damage in children and youth. These perceptions, along with the understandable wish of all parents to minimize the severity of an injury and illness for their child, often lead to situations where parents do not understand or grasp the extent of the potential long-term problems. They have lived through a catastrophic insult to their child and impact on their family and have been terrified about basic survival. When their child then lives through that first 48–72 hours and begins to improve, the questions begin to relate to the child's likelihood of walking, talking, returning to home and school, and the return to normalcy. The neurosurgeon must counsel about the possible negative outcomes in each of these areas, and when the child is able to progress to these basic levels of function in a stepwise pattern, the pattern of the child's actual recovery exceeding the doctors' prediction is established in those children with severe but non-fatal TBI who make it to rehabilitation.

'The surgeon said that he might die in the first two days and then he lived. Next I was told that he might never wake up from the coma and be a 'vegetable', and he woke up and began to respond. Then I was told he might not be able to stand or walk, and he is now up in therapy with a walker and his therapist taking his first steps. He has not had any seizures, he is beginning to talk more normally and you tell me that he cannot safely swallow liquids and has had severe damage to his memory, thinking and behaviour!?! I think that this is all because he hates being in hospital and is away from his friends. He has proved the specialists all along that they were wrong, and he will prove you wrong too!'

(personal communication)

This is a recurring pattern of thinking and comment encountered among parents and family members about their recovering child, and it can easily be seen how this thought pattern can be established. To try to inform families about the natural recovery process post TBI, it is necessary that they have regular contact with the treating staff to update them on progress and to properly frame the changes and functional improvements noted. It is difficult to provide accurate information and reasonable hope about a child's recovery while ensuring that the family fully see the significant impact of the injury and the likely ramifications. Although it is impossible to expect any family member to grasp the depth and breadth of the possible effects of the injury for the individual and their family in these early stages, it is extremely important that they see their care providers and therapists as sources of reliable, accurate and balanced information. Opportunities to meet with the surgeons and specialists to discuss the effects of a traumatic brain injury are usually brief in the acute care environment, but this part of their role can be well supplemented by nurses, nurse educators and therapists working with the patient, both at the bedside and in more structured therapy or teaching sessions.

Parent educational resources are currently available in a number of forms – pamphlets, binders, books, videos, computer interactive and online, parent support groups, and one-to-one support from local head injury or brain injury associations. Matching the individual with the locally available resources and the media format they are most comfortable with is well worth the time and effort. Early investment in proper information provides families with a better understanding and sense of control with respect to the issues and usually improves compliance with the therapeutic regimen proposed by the treatment team.

ASSESSMENT OF OVERALL SEVERITY

A review of the literature clearly shows that there are a number of clear indicators regarding the severity of a traumatic injury in children as well as adults. The key indicators are the length of time during which consciousness was lost, the duration of the subsequent post-traumatic amnesia (PTA), and whether there were confounding factors at the time of injury, including penetration of the skull and an open head injury or a projectile involved, secondary hypovolemia and shock or anoxia. In addition, the complicating factors of infection and metabolic instability and the effects of toxins at the time of trauma all add to the impact of the physical assault to the brain. All of these factors are reviewed in Chapter 4 of this volume, on acute and emergency management. Bruce reviews these issues in his discussion of the early assessment and management of the child with TBI and summarizes the situation in the following way: 'The lower the GCS score and the longer the duration of coma, the greater the risk of permanent neurologic or cognitive damage'(1990: 521–538). This is clearly our clinical experience and we feel certain in informing each parent that when their child has been in coma for more than 24 hours, be it pharmacologically sustained or spontaneous, and/or post-traumatic amnesia of more than 48 hours, then their child has sustained a severe traumatic brain injury and will have some measure of long-term change in thinking, cognition, behaviour or physical function.

Ponsford et al. (2004) recently discussed the use of the Westmead PTA scale as a reliable measure of the indication of severity of TBI in children, but also described its shortcomings in that it is unreliably used in acute care centres in a prospective way, and in that the retrospective assessment of PTA – i.e. by history – is far less reliable. They used a revised Westmead scale of 12 questions on an hourly basis in the emergency room to evaluate a cohort of 147 adults to look at correlation with other measures of mild head injury and cognitive function, especially memory. The closest analogue we have at present is the Children's Orientation and Amnesia Test (COAT) (Ewing-Cobbs et al. 1990) utilized on the neurosurgical floor of the Hospital for Sick Children by the occupational therapy staff to help evaluate the orientation of children on the day after admission. It has norms which help to discriminate those with more lasting effects and at highest risk for long-term problems.

The other key factor we have learned in the discussion of clinical cases with Dr Russell Schachar, Dr Maureen Dennis and Dr Harvey Levin in their collaborative study of outcomes in children with TBI is that those seen to be moderate in severity by virtue of GCS score (9–12) or length of coma (1–23 hours) are equivalent to children in the severe category with respect to their outcomes at six months and a year if they have any positive findings on their admission CT scans (personal communication 1996).

ADMISSION TO THE REHABILITATION PROGRAM

Whether the child begins rehabilitation in an inpatient or outpatient program at a rehabilitation facility or hospital, or through home-based care rehabilitation, at this point the process of transition and entry into the rehabilitation system begins. There is evaluation by the various specialties and therapists, and then the establishment of treatment goals and the setting up of therapy programs, which may be short or long, professionally driven or family applied. It is impossible to address all of the various protocols available but an overview of the most intense and involved may be instructive.

The intake process begins before the patient/client is admitted to the rehabilitation setting in order to establish whether they have the type of injury and problems that can be addressed by the team and facility. This involves review of the presenting diagnosis, medical and psychological complications, and the psychosocial milieu from whence the child comes.

In screening all the referrals for appropriateness, the rehabilitation staff must ensure that the patient is medically stable, as most rehabilitation facilities do not have 24-hour access to acute care nursing, medical care with all the necessary consultant specialty services, or diagnostic facilities of laboratory and medical imaging modalities. It is also necessary to rule out any ongoing degenerative disease process. Progress cannot be made until deteriorating neurological and physical problems have been halted or reversed.

The person to be treated must also be at a Rancho level of 3 (Rosenthal et al. 1990) or better. Cognitively this means that in order to benefit from the rehabilitation effort the patient must show some ability to respond to the environment and stimuli around them. Individuals who remain in a persistent coma vigil (persistent vegetative state) have no reliable response to tactile/verbal/visual stimuli and drift into a sleep/eyes open–wake cycle.

As a child progresses through the recovery stages described by the Rancho Los Amigos Group (Rosenthal et al. 1990), they first show generalized and non-specific responses to stimuli both noxious and neutral in nature. At Rancho level 3, the individual demonstrates specific responses to specific stimuli – for example, pulling the hand away while it is being washed – and not a generalized flexor posturing, and it is accepted that the child will benefit from therapeutic interactions with focused rehabilitation. Coma stimulation programming may be sensory-based (Gill-Thwaites and Munday 1999), dependent upon pharmacologic stimulation (Patrick et al. 2003), or based on electrophysiologic stimulation.

Our experience with individuals admitted to our Complex Continuing Care Ward at Rancho level 1 or 2 is that some stay at that level. Most children, however, then progress gradually to higher levels of cognition. Similar data are reported from the NIH Trauma Coma Databank (Multi-Society Task Force 1994) for pediatric survivors.

TABLE 5.1
Rancho Los Amigos Scale

Level 1	No response to stimuli. Appears in a deep sleep.
Level II	Generalized response. Has delayed, inconsistent responses.
Level III	Localized response. Inconsistent responses, but reacts in a more specific manner to stimulus. Might follow simple commands.
Level IV	Confused/agitated. Reacts to own inner confusion, fear, disorientation. Excitable behaviour, may be abusive.
Level V	Confused/inappropriate. Usually disorientated. Follows tasks for 2–3 minutes, but easily distracted by environment. Frustrated.
Level VI	Confused/appropriate. Follows simple directions consistently. Memory and attention increasing. Self-care tasks performed without help.
Level VII	Automatic/appropriate. If physically able, can carry out routine activities. Appears normal. Needs supervision for safety. Supervision is based on the nurse's assessment of the client's cognition and behaviour and determines the frequency of observation required and the degree of independence awarded to the client.
Level VIII	Purposeful/appropriate. May have decreased abilities compared to premorbid state.

Source: Professional Staff Association, Rancho Los Amigos Hospital, Inc., Downey, California, 1990.

Rancho Los Amigos has developed the eight level descriptors of cognitive communication patterns seen in the child or adult as they recover from significant TBI (see Table 5.1). These levels are quite helpful in communication from one caregiver to another about the general level of response of a child as they emerge from coma, and can be helpful for rehabilitation staff in the development of care plans for the individual client, but are not helpful in the assessment of ultimate outcome or function.

Children who are ready to participate in intensive rehabilitation programs have some basic ability to communicate. This may mean a system which is non-verbal or gestural in nature and may need to be augmented by technology (either high- or low-level).

Older children and adolescents must also be ready to benefit from the rehabilitation process. This means that they must not have an overriding drug/alcohol dependency and abuse that will interfere with their cognition and compliance with therapy. The individual must not be acutely psychotic as this has the same blocking affect on new learning and cognitive retention. There will be similar problems with depression and suicidality or self-harm or frank mania. These problems must be stabilized before active rehabilitation can be effective.

Another key issue is the knowledge that there is an appropriate discharge environment post-initial rehabilitation. Many decisions regarding home adaptation, school environments and programs and recreational settings are dependent upon the home discharge environment and local resources available.

In certain cases the question arises as to whether the family or guardian is capable of providing care for the individual once they are discharged. This situation may occur when a sole parent survives a motor vehicle collision and has problems of his/her own relating to cognition, mental health stability, drug or alcohol dependency or severe financial straits. Often involvement of the child protection services or public advocacy system must be arranged to ensure that appropriate planning on behalf of the child can begin.

When it has been determined that the individual is ready for pediatric rehabilitation, the process of assessment and initial discharge planning begins. The program available at Bloorview Kids Rehab focuses on return to home community and school for the child and their family. We begin the physical rehabilitation and cognitive assessment by evaluating the functional limitations of the child in current activities of daily living, with emphasis on the return to educational programming and school. If an adolescent has left school and begun a vocational career we ensure that the referral to rehabilitation services is sent to adult service providers in the community who are better equipped to meet these needs.

If the child or youth has behaviour that is currently manageable – meaning agitation or aggression that is stimulus-dependent – at Rancho level 4 and not psychopathological in origin, then therapy can begin. Children functioning at a higher level – Rancho level 5 or greater – must demonstrate some interest in the rehabilitation process and this must be met equally by guardians or family members. Rehabilitation is not a therapy that can be applied without the individual's consent and collaboration.

The family and the survivor must learn about the rehabilitation program, including benefits and limitations, prior to acceptance of their service providers. The focus is one of returning the child to their home, community and family. This demands commitment and involvement of the family members throughout the inpatient or day-patient admission. No program can provide 24-hour therapy and intervention; therefore true progress is gained with the integration of therapy interventions throughout the day in a number of different functional activities.

TBI leads to increased challenges of carry-over and generalization of new learning (Ylvisaker 1998). Learning of skills in a functional environment is naturally the best solution for successful rehabilitation. Teaching parents and caregivers about strategies and exercises focused in real time permits successful repetition and carry-over into other environments (home and community).

The other key feature that is required to ensure success is compliance. This can be improved by ensuring that the goals set for rehabilitation are realistic and that the patient and their family see these goals as necessary and important. Family-centred goal setting is a strategy that has been well described in the literature (AAP Task Force on the Family 2003, Geller 2004). Goals must be set collaboratively after an initial period of evaluation and must be measurable, objective and in most cases time limited to a reasonable time frame (for example, six to eight weeks).

Family-centred care also means that the complete family unit (both biological and social) needs to be involved in the rehabilitation process. This may include educational sessions for the parents about the effects of the TBI on their child currently and in the long term, but it may also include educational sessions for the siblings and grandparents to ensure that they understand and do not undermine the efforts of caregivers due to lack of knowledge or feelings of frustration and abandonment. Sessions should be structured in informal one-on-one sessions as well as larger group support sessions so that learning may occur in an optimal way.

Creative collaboration by the various therapists and team members is essential to ensure success. The process of rehabilitation is one that involves not only retraining motor patterns and strengthening functions, but also teaching the individual and their caregivers how to work with and around the current limitations and challenges using strategies, manoeuvres and equipment. Having family members and the patients working together on the same target goals improves compliance and mutual satisfaction in the family members and the staff involved in the rehabilitation.

STRUCTURE OF THE REHABILITATION TEAM

The use of a comprehensive team model to address the multifaceted issues of acquired brain injury is optimal. Team dynamics can be variable – whether they are multidisciplinary or transdisciplinary – but each team must develop its own specifics of communication, problem solving and role development dependent upon the skill set and personality strength of the individual team members.

At Bloorview Kids Rehab, we have all of the traditional therapies represented: nursing, occupational therapy, physiotherapy, psychology, recreational therapy, speech language pathology, and social work. We also draw upon the expertise of other psychosocial support experts such as creative arts therapists, child life specialists, child and youth workers and chaplaincy. These team members become the key behavioural/developmental therapists working with psychology and social work to allow children to express and cope with their feelings of loss, anger, frustration and despair, with a broader range of methods than in the traditional psychotherapeutic modalities usually offered in adult-based programs. This often ensures that the child will identify with one of the team members as their key contact and advocate within the larger group.

Another key service provider within the program is the teacher/educator. The teacher, in the setting of a smaller resource classroom, begins the process of educational assessment and provides one-to-one or small-group remediation for lost or impaired skills prior to return to school. The school record is requested (the file of the student's history and progress through school to date) and there is contact with the home school and classroom teacher to learn about the student and his or her skill sets and strengths prior to the recent ABI. The educator's assessment, together with the reports of the neuropsychologist, speech language pathologist and occupational therapist, has a robust validity when describing the patient/student at the time of discharge and can highlight their current learning needs. Teachers are often the first professional working with the student who sees how the ABI has affected their learning style and capacities in a real world environment. It must be determined if the child is capable of working through distractions, can cope with frustration, can retain new information in a multitude of modalities and can synthesize the salient points of information and create a coherent report or synopsis. None of the standard assessment tools used in psychology, or other therapies, properly evaluates these activities. Academic assessment in the classroom provides a useful window on the patient's daily cognitive function.

STRUCTURE OF THE REHABILITATION TEAM'S INTERVENTION

Interactions of the therapists have to be mutually complementary to achieve maximal impact and carry over in the transdisciplinary/multidisciplinary service. This model, however, only demonstrates the individual's capabilities in the optimal environment of the small, quiet assessment room, with minimal distracters and the structured presentation of information. In addition, group assessment and therapy opportunities must be available for the child or youth, including a cognitive group (cognitive remediation skills), recreational groups for activities of daily living, and social skills groups, as well as the more traditional educational venue of the classroom.

Recreational therapy is another component of the program, allowing the social skills of the child or youth to be evaluated in a less structured situation. Recreational therapists involved in these programs help with initiation of tasks and supervision of the children and youth to foster inclusion and avoid emotional and physical harm. Therapists can then assist the team in the clinical rounds with respect to the individual's challenges and retained skills, and aid in shaping further rehabilitation goals and targets. It is this psychosocial skill set and adaptability of the individual in the community that relates to success at reintegration rather than individual cognitive skills or measurable intellectual function (Ewing-Cobbs et al. 1997, Lannoo et al. 2001, Viguier et al. 2001).

CONTINUUM OF SERVICE AND CARE

To provide for the wide range of therapy needs and intensities, there must be various levels of intervention and support for the individual and their family after discharge from an acute care setting. Inpatient rehabilitation should be available for those who need observation and nursing care along with the intensive rehabilitation therapy. Day-patient programming is available if there is no requirement for 24-hour nursing intervention and the child lives within a reasonable commute of the facility and has sufficient endurance to be able to tolerate the travel and the full-day rehabilitation program. Some children must remain as inpatients during the working week if there are transportation issues, if they cannot receive the level of rehabilitation intensity that they need in their local community initially, or if a specific service is not available in their local treatment centre (for example, neuropsychological assessment, higher-technology augmentative communication services or unique seating needs).

Outpatient services are available for less intensive intervention, including weekly physical or occupational therapy or speech language pathology services. This team of service providers offers traditional outpatient clinic services, but also as much community-based rehabilitation as is possible, as this provides the therapy in a more ecologically valid environment to assist in learning retention and carry-over (Ylvisaker 1998). There is a shift in the needs of these children toward psychosocial demands and needs relating to adjustment, behaviour and education, and so the outpatient team reflects this with a higher proportion of appropriate service providers in these areas, specifically social work, psychology and child and youth workers.

The advantage that this team has over individual service providers (public or private) in the community is that there is the opportunity to collaborate with one another and the consultant physician about the goals established by the client and their family. The team also collaborates with service providers in the community to offer groups for patients addressing needed skills and accessing resources in the community. Support groups are held to provide information for the patients, their parents, their siblings and occasionally other friends in the community. One successful approach is offering all of these groups at one site at the same time so that all family members can participate while avoiding the need for additional child supervision costs and multiple transportation costs.

Information and advocacy sessions are also offered to community service providers and groups regarding the issues of ABI and the effect on children and their families. The purpose is to improve the overall knowledge base in the community and provide comfort and flexibility within these groups to offer assistance to an ABI survivor. The team members must visit homes, schools, and community centres to provide information and support.

Children and adolescents with severe ABI who are slow to recover may remain in the lower Rancho levels 1–3. There are often few programs for these children and waiting lists for services may be as long as 6–12 months. Return to community hospitals, nursing homes or parental homes may be the only option in this situation.

Children and youth with significant neurobehavioural problems post-ABI are often refused services due to their level of aggression, agitation or psychosis. With these significant levels of disruptiveness and issues related to safety for the individual or others, they are refused admission to rehabilitation services or are expelled from educational settings as there are 'zero tolerance' policies adopted by school boards. In the acute crisis of depression and suicidal ideation or aggression, an acute psychiatric assessment must be arranged. Often no appropriate service (either inpatient or outpatient) exists to address the needs of children and youth with ABI and significant psychiatric diagnoses. The families and individuals are trapped in the psychiatric–rehabilitation 'dual diagnosis' situation where each service provider points to the issue that is relevant to the other service or facility and notes that intervention and therapy in that area are necessary before the other can intervene successfully with the client. Co-assessment and treatment with neurobehavioural experts in acquired frontal lobe pathology and intensive neuropsychiatric intervention represents the ideal approach.

FAMILY ISSUES AND CHALLENGES

It is a well recognized principle in family therapy that the person presenting with the symptoms may only be manifesting them on behalf of the family system and that the real crisis may exist within another component of the family system. The adaptation to the disability is as important as learning to recognize the disability and overcome physical dysfunction and social handicap. Parents must learn to adapt their expectations of the individual, provide appropriate discipline to the child and ensure fairness of attention is established within the family, particularly with other siblings and between the parents themselves. The demands of the medical and rehabilitation system are often onerous and disruptive to normal family life. There may be times when the optimal rehabilitation prescription may be too overwhelming to the family and impossible to achieve. Collaborative goal setting with the family and the child is helpful and avoids unnecessary conflict. With agreed-upon goals and outcomes, issues of miscommunication and non-compliance are minimized.

Kreutzer et al. (2002) provide a model that can be used to achieve collaborative goal setting. It uses a questionnaire to assess the importance of numerous needs for the family members with respect to their injured member. The questionnaire determines whether or not the need as identified has been met in part or in whole. Having identified those high-priority needs that have not been met, a rehabilitation team can use this information for setting realistic and achievable goals with the family. The major areas of need as described by the questionnaire include health information, emotional support, instrumental support, professional support, community support and involvement with care. There is then a process of family assessment and intervention after the initial evaluation, through anticipating issues, preventing foreseeable challenges and problem solving. The skilled family worker or therapist will listen, normalize, reframe and teach the various family members and identify positive attributes and accomplishments within the family using a number of different treatment methods. The ability to identify and refer to community resources and treatment programs is important, and is a key skill for the effective clinician.

REFERENCES

AAP Task Force on the Family (2003) Family pediatrics; report of the Task Force on the Family. *Pediatrics* 111(6 Pt 2): 1541–1571.

Bruce D (1990) Scope of the problem – early assessment and management. In: Rosenthal M, Griffith E *et al.* (eds) *Rehabilitation of the Adult and Child with Traumatic Brain Injury, 2nd edn.* Philadelphia: FA Davis Co.

Cooper EB, Cooper JB (2003) Electrical treatment of coma via the median nerve. *Acta Neurochir Suppl* 87: 7–10.

Cooper EB, Scherder EJ, Cooper JB (2005) Electrical treatment of reduced consciousness: experience with coma and Alzheimer's disease. *Neuropsychol Rehabil* 15(3–4): 389–405.

DiScala C, Grant CC (1992) Functional outcome in children with traumatic brain injury. *Am J Phys Med Rehab* 71(3): 145–148.

Ewing-Cobbs L, Levin HS, Fletcher JM (1990) The Children's Orientation and Amnesia Test: relationship to severity of acute head injury and recovery of memory. *Neurosurgery* 27: 683.

Ewing-Cobbs L, Fletcher JM, Levin HS, Francis DJ, Davidson K, Miner ME (1997) Longitudinal neuropsychological outcome in infants and preschoolers with traumatic brain injury. *J Int Neuropsychol Soc* 3: 581–591.

Geller G (2004) Toward an optimal healing environment in pediatric rehabilitation. *J Altern Complement Med* 10(Suppl 1): S179–S192.

Gill-Thwaites H, Munday R (1999) The sensory modality assessment and rehabilitation technique. *Neuropsychol Rehabil* 9(3/4): 305–320.

Hugh Macmillan Rehabilitation Centre predictor analysis of factors relating to inpatient stay (1994) (unpublished).

Kalisky Z, Morrison DP et al. (1985) Medical problems encountered during rehabilitation of patients with head injury. *Arch Phys Med Rehabil* 66: 25–29.

Kreutzer JS, Kolakowsky-Hayner SA, Demm SR, Meade MA (2002) A structured approach to family intervention after brain injury. *J Head Trauma Rehabil* 17(4): 349–367.

Lannoo E, Colardyn F, Jannes C, de Soete G (2001) Course of neuropsychological recovery from moderate to severe head injury: a 2 year follow-up. *Brain Inj* 15(1): 1–13.

McLean DE, Kaitz ES, Keenan CJ, Dabney K, Cawley MF, Alexander MA (1995) Medical and surgical complications of pediatric brain injury. *J Head Trauma Rehabil* 10(5): 1–12.

Max J, Roberts MA, Koele SL, Lindgren SD, Robin DA, Arndt S, Smith WL Jr, Sato Y (1999) Cognitive outcome in children and adolescents following severe traumatic brain injury: influence of psychosocial, psychiatric and injury related variables. *J Int Neuropsychol Soc* 5: 58–68.

Moscato BS, Trevisan M, Willer BS (1994) The prevalence of traumatic brain injury and co-occurring disabilities in a national household survey of adults. *J Neuropsychiatry Clin Neurosci* 6(2): 134–142.

The Multi-Society Task Force on PVS (1994) Medical aspects of the persistent vegetative state, Parts 1 & 2. *N Engl J Med* 330(21): 1499–1508, 1572–1579.

Patrick PD, Buck ML, Conaway MR, Blackman JA (2003) The use of dopamine enhancing medications with children in low response states following brain injury. *Brain Inj* 17(6): 497–506.

Peri CV, Shaffrey ME, Farace E, Cooper E, Alves WM, Cooper JB, Young JS, Jane JA (2001) Pilot study of electrical stimulation on median nerve in comatose severe brain injured patients: 3–month outcome. *Brain Inj* 15(10): 903–910.

Ponsford J, Willmott C, Rothwell A, Kelly AM, Nelms R, Ng KT (2004) Use of the Westmead PTA scale to monitor recovery of memory after mild head injury. *Brain Inj* 18(6): 603–614. Erratum in: (2004) *Brain Inj* 18(10): 1065.

Rosenthal M, Griffith ER, Bond MR, Miller JD (1990) *Rehabilitation of the Adult and Child with Traumatic Brain Injury, 2nd edn.* Philadelphia: FA Davis Co.

Sirios MJ, Lavoie A, Dionne CE (2004) Impact of transfer delays to rehabilitation in patients with severe trauma. *Arch Phys Med Rehabil* 85: 184–191.

Viguier D, Dellatolas G, Gasquet I, Martin C, Choquet M (2001) A psychological assessment of adolescent and youth adult inpatients after traumatic brain injury. *Brain Inj* 15(3): 263–271.

Wohlrab G, Boltshauser E, Schmitt B (2001) Neurological outcome in comatose children with bilateral loss of cortical somatosensory evoked potentials. *Neuropediatrics* 32(5): 271–274.

Ylvisaker M (1998) *Traumatic Brain Injury Rehabilitation: Children and Adolescents.* Boston, MA: Butterworth-Heinemann.

6
OVERVIEW OF OUTCOMES

Peter Rumney

> Traumatic brain injury (TBI) in children and adolescents is a major public
> health problem in the United States, with an incidence of approximately
> 180 per 100,000 children per year (Kraus 1995). Between 5 and 8% of children
> treated at hospitals for TBI have severe TBI (Kraus 1995). About 50% of these
> children have major neurological sequelae; these deficits result in a lifetime of
> severe disability for 2 to 5% (Di Scala et al. 1991).
>
> (Max et al. 1998)

This statement is as true in Canada and Europe as it is in the United States. Our
society, however, continues to view traumatic brain injury (TBI) as inconsequential
since 'kids recover better than adults'. This viewpoint is inaccurate, as is illustrated
by a review of the scientific evidence and current clinical opinion.

It is clear in the medical and psychological literature that children and youth
with traumatic brain injury of a severe nature have long-term outcomes that
are worse from a cognitive and behavioural standpoint than those of their adult
counterparts, although the basic physical function recovery seems to be excellent.
The Kennard Principle (Kennard 1938) (based on research in the 1930s) describes
how, from a physical function standpoint, young primate recovery from a
reproducible TBI surpassed that of older primates, but from a social and behavioural
standpoint the younger primates had more difficulty returning to the larger group in
comparison to their older adult peers.

In the analysis of our own outcome data from Bloorview Kids Rehab, children
with moderate and severe TBI have worse outcomes at three to five years post-
discharge than their older peers with a similar array of injuries and severity.

Children with concussion and mild TBI have been reported to do well in
general and have good long-term outcomes (Behrman 1992). Current research, however, demonstrates that the outcome of mild TBI is more complex than first thought
and not as optimistic.

Teasdale and Engberg (2003) evaluated retrospective data of 3091 men entering
the Danish military (compulsory service) who had been injured prior to the age of
18 years, and assessed those with two concussions with hospitalization. Admission
of one day each (N = 521) led to an odds ratio >1.4 over that of the general
population of having a statistically increased rate of cognitive dysfunction barring

enrolment in the military. The severity of injury, as measured by associated skull fracture or cerebral lesion, also had a predictive effect in those males injured after 11 years of age.

Hawley et al. (2004) reported a population study of childhood head injury using a mailed survey to families whose children were admitted to a National Health Service trust (England) from 1992 to 1998. These children were 5–15 years of age at the time of injury, and 526 parents participated and 45 controls were surveyed. Mean time of follow-up was 2.2 years. There was a high prevalence of problems with memory, attention, emotional changes and behavioural changes in the survey responses: 33% in the severe TBI group, but also 25% in the moderate group and 10–18% in the mild group (using the King's Outcome Scale for Childhood Head Injury – Crouchman et al. 2001). The frequency of medical follow-up for this group was poor, with 64% of those with moderate disability having no medical follow-up at two years. It was stated that 'no evidence was found to suggest a threshold of injury severity below which the risk of late sequelae could safely be discounted'.

There was also discussion regarding the additive effects of social deprivation on the longer-term outcome. Anderson et al. (2005) studied child and family outcome 30 months post-TBI prospectively in 150 children aged 3–12 years admitted to hospital with a TBI diagnosis, with cohorts of 42 mildly injured, 70 moderately injured and 38 severely injured children. They reported a 'dose dependent' effect on outcome from a physical and cognitive standpoint, but where behavioural problems were noted, little recovery occurred from 6 to 30 months in follow-up. Family function and child behavioural issues were predicted by psychosocial and premorbid factors.

Longitudinal follow-up of families and children post-TBI has been described by Keenan et al. (2006). They looked at the two years after TBI for those children hospitalized and admitted to an intensive care unit with a head injury in 2000 in a region in North Carolina. They found that these children had stable functional outcomes at one to two years post-injury, using the Pediatric Overall Performance Category score (Fizer 1992). They also assessed ongoing health status using the Stein–Jessup Functional Status II (revised) (Stein and Jessup 1990) and the Global Health Index (2001). Family characteristics were gathered and categorized using the Social Capital Index (1998). Their conclusions were telling in that many of the children treated were from socially disadvantaged families (~50%), with their regional norm closer to 12.3%, and they raised questions about the future developmental trajectory of those children followed post-TBI and underscored the need for consistent long-term follow-up and staged intervention when problems are identified, especially in those families with the least economic and social resources to advocate for their needs.

McKinlay et al. (2002) noted long-term poor psychosocial outcomes after mild TBI in early childhood. A birth cohort was followed prospectively. Children with mild TBI who had inpatient or ambulatory/outpatient care after their injury were examined before the age of 10 years. It was reported that the inpatient group displayed increased hyperactivity/inattention and conduct disorder measured at ages 10–13 years, compared to their pre-injury status and controls. A higher prevalence of psychosocial deficits was also seen in the inpatient group injured before the age of 5 years, compared to peers.

The adult literature has also focused on predictive factors for intracranial pathology with minor head trauma (Dunning et al. 2004), to assist in the process of more thoroughly screening those presenting in the office or the emergency room with mild TBI.

Predicting outcomes in children with TBI in general has been difficult. Prasad et al. (2002) looked prospectively at 60 cases of childhood TBI. In those less than 6 years of age they noted that the best predictors remained the modified Glasgow Coma Scale score, the duration of impaired consciousness, and the number of lesions seen on neuroimaging. If the TBI was inflicted, as opposed to accidental, there were poorer outcomes for the children, measured by the Glasgow Outcome Scale and cognitive measures. Pupillary changes also predicted poorer motor outcomes.

A study (Klonoff et al. 1977) of a five-year follow-up of two groups of children and youth was reported in 1977. Four domains of function were assessed including physical/medical, cognitive, behavioural, and educational. There were differential recoveries over time for the four domains and more educational problems in the younger group. Over 23.9% of those followed had neurological sequelae.

Another study (Levin and Eisenberg 1979) reported on a sample of 45 children with TBI, with three levels of severity (mild, moderate, severe). The study was stratified into three age groups: 0–5, 6–12 and 13–18 years. There was a relationship between severity and age at time of injury, with worse outcomes in the younger patients.

Older children have better outcomes (Kriel et al. 1989), as was demonstrated in a study involving 97 children with severe closed head injury. Worse outcomes are seen in a direct relationship to distance of referral from the trauma centre. This would imply that faster definitive therapy post-trauma has lasting positive effects with respect to ultimate outcome.

A report of a study of 84 children (Tompkins et al. 1990) followed after rehabilitation for moderate to severe TBI in the first year post-injury (using three separate evaluations of language, memory skills, visuomotor and speeded performance) indicated that injury severity and pre-injury intellectual challenges were the best predictors of timing of discharge in older children, over 9 years of age. In the younger children followed, parental marital status was the best predictor of cognitive performance early in recovery.

Klonoff et al. (1993) have reported long-term outcome of head injuries with a one-year follow-up study. The study assessed 159 individuals with a mean age of 31.4 years. In this group, 91% had been admitted to hospital with a diagnosis of mild TBI. General IQ scores at discharge were a good predictor of long-term outcome. In this largely mildly injured group there was a high frequency of long-term challenges: 32.7% had physical complaints that persisted and were attributed to the earlier injury, and 17.6% psychological and psychiatric problems. The authors also noted that the severity of the head injury was the primary contributory factor in affecting long-term outcome in these patients.

There is evidence of age-related differences in outcome (Taylor and Alden 1997), depending on age at injury, time since injury, and age at testing. Development is more adversely affected the younger the child at the time of injury.

Long-term studies have been possible since the new era in trauma care was instituted in the 1970s, with significantly improved trauma survival and newer methods of diagnostic imaging (Himanen et al. 2005). There is a relationship between long-term cognitive effects of a remote traumatic brain injury (TBI) which can be correlated to MRI findings and the clinical evaluation of severity of injury. In a report on 61 patients assessed on average 30 years after TBI of variable severity, there were reductions in hippocampal volumes and lateral ventricular enlargement. These were significantly associated with impaired memory functions, memory complaints and executive functions. The best predictor of cognitive outcome is thought to be the volume of the lateral ventricle. This would suggest that the degree of diffuse injury with atrophic changes is prognostically more important than the initial severity of the brain injury.

Another study (Max et al. 1999) assessed the psychosocial and psychiatric factors after TBI in a series of children aged 5–14 years. The patients were followed for two years post-trauma. Severe TBI was associated with significant decrease in intellectual and memory function. Post-injury psychiatric disorders added significantly to severity indices. These factors may help to define subgroups of children requiring more intensive services.

The injury to the brain is 'dose dependent' and compounded by a number of aggravating factors. The younger the child at the time of injury the worse the outcome is in the long term in the realms of learning and cognition. Family factors as well as pre-injury factors have a dramatic impact on functional outcome. In moderate and severe traumatic brain injury in children, recovery continues for three to five years, but even then it is less than complete.

There is a significant increase in the lifetime frequency and novel presentation of psychiatric disorders in individuals after pediatric TBI (Bloom et al. 2001). A study of 46 youth who were injured between 6 and 15 years of age, at one year or more post-TBI, reported that 48% of the children had novel psychiatric disorders and that problems persisted in 74% of these patients. Attention deficit/hyperactivity disorder and depressive disorders were the most common diagnoses. There were a significant number with subsequent explosive dyscontrol associated with frontal lobe trauma as well as mania post-injury. Obsessive compulsive disorders and anxiety spectrum disorders which occur post-trauma may persist lifelong in a significant number of patients.

The program at Bloorview Kids Rehab has developed a clinical database to track the individuals admitted to the rehabilitation program and the follow-up clinic over a time frame of five years. These data have been evaluated and utilized for further outcome research and evaluation. The study used the Mayo-Portland Adaptability Inventory (MPAI) scores. Clinical information was entered at the time of admission, at discharge and at regular follow-up clinics. MPAI data have been collected on 335 clients from five months to five years post-discharge.

Because of its broader design, the Mayo-Portland Adaptability Inventory (MPAI), created by and published by Malec and Thompson (1994), is useful for rating the severity of emotional behaviour, functional skills (including social skills) and physical disability following traumatic brain injury in adults. As an outcome measure, it is easily administered in a 20–30-minute follow-up assessment by the evaluating clinician and can be used as a framework for a clinical visit with little need for modification. The actual scoring time is 1–2 minutes. The inventory can yield a raw total score as a measure of disability post-acquired brain injury (ABI). The tool contains 30 questions divided into six domains including: physical/medical, cognition, emotion, everyday activities, and social behaviour.

As the original measure was developed for adults and there is no comparable measure for children and youth, the MPAI was adapted for use in pediatric TBI. Most items can be given with no modification. A few key questions were modified to reflect developmental issues for the pediatric population, including assessment of normal walking for a 1-year-old rated as impaired for a 3-year-old (stability and rate, but with assessment of the quality of gait and mobility).

The modified MPAI was evaluated and demonstrated a reasonable inter-rater reliability ($r = 0.83$). Concurrent validity was established by examining correlations between scores in the activity, cognitive, emotional and physical domains and real world function as reported to us by parents at the time of clinic follow-up. There was a significant test–retest reliability ($p<.001$) with correlation of the MPAI scores over time (average eight months follow-up), which were significant on all domains ($p<.001$). The change between first and last follow-up appointments was generally positive (64% improvement). With clinical complications, including problems with illness, depression or worsening behaviour, the scores deteriorated.

The demographic profile of the subjects in the study was consistent with the typical profile described in the literature and seen in our client population:

- Clients had moderate to severe TBI.
- GCS scores ranged from 3 to 15.
- Clients were aged between 1 and 19 years (M = 9.7 years).
- 64% of clients were male.

- Motor vehicle accidents were the most common cause of injury (46%).
- Strokes accounted for 11%.
- Tumours accounted for 8%.
- Sports injuries accounted for 6%.

PATTERNS OF RECOVERY

Our analysis of the data showed some consistent patterns. Older children showed more impairment at admission to the rehabilitation program and this may reflect bias of the scoring procedure for adapted MPAI as young children are scored as having 'no impairment' on four questions when it is developmentally inappropriate. The patients were seen in a second follow-up visit (one year post-discharge) and at that time this relationship was no longer seen. Older children then showed more recovery but both age groups showed that overall improvement only occurred in the presence of significant cognitive improvements.

Difficulties with anger, endurance, initiative, sleep, and processing speed were not associated with recovery. Children injured younger than 5 years showed the least recovery and, over time, for this age group, impairments in the social behaviour domain increased.

Although most recovery was noted in the first two years after injury, some children showed no improvement in MPAI scores over the first two years, but 65% of these children did show positive change in years 3 and 4 post-discharge. It cannot be predicted which children will fall into which group. In most cases, improvement does not lead to complete freedom from impairments in the group of more severely injured children, even five years after injury. Younger children (those under 6 years at the time of injury) demonstrated less improvement than older children after five years of recovery.

In evaluation of activities in the community post-discharge, poor MPAI scores (worsened functional outcomes) did not reliably predict the requirement for or extent of school support. Factors that did correlate with the provision of school-based help were mobility difficulties and obvious speech impairment. The correlation of visible disability seemed to be the best predictor of provision of school support. There were other correlations of interest. Poor MPAI scores in the behaviour domain predicted the need for speech therapy and special education/resource class support. Poor MPAI scores in the social domain did not predict requirement for speech therapy services although pragmatic skill impairment is often a feature of TBI.

Ten years post-TBI, approximately 50% of parents reported significant concerns about their children's anger and resultant behaviour. For children and adolescents over 10 years of age at the time of injury, reports of anger peaked two years post-discharge, with 23% of those seen reporting a serious episode. Verbal anger was more common than physical outbursts initially (4:1), but four years after discharge, reports of verbal and physical anger are equal.

In other areas, children under 5 years of age at the time of injury were seen to be differently affected. They had fewer sleep limitations than the older children (7% versus 15%). Younger children demonstrated more mobility limitations and clinically evident spasticity, with more speech problems (50%) – dysarthria being the most commonly observed problem. A slowed speech rate was an issue with all age groups. Children with impaired social skills at the time of discharge had not developed those skills at the time of most recent follow-up assessment.

Children and adolescents over the age of 5 years at the time of injury had a high incidence of learning disabilities (13–17%). Four years post-injury older adolescents had a high school drop-out rate of 16%.

PROSPECTIVE STUDY

Our research group has studied outcome information on pragmatic language skills and quality of life measures with a longer-term follow-up. This study investigated the relationship between functional outcomes for the TBI children/youth and family stress levels.

The study population consisted of children and adolescents aged 5–18 years with a moderate to severe TBI as assessed by GCS score, between three and five years post-injury. In total, 64 children/adolescents and families participated in the study. Measures included the MPAI-3, the Family Burden of Injury Interview (FBII), the Children's Communication Checklist-2 (CCC-2), the Pragmatics Test of the Comprehensive Assessment of Spoken Language (CASL) and the PEDS QL (a quality of life measure). The MPAI-3 had been revised by Malec et al. (2003) and changed to 34 questions, and reduced from six domains to three subscales: physical/cognitive, pain/emotion and social participation.

The Family Burden of Injury Interview (Wade et al. 1998) was designed to measure the impact of childhood traumatic brain injuries on the family. The Children's Communication Checklist-2 (Bishop 1998) is a checklist for parents of children aged 4–17 years evaluating language and communication skills and screening for issues of concern. It is designed to assess aspects of communication that are not easily evaluated in more traditional one-to-one assessments (for example, pragmatic skills). This tool screens for specific language impairments and assists in identifying children who have an autistic spectrum disorder. Seven individual scales are tested and then collapsed into two composite scores. The General Communication Composite score is based on all communication scales, and the Social Interaction Deviance Composite is designed to discriminate children with disproportionate pragmatic difficulties, such as autistic spectrum disorders, from those with specific language impairments. This measure assesses the challenges experienced by TBI patients as the pragmatic assessment component is well developed and more sensitive.

We also utilized the Comprehensive Assessment of Spoken Language (CASL) (Carrow-Woolfolk 1999). This is a normative-referenced oral language assessment battery of tests for children and young adults aged 3–21 years. It contains several language tests. Each test is scored and normed separately. The Pragmatics Test measures a child's knowledge and use of pragmatic language rules such as recognizing appropriate topics for conversation and selecting relevant information for requests/replies, as well as adjusting communication according to the situation (for example, age and relationships).

The PEDS QL (Varni 1998a, 1998b) assesses health-related quality of life through an interview format, with two versions available – one for parents and one for children and adolescents to complete. Questions are in four domains:

- Physical functioning
- Emotional functioning
- Social functioning
- School functioning

In assessing speech and language pragmatics, the CCC-2 identified 59% of the sample (n = 59) as having communication impairments, while the CASL identified only 27% of the sample as having pragmatic impairments. The two tests were in 77% agreement (p = .01) in identification of pragmatic impairments. The CCC-2 General Communication Composite score was significantly correlated with the CASL standard scores (p<.0001), which means that parents are accurate reporters of their child's communication/pragmatic skills.

The Social Interaction Deviance Composite score of the CCC-2 did not correlate with the CASL score (but was not significant). This score and subscale was originally intended for research purposes as a possible screening tool for autistic spectrum disorders. Children with TBI experience different pragmatic difficulties from children with autism, and this tool did not detect the TBI-specific nature of communication breakdown.

The CCC-2 General Communication Composite (p<.0001) and the CASL scores (p<.01) significantly correlated with functional outcome as measured by the MPAI-3, and there was a strong relationship between pragmatic/language skills and the physical/cognition (p<.0001) and pain/emotion scales (p<.0001) of the MPAI-3.

The General Communication Composite score of the CCC-2 strongly correlated with PEDS QL (p<.0001) as reported on the parent forms. High scores on the CCC-2 General Communication Composite (identified language difficulties) correlated with higher levels of family stress as measured by the Family Burden of Injury Inventory (p<.0001). Pragmatic language difficulties predict functional disability in the children and youth as measured by the MPAI-3, and quality of life issues as described by the children's parents, and are a positive predictor of family stress.

These tools and their resultant scores correlated more with functional disability than simple GCS scores, severity measures of the TBI or the concurrent use of school support in the community.

The PEDS QL parent (p<.0001) and child (p<.05) forms significantly correlated with the CCC-2 General Communication Composite score. The PEDS QL parent form also significantly correlated (p<.0001) with CASL scores, but the child form did not correlate with CASL scores. Both parent (p<.0001) and child (p<.01) PEDS QL forms significantly correlated with functional outcome scores (MPAI-3). There was a strong relationship between quality of life and the physical/cognition (p<.0001) and pain/emotion scales (p<.0001) of the MPAI-3. The correlations were all stronger for the parent form of the PEDS QL than for the child form. There was a clear difference in perception in the children and youth compared to their parents. The PEDS QL parent form significantly correlated (p<.0001) with the family stress measure; however the PEDS QL child form was not correlated with family stress scores. This may relate to differing levels of insight by the survivors, as opposed to that of their caregivers/parents.

Pragmatic language skill difficulties and quality of life challenges after TBI are significantly correlated. Quality of life changes post-pediatric TBI and problems in a child's pragmatics/communication skills predict levels of functional disability and correlate with reported levels of family stress at a point three to five years post-injury. By this time most anticipated physical recovery has occurred.

Appropriate psychosocial support in the medical/rehabilitation system is absolutely essential for families. Much of the pathology that is experienced by individuals and their families relates to the cognitive and behavioural changes that persist. Early intervention by social work and psychology service providers is a key component of a rehabilitation program and may have positive effects on longer-term outcomes. Outpatient rehabilitation services for the hospital-based team and the community outreach service from a family support service must focus on the psychosocial adaptation issues for the child and family. As time post-injury passes and the process of physical recovery slows, the need for adaptation to the new long-term issues increases and psychosocial support services need to be readily available.

Yeates and colleagues (1997) noted that the family's pre-injury environment was a strong predictor of recovery of function in children post-TBI. High-functioning families seemed to significantly moderate the effects of more severe TBI when compared to those who are low-functioning (Anderson et al. 2005). This effect is seen when socio-economic status, age at time of injury and family environment are controlled for.

This information is helpful for prognostically evaluating potential outcomes for individuals and their families, but does not help in planning interventions with those families who have a poorer prognosis. Skilled social work/psychology staff are invaluable in intervening with families in these circumstances. Helping individuals and the family system explore and marshal their innate coping strategies to address the challenges is the first step. Giving families structured supportive counselling and providing details of the available resources in the community, both financial and emotional, is crucial (Sander et al. 2003).

It is helpful to utilize tools such as the Family Assessment Measure (FAM-III) (Skinner and Steinhauer 1995). Studies have shown that those families with more structured role definitions and a tendency to be more rigid in rule application and problem solving seem to do better over the long term with intervention (Gates et al. 1990, Gan et al. 2002) than those leaning towards more flexible roles, looser patterns of behaviour and more relaxed or laissez-faire boundaries. There needs to be organization and consistency for more successful post-TBI return to the community.

Studies assessing family needs after TBI (Minnes et al. 2000, Armstrong and Kerns 2002, Benn and McColl 2004) have indicated that the needs for health and medical information, professional support and community support were not met, in comparison to those families whose children had purely orthopedic injuries. Benn (2000) demonstrated that the coping strategies utilized by parents were focused on changing the perceptions of others after the TBI and that mothers tended to use a broader array of strategies than the fathers. Maternal and paternal coping strategies were often complementary in nature, and 'a relationship existed between instrumental or practical support and emotional focused coping, as well as between family cohesion and perception focused coping'. Minnes et al. (2000) documented the stresses reported by Canadian caregivers of persons with TBI and reported that the highest scores related to lifespan care and personal burden. Correlations were seen between higher stress and issues of cognitive impairment, physical limitation, lifespan care, terminal illness, limits on family opportunities, and personal burden. Stress did not correlate with time post-injury and other client characteristics. Coping strategies of reframing and seeking spiritual support made 'important contributions to stress reduction'.

Time does not appear to reduce stress or burden with some individuals with TBI. 'Mobile mourning' (Muir et al. 1990) is a well reported process in the adult literature, describing the process of prolonged but incomplete adaptation to the person with TBI, who develops in a new life trajectory, deviating from the expected. The difference is regularly reinforced by the more 'normal' path being followed by peers and family members. Parents see their children returning to school after TBI only to gradually fall behind their peers academically and socially. When teens start dating, their child often becomes socially isolated. As the peer group graduates from school and goes on to college, university or work, the TBI survivors are later in graduating and have fewer options open to them. Thomsen (1992) reports in her long-term follow-up study that the issues of anger, memory dysfunction, immature behaviour and social problems persist for 15 to 30 years post-severe TBI.

Prigatano (2002) discusses the problems with interpersonal relationships which continue after TBI. Recurring therapeutic alliances with psychological service providers are shown to be helpful. A more supportive counselling role on an intermittent basis, not psychotherapy, is both needed and effective. The key issue is to learn to accommodate to long-term disabilities and to restore and maintain meaning to life over the longer term.

Kreutzer et al. (2002) discuss the issue of family stresses and challenges in research on the effects of TBI on the mothers and wives of injury survivors. Challenges to the family include less free time, greater financial insecurity, guilt issues and lack of respite. Reactions to these challenges often lead to maladaptive behaviours and mothers reported family reactions of anger (45%), verbal abuse (36%), and being physically threatened (18%). Depression was seen in 45% of the mothers and 55% of survivors.

Condeluci (1991) has written extensively about the need for individuals to reconnect with their community, with issues related to interdependence, overcoming differences and the process of cultural shifting in building bridges with the local groups and community.

PEDIATRIC TEST OF BRAIN INJURY

In an effort to improve the functionality of outcome measures in the area of pediatric ABI rehabilitation, Hotz et al. (2001) published the Pediatric Test of Brain Injury. In their article they describe the measure and its strengths. It was devised to measure the cognitive-linguistic skills of school-aged children after TBI and then to track the changes or recovery in these areas over time. This functionally focused measure taps into those skills necessary for the successful reintegration into school – the closest measure to vocational outcome for children and an area of measurement that to date has been lacking. At present the return to school is not a measure of success – it is compulsory for all children of a certain age in western society. The successful advancement from one grade to another may speak more to the accommodations available in a particular school board, and, to date, no well utilized quality of life measures exist for children in school.

It is also clear that focused psychological testing targeting academic achievement assesses old learning such as the WRAT and Woodcock-Johnson, and the isolated skill testing done in neuropsychological evaluation is helpful in the analysis of isolated skill sets but translates poorly into functional outcomes if they are stand-alone assessments (Ylvisaker 1998). Hotz and her colleagues (2001) are approaching the outcome measurement task from a functional standpoint which will complement other more physically focused measures, such as the Glasgow Outcome Scale, the Rappaport Disability Rating Scale and the Pediatric Evaluation of Disability Inventory, quite nicely.

HEALTH CARE UTILIZATION

Slomine and colleagues (2006) looked at the short-term health care needs of children after moderate to severe TBI for one year and found that the unmet or unrecognized health care needs of these children were not predicted by the severity of the TBI but rather by the insurance status of the individual, and by the level of family functioning as measured by the General Functioning Scale of the Family Assessment Device (1985). They reported that they were the first to demonstrate 'a protective effect between normal family function and unrecognized need'. This is clearly our clinical experience over the last 18 years and I would propose that this may be the *key* factor in influencing the outcome of a child post-ABI after the severity of the original insult has been taken into account.

CONCLUSION

There is a paucity of long-term outcome studies in pediatrics. An accurate long-term study of the outcome of pediatric TBI needs to account for the individual developmental effects and should follow a trauma cohort, with controls, for 10 to 20 years after their injury into adulthood. There should also be consideration of possible early-onset Alzheimer's disease and dementia. This kind of study is not one easily supported by current funding opportunities or individual institutions in Canada. A multicentred approach is clearly indicated for this type of evaluation and outcome research.

It is clear from the literature, however, that we must be clear in the education of our colleagues, our society and our patients that children and adolescents progress differently in their recovery trajectory compared to young and old adults. The earlier the child or youth sustains an acquired brain injury, the more severe the long-term outcome is with respect to cognition, learning and behaviour, when the dose/severity factors are taken into account. This factor alone is potent enough to compel us to advocate strongly for preventative measures in our society regarding injury, violence, helmet legislation and gun control. Prevention is our only sufficiently effective tool in this domain of health maintenance for children and their families.

REFERENCES

Anderson VA, Catroppa C, Haritou F, Morse S, Rosenfeld JV (2005) Identifying factors contributing to child and family outcome 30 months after traumatic brain injury in children. *J Neurol Neurosurg Psychiatry* 76: 401–408.

Armstrong K, Kerns KA (2002) The assessment of parent needs following paediatric traumatic brain injury. *Pediatr Rehabil* 5(3): 149-160.

Behrman RE (ed) (1992) *Textbook of Paediatrics, 14th edn.* Philadelphia: WB Saunders, pp 1521–1524.

Benn KM, McColl MA (2004) Parental coping following childhood acquired brain injury. *Brain Inj* 18(3): 239–255.

Bishop DVM (1998) Development of the Children's Communication Checklist (CCC): a method for assessing qualitative aspects of communicative impairment in children. *J Child Psychol Psychiatry* 39: 879–891.

Bloom DR, Levin HS, Ewing-Cobbs L, Saunders AE, Song J, Fletcher JM, Kowatch RA (2001) Lifetime and novel psychiatric disorders after pediatric traumatic brain injury. *J Am Acad Child Adolesc Psychiatry* 40(5): 572–579.

Carrow-Woolfolk E (1999) *Comprehensive Assessment of Spoken Language (CASL)*. Textbook. Circle Pines, MN: American Guidance Services.

Cascella PW (2006) Standardised speech language tests and students with intellectual disability: a review of normative data. *J Intellect Dev Disabil* 31(2): 120–124.

Condeluci A (1991) *Interdependence: The Route to Community*. Orlando, FL: Paul M Deutsch Press.

Crouchman M, Rossiter L, Colaco T, Forsyth R (2001) King's Outcome Scale for Childhood Head Injury: a practical outcome scale for paediatric head injury. *Arch Dis Child* 84(2): 120–124.

De Kruijk JR, Leffers P, Menheere PP, Meerhoff S, Rutten J, Twijnstra A (2002) Prediction of post-traumatic complaints after mild traumatic brain injury: early symptoms and biochemical markers. *J Neurol Neurosurg Psychiatry* 73(6): 727–732.

Dunning J, Stratford-Smith P, Lecky F, Batchelor J, Hogg K, Browne J, Sharpin C, Mackway-Jones K, Emergency Medicine Research Group (2004) A meta-analysis of clinical correlates that predict significant intracranial injury in adults with minor head trauma. *J Neurotrauma* 21(7): 877–885.

Ewing-Cobbs L, Barnes MA, Fletcher JM (2003) Early brain injury in children: development and reorganization of cognitive function. *Dev Neuropsychol* 24(2–3): 669–704.

Fizer DH (1992) Assessing the outcome of pediatric intensive care. *J Pediatr* 121: 68–74.

Gan C, Schuller R (2002) Family system outcome following acquired brain injury: clinical and research perspectives. *Brain Inj* 16(4): 311–322.

Gates R, Gemeinhardt M, Gan C (1990) Family support service internal review – Bloorview MacMillan Rehabilitation Centre, Toronto, Canada.

Geurts HM, Verte S, Oosterlaan J, Roeyers H, Hartman CA, Mulder EJ, Berckelaer-Onnes IA, Sergeant JA (2004) Can the Children's Communication Checklist differentiate between children with autism, children with ADHD, and normal controls? *J Child Psychol Psychiatry* 45(8): 1437–1453.

Haley SM, Ni P, Ludlow LH, Fragala-Pinkham MA (2006) Measurement precision and efficiency of multidimensional computer adaptive testing of physical functioning using the pediatric evaluation of disability inventory. *Arch Phys Med Rehabil* 87(9): 1223–1229.

Hawley CA, Ward AB, Magnay AR, Long J (2004) Outcomes following childhood head injury: a population study. *J Neurol Neurosurg Psychiatry* 75(5): 737–742.

Himanen L, Portin R, Isoniemi H, Helenius H, Kurki T, Tenovuo O (2005) Cognitive functions in relation to MRI findings 30 years after traumatic brain injury. *Brain Inj* 19(2): 93–100.

Hotz G, Helm-Estabrooks N, Nelson NW (2001) Development of the Pediatric Test of Brain Injury. *J Head Trauma Rehabil* 16(5): 426–440.

Keenan H, Runyan D, Nocera M (2006) Longitudinal follow-up of families and young children with traumatic brain injury. *Pediatrics* 117: 1291–1297.

Kennard M (1936) Age and other factors in motor recovery from precentral lesions in monkeys. *Am J Physiol* 115: 138–146.

Kennard M (1938) Reorganization of motor function in the cerebral cortex of monkeys deprived of motor and premotor areas in infancy. *J Neurophysiol* 1(6): 477–496.

Kirkwood M, Yeates KO, Wilson P (2006) Pediatric sport-related concussion: a review of the clinical management of an oft-neglected population. *Pediatrics* 117: 1359–1371.

Kliegman R, Nelson W, Vaughan V (1992) Head injuries. In: Behrman RE (ed) *Textbook of Paediatrics, 14th edn*. Philadelphia: WB Saunders, pp 1521–1524.

Klonoff H, Low MD, Clark C (1977) Head injuries in children: a prospective five year follow-up. *J Neurol Neurosurg Psychiatry* 40(12): 1211–1219.

Klonoff H, Clark C, Klonoff PS (1993) Long-term outcome of head injuries: a 23 year follow up study of children with head injuries. *J Neurol Neurosurg Psychiatry* 56(4): 410–415.

Kreutzer JS, Kolakowsky-Hayner SA, Demm SR, Meade MA (2002) A structured approach to family intervention after brain injury. *J Head Trauma Rehabil* 17(4): 349–367.

Kriel RL, Krach LE, Panser LA (1989) A comparison of children younger and older than 6 years. *Pediatr Neurol* 5(5): 296–300.

Levin HS, Eisenberg HM (1979) Neuropsychologic outcome in children and adolescents. *Childs Brain* 5(3): 281–292.

McKinlay A, Dalrymple-Alford JC, Horwood LJ, Fergusson DM (2002) Long term psychosocial outcomes after mild head injury in early childhood. *J Neurol Neurosurg Psychiatry* 73(3): 281–288.

Malec JF, Thompson J (1994) Relationship of the Mayo-Portland Adapability Inventory (MPAI) to functional outcome and cognitive performance measures *J Head Trauma Rehabil* 9(4): 1–15.

Malec JF, Kragness M, Evans RW, Finlay KL, Kent A, Lezak MD (2003) Further psychometric evaluation and revision of the Mayo-Portland Adaptability Inventory in a national sample. *J Head Trauma Rehabil* 18(6): 479–492.

Max JE, Roberts MA (1999) Cognitive outcome in children and adolescents following severe traumatic brain injury: influence of psychosocial, psychiatric, and injury-related variables. *J Int Neuropsychol Soc* 5: 58–68.

Max JE, Robin DA, Lindgren SD, Smith WL Jr, Sato Y, Mattheis PJ, Stierwalt JA, Castillo CS (1998) Traumatic brain injury in children and adolescents: psychiatric disorders at one year. *J Neuropsychiatry Clin Neurosci* 10(3): 290–297.

Miller I, Epstein N, Bishop D, Keitner G (1985) The McMaster Family Assessment Device: reliability and validity. *J Marital Fam Ther* 11: 345–356.

Minnes P, Graffi S, Nolte ML, Carlson P, Harrick L (2000) Coping and stress in Canadian family caregivers of persons with traumatic brain injury. *Brain Inj* 14(8): 737–748.

Minnes P, Buell K, Nolte ML, McColl MA, Carlson P, Johnston J (2001) Defining community integration of persons with brain injuries as acculturation: a Canadian perspective. *NeuroRehabilitation* 16(1): 3–10.

Muir C, Rosenthal M, Diehl L (1990) Methods of family; mobile mourning. In: Rosenthal M, Griffith ER, Bond MR, Miller JD (eds) *Rehabilitation of the Adult and Child with Traumatic Brain Injury, 2nd edn.* Philadelphia: FA Davis Co., pp 436–437.

Prasad MR, Ewing-Cobbs L, Swank PR, Kramer L (2002) Predictors of outcome following traumatic brain injury in young children. *Pediatr Neurosurg* 36(2): 64–74.

Prigatano G (2002) What do patients need several years after brain injury? *Barrow Neurologic Institute Quarterly* 18(2): 1–11.

Rancho Los Amigos Cognitive Scale – Professional Staff Association, Rancho Los Amigos Hospital, Inc., Downey, CA (1990) In: Rosenthal M, Griffith ER, Bond MR, Miller JD (eds) *Rehabilitation of the Adult and Child with Traumatic Brain Injury, 2nd edn.* Philadelphia: FA Davis Co.

Rappaport M (2005) The Disability Rating and Coma/Near-Coma scales in evaluating severe head injury. *Neuropsychol Rehabil* 15(3–4): 442–453.

Rappaport M, Hall KM, Hopkins K, Belleza T, Cope DN (1982) Disability rating scale for severe head trauma: coma to community. *Arch Phys Med Rehabil* 63(3): 118–123.

Runyan DK, Hunter WM, Socolar RR et al. (1998) Children who prosper in unfavorable environments: the relationship to social capital. *Pediatrics* 101: 12–18.

Sander AM, Sherer M, Malec JF, High WM Jr, Thompson RN, Moessner AM, Josey J (2003) Preinjury emotional and family functioning in caregivers of persons with traumatic brain injury. *Arch Phys Med Rehabil* 84(2): 197–203.

Skinner HA, Steinhauer PD, Santa-Barbara J (1995) *FAM-III Manual.* Toronto: Multi-Health Systems.

Slomine B, McCarthy M et al. (2006) Health care utilization and needs after pediatric traumatic brain injury. *Pediatrics* 117: 663–674.

Stein RE, Jessup DJ (1990) Functional Status II(R): a measure of child health status. *Med Care* 28: 1041–1055.

Steinhauer PD, Santa-Barbara J, Skinner H (1984) The process model of family functioning. *Can J Psychiatry* 29(2): 77–88.

Taylor G, Alden J (1997) Age-related differences in outcomes following childhood brain insults: an introduction and overview. *J Int Neuropsychol Soc* 3: 555–567.

Teasdale TW, Engberg AW (2003) Cognitive dysfunction in young men following head injury in childhood and adolescence: a population study. *J Neurol Neurosurg Psychiatry* 74(7): 933–936.

Teasdale GM, Pettigrew LE, Wilson JT, Murray G, Jennett B (1998) Analyzing outcome of treatment of severe head injury: a review and update on advancing the use of the Glasgow Outcome Scale. *J Neurotrauma* 15(8): 587–597. (Review.)

Thomsen IV (1992) Late psychosocial outcome in severe traumatic brain injury. Preliminary results of a third follow-up study after 20 years. *Scand J Rehabil Med Suppl* 26: 142–152.

Tompkins CA, Holland AL, Ratcliff G, Costello A, Leahy LF, Cowell V (1990) Predicting cognitive recovery from closed head-injury in children and adolescents. *Brain Cogn* 13(1): 86–97.

Varni JW, Katz ER, Seid M, Quiggins DJ, Friedman-Bender A, Castro CM (1998a) The Pediatric Cancer Quality of Life Inventory (PCQL). I. Instrument development, descriptive statistics, and cross-informant variance. *J Behav Med* 21(2): 179–204.

Varni JW, Katz ER, Seid M, Quiggins DJ, Friedman-Bender A (1998b) The Pediatric Cancer Quality of Life Inventory-32 (PCQL-32): I. Reliability and validity. *Cancer* 15; 82(6): 1184–1196.

Wade SL, Taylor HG, Drotar D, Stancin T, Yeates KO (1998) Family burden and adaptation during the initial year after traumatic brain injury in children. *Pediatrics* 102(1 Pt 1): 110–116 (The family burden of injury.)

Yeates KO, Taylor HG, Drotar D, Wade SL, Klein S, Stancin T, Schatschneider C (1997) Preinjury family environment as a determinant of recovery from traumatic brain injuries in school-age children. *J Int Neuropsychol Soc* 3(6): 617–630.

Ylvisaker M (ed) (1998) *Traumatic Brain Injury Rehabilitation: Children and Adolescents, 2nd edn.* Boston, MA: Butterworth-Heinemann, pp 5–10.

7
NEUROPSYCHIATRIC OUTCOMES

Chanth Seyone, Babita Kara and Nicola Hunt

INTRODUCTION

Often described as a 'disease of modernity', the incidence of neuropsychiatric sequelae resulting from trauma or brain injury is increasing. While better treatments and assessments have increased survival rates from childhood head injuries, these advances have also meant that the chronic outcomes of these injuries (physical, cognitive and psychosocial) have even greater implications for families, clinicians and the health care system.

To gain a clearer picture, this chapter will first briefly examine the epidemiology and pathophysiology of acquired brain injury in Canada. Much of the significance of childhood head injuries may not immediately be realized, as some sequelae are not apparent until later stages of development. Thus, it is crucial to consider all the outcomes to better educate clinicians and pediatric health care workers that behavioural problems in individuals may be linked to acquired brain injury.

There are various designations that are used interchangeably in regard to brain injury. However, this chapter will employ the term traumatic brain injury (TBI), which is more specific than head injury. Acquired brain injury (ABI) refers to any acquired damage to the brain after birth either by external physical forces or internal causes. External forces include collisions, falls, assaults, and sports injuries that are grouped under TBI. Internal or non-traumatic causes may be vascular lesions and neurological diseases (Provincial Acquired Brain Injury Advisory Committee 1999, Walker et al. 2002).

EPIDEMIOLOGY

INCIDENCE

Approximately 1.5 million people incur a traumatic brain injury every year in the United States alone. This is eight times the number diagnosed with breast cancer and 34 times the number of new cases of HIV/AIDS. The Canadian Institute for Health Information (CIHI) reports that the average national rate of head injury in 2001/2002 was 72.86 per 100,000 people (Fraser Health Authority 2003).

According to the World Health Organization, child mortality rates following TBI are low, ranging from 0 to 0.25% (Carroll et al. 2004). However, among young Canadians, brain injury is the leading cause of mortality and disability: 90% of new cases of ABI in children result from traumatic injuries, 20% of which are terminal

(Fraser Health Authority 2003). Children under the age of 14 account for approximately 3000 deaths, 29,000 hospitalizations, and 400,000 emergency visits due to TBI (Fraser Health Authority 2003). Also, TBI is the leading reason for trauma admission in pediatric populations (Campbell et al. 2004). Of the total number of children admitted into hospitals, 10% suffer from mild brain injuries while an additional 1% suffer from severe head injuries. The prognosis for children who experience mild TBI is quite good, with most recovering completely (Fraser Health Authority 2003).

PREVALENCE

Now more than ever, children are surviving brain injuries because of advances in medical and trauma care, as well as improved safety in motor vehicles, workplace and sporting equipment. This has been accompanied by a general increased awareness of the importance of maintaining safety equipment in various venues. Many of those who previously would have died from their injuries now survive with diminished capacity for living. For instance, it has been shown that child safety seats have drastically reduced the number of moderate to severe head injuries among all pediatric age categories. The greatest difference is seen in the infant group where previously there was a 7% risk; there is now a 0.5% risk of head injury with proper use of child safety seats (Muszynski et al. 2005).

Currently, an estimated 2% of the American population, or 5.3 million people, are living with disabilities resulting from TBI (Walker et al. 2002). The survival rate is 80% from TBI, with that from mild injuries accounting for 88%, while only 12% live with moderate to severe injuries. Each year 1260 new injury cases require post-injury rehabilitation. Long-term disability resulting from TBI among individuals 15–24 years of age is 39 per 100,000; and 40–86 per 100,000 children aged 0–19 must cope with disabilities due to TBI (Fraser Health Authority, 2003). Moreover, all pediatric rates may be underestimated because government and hospital data do not reflect the many children who receive private rehabilitation and treatment (Walker et al. 2002).

PATHOPHYSIOLOGY

The neuropsychiatric outcomes of ABI are unique to each incident and are determined by variables associated with the injury and the child (Middleton 2001). The cause, type and severity of injury, as well as the child's age, premorbid functioning and developmental level, all affect the pathophysiology of TBI (Anderson et al. 2004).

INJURY VARIABLES

As can be seen in Fig. 7.1, the causes of TBI in pediatric populations are mainly falls, pedestrian accidents, and motor vehicle accidents (MVAs) (CIHI 2004). Secondary

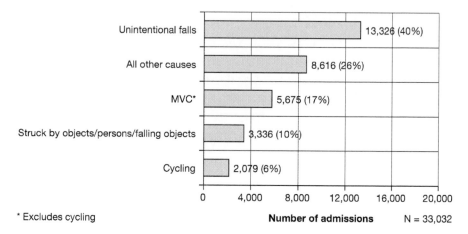

Fig. 7.1 Causes of injury – persons under 20 years of age, 2001–2002.

Source: National Trauma Registry/CIHI 2004.

causes include child abuse, assaults, and sports injuries. While MVAs are the most frequent cause of ABI in all populations, the most common causes of TBI in pediatric populations may differ when stratified by age. For instance, babies under 2 years of age are least likely to incur a head injury by accident. Conversely, young children mainly sustain injuries through falls, while older children tend to incur injury through traumatic means such as pedestrian, bicycle and sports-related accidents (Provincial Acquired Brain Injury Advisory Committee 1999, Walker et al. 2002, Fraser Health Authority 2003).

Injury severity is a good predictor of a child's long-term prognosis post-injury, but is by no means conclusive. Acquired brain injuries are categorized into three groups (mild, moderate and severe), dependent upon the period of unconsciousness. Post-traumatic amnesia (PTA), which is a gradual stage of regaining consciousness, may last from a few hours to a few days and can be used as a guide to injury severity. Generally, the more severe the head injury or the deeper the coma, the more likely it is that the patient will present neuropsychological and psychiatric sequelae later (Goldsmith and Plunkett 2004).

There are exceptions to this statement. In post-concussion syndrome, a commonly mild cerebral injury, there may be no loss of consciousness, external bruises, or tangible evidence, as the parent may not take their child to the hospital to be diagnosed (Goldsmith and Plunkett 2004). Although the injuries are minor, the individual appears to be slowed and may suffer from cognitive and psychosocial deficits. Injury severity can also be heightened by post-traumatic syndrome, characterized by the presence of persistent headaches, dizziness, fatigue, insomnia, poor memory, irritability and emotional lability, and aggravated by stress, tension or depression. Studies show that although physical causes are the initial reason for these symptoms, with time psychogenic causes may become evident, including the individual's premorbid personality (Kushner 1998).

CHILD VARIABLES

The pediatric head injury population is significantly self-selecting. Research has shown that children who sustain brain injuries often also present with premorbid behavioural difficulties such as poor attention, impulsivity and overactivity (Middleton 2001). Experimental animal models have demonstrated that repeated injury to the head, even after periods of assumed recovery, magnifies neuropsychiatric outcomes to a greater extent than previously assumed (Goldsmith and Plunkett 2004). These observations imply that premorbid functioning may influence the severity and pathophysiology of TBI.

It is also very important to consider the developmental level of the child at both the time of injury and the time of assessment. This is closely linked to another variable, namely age. On average, those children who die from TBI are much younger than those who survive (Greenwald et al. 2003). Studies have demonstrated that younger children are more at risk of developing global problems than focal ones, because at the time of injury the affected brain regions may be taking over new functions. Children under the age of 5 with severe TBI commonly have difficulties with motor and cognitive skills. In later childhood or adolescence more specific problems with behaviour are seen, such as impaired attention. School performance tests have documented that, in comparison to older children who have been in a coma for the same period, those under 8 years have more reading problems. Also, adolescents have less difficulty with written language than children (Middleton 2001).

DIFFERENCES BETWEEN ADULT AND CHILD POPULATIONS

There are some differences in how a head injury will affect a child compared to an adult, as the immature brain is more vulnerable to damage than the mature one. It has been noted that children more often present with diffuse axonal injuries (DAI) than adults, due to physical differences such as greater head to body ratios and weaker neck muscles (Kushner 1998, Thompson and Irby 2003). Additionally, a young child's skull is often soft and the bones are not yet fully fused; therefore there is a greater movement of the brain upon impact.

Recovery from a focal lesion is often much more satisfactory in a child than in an adult because of the plasticity of a child's brain (recovery in teenagers is similar to that in adults) (McKinlay et al. 2002). On the other hand, diffuse injury produces more severe and longer-lasting sequelae in children than in adults, especially with regard to memory deficits, intelligence, conduct and behavioural disturbance (Kushner 1998). It appears that the extent of neuropsychological sequelae varies directly with the volume of frontal lobe lesions (Hanten et al. 2004). The frontal lobe is associated with disorganized narrative speech and executive functions as the child develops; thus injuries to this brain region in a child can cause greater chronic disability than in an adult (Limond and Leeke 2005).

NEUROPSYCHIATRIC OUTCOMES

The long-term effects of TBI are hard to predict and are different for every individual because of the uniqueness of each injury. In general, however, most will experience some of the deficits listed (Table 7.1). The number of symptoms experienced will depend on the nature, location and intensity of the brain damage sustained. Table 7.1 is a list of the physical, cognitive and psychosocial deficits and common psychiatric syndromes that occur. This list is by no means exhaustive (APA 1994).

COGNITIVE OUTCOMES

The majority of cognitive deficits present in older age groups, although an explanation for this remains elusive. One hypothesis proposes that developing skills are more at risk than established skills during head injury in children. If myelination is disrupted, for example, cognitive skills may not develop or may be constrained. Since the frontal lobe comes into maturation in late childhood and adolescence, impairments in processes such as attention, working memory and verbal learning, which are mediated by this region, present in older children due to arrested development (Aaro Jonsson et al. 2004). Research supporting this theory asserts that the volume of frontal lobe lesions is proportional to the scale of neuropsychological sequelae (Middleton 2001).

Short-term recovery is seen one year from the injury; however, progress appears to plateau two to four years later (Anderson et al. 2004). Even after many years, problems in attention capacity, memory and learning, psychomotor skills, linguistic abilities, and executive functions persist (Anderson et al. 2004). Development of motor and visuo-spatial skills is delayed in children with severe TBI compared to that in mild TBI groups and older children (Anderson et al. 2004). Statistical analysis has revealed that those who have been comatose for longer than a week due to their injury have reduced cognitive functioning (Middleton 2001). The outcomes of several key cognitive areas will be discussed in depth: intelligence; attention; memory and recall; and executive functioning.

Intelligence/academic outcomes

Intelligence among TBI populations may be limited as new cognitive processes cannot develop completely during growth (Aaro Jonsson et al. 2004). Mild head injury (MTBI) is often thought to have inconsequential effects on general intelligence and academic skills, although this is somewhat unfounded as children with mild to moderate injuries do not always recover as predicted (McKinlay et al. 2002).

TABLE 7.1
Possible injury outcomes and affected brain regions

Physical deficits	Cognitive deficits	Psychosocial deficits	Common psychiatric syndromes*
• Weakness & fatigue • Fine & gross motor coordination • Balance & gait (C) • Vision (P) • Motor speech • Taste & smell • Seizure disorders • Sexual dysfunction (can be physical or psychosocial)	• Attention & concentration (F) • Memory & recall (F) • Problem solving & decision making (F) • Alertness (F) • Learning (F) • Speed of processing new information (F) • Organization & planning (F) • Sequencing (F) • Preservation (F) • Concept formation & abstraction (F) • Perception (F) • Intelligence (F) • Auditory/visual processing abilities (T) • Judgment & insight (F)	• Emotionally overactive (F) • Disinhibition (F) • Inappropriate behaviour (F) • Poor initiation (F) • Anger & aggression (T, F) • Antisocial behaviour (F) • Personality change (F) • Substance abuse & dependence • Flat effect (F) • Social insensitivity (F) • Lack of response to social/environmental cues (F) • Impulsivity (F) • Dependency • Manic behaviour • Sexual precociousness (F) • Mood swings (F) • Exaggeration of pre-injury behaviour • Paranoid/suspicious (P, T) • Stress, anxiety & frustration (F, T) • Suicidal ideation (F) • Difficulty forming & maintaining relationship (F) • Reduced self-esteem • Depression (F)	• **Mood disorders** Major depressive disorder Bipolar I & II disorder Substance-induced mood disorder • **Anxiety disorders** Panic disorder with/without agoraphobia Generalized anxiety disorder Phobia (social & specific) Obsessive compulsive disorder Post-traumatic stress disorder Substance-induced anxiety disorder • **Personality disorders (cluster B)** Antisocial personality disorder Borderline personality disorder Narcissistic personality disorder Avoidant personality disorder

continued

TABLE 7.1 (continued)
Possible injury outcomes and affected brain regions

Physical deficits	Cognitive deficits	Psychosocial deficits	Common psychiatric syndromes*
		• Visual & auditory hallucinations (F) • Sexual dysfunction (F) (can be physical or psychosocial)	• **Conduct disorders** Oppositional defiant disorder Attention deficit hyperactivity disorder (ADHD) • **Somatoform disorders** Conversion disorder Somatization disorder • **Psychotic disorders** • **Sleep disorders** Dysomnias Parasomnias • **Impulse control disorders** • **Adjustment disorders** *all disorders except for conduct disorders are diagnosed essentially in late adolescence and in adults*

Associated brain regions: frontal lobe (F); temporal lobe (T); parietal lobe (P); cerebellum (C).

Long-term outcomes show a decline in the speed of information processing, which leads to impairments in communication, language, visuo-perceptual functions, and motor capabilities (Middleton 2001).

Long-term recovery of language skills in young children with severe TBI is delayed compared to older or less severe categories (Aaro Jonsson et al. 2004). Among school-aged children and adults, non-verbal skills improve along with psychomotor and executive functions, except in children who sustained injury early

(Anderson et al. 2004). Follow-up studies conducted ten years after brain insult concluded that approximately 50% of children with TBI do not make normal progress in school. Reading goals were not met in more than half of those with unilateral, depressed skull injuries. Furthermore, children under 8 years who experienced long periods of coma were found to have greater difficulties with reading (Middleton 2001).

Expressive language, receptive language and verbal knowledge may all be reduced (Aaro Jonsson et al. 2004). During the sub-acute phase post-injury, there can be problems with naming, expressing, writing, sentence repetition and verbal fluency (Middleton 2001). Word fluency issues are more prevalent in younger children who have incurred severe injuries. The exception is if the injury damages the left frontal lobe, in which case word fluency weaknesses appear in older children. Research has demonstrated that from 12 months to even 14 years post-injury, verbal skills will have recovered very little. In fact, verbal intellect can decrease and there may be major deficits in verbal learning. In severe cases, receptive language capabilities may never improve (Aaron Jonsson et al. 2004, Anderson et al. 2004).

Similar to verbal skills, spatial abilities have poorer outcomes for those who sustain early childhood injuries. Research has shown that older children are less impaired in spatial layout learning tests than younger victims. Despite severe trauma, spatial learning has been found to recover several years later. However, cognitive mapping deficits remain (Aaro Jonsson et al. 2004).

Attention

There are several forms of attention that are impacted by childhood TBI since these forms emerge during adolescence: sustained attention, divided attention, and response inhibition (Aaro Jonsson et al. 2004). By contrast, focused attention remains intact because it matures around mid-childhood (Aaro Jonsson et al. 2004). Specifically, children will appear distracted or unaware, they will go off on tangents in school, or wander away. Younger children have more difficulty in inhibiting responses related to attention issues. As such, failure to concentrate and monitor the stimuli in their environment compromises behavioural, memory and learning objectives. It can also affect social relationships or interactions with family, friends and teachers (Middleton 2001).

Memory and recall

Actual deficits in memory may be difficult to identify because they can be masked or dismissed as absent-mindedness or forgetfulness (Middleton 2001). Consequently, achievements on memory tasks can be overestimated. A comparison of memory outcomes across different age groups reveals that teenagers make better advances in organization of memory strategies, but continue to have a number of verbal memory deficits (Aaro Jonsson et al. 2004).

A series of learning tests may help detect memory deficits. Middleton maintains that children with TBI do learn, but their acquisition of knowledge and skills is protracted and may be forgotten in a day (Middleton 2001). For example, severe TBI patients assessed at 12 and 30 months post-injury displayed decreased verbal learning skills. Further analysis discovered that these individuals actually had difficulty in recalling the story due to ongoing memory problems (Anderson et al. 2004).

Explicit memory develops after implicit memory and is thus more vulnerable to injury. In addition, implicit memory functions are believed to be more 'protected' since they are governed by inferior and posterior areas of the brain less prone to damage from TBI (Aaro Jonsson et al. 2004).

Executive functioning and problem solving

Late outcomes of TBI (more than 20 years post-injury) that are often reported are intellectual (e.g. difficulties with learning, memory, intellectual functioning and slowed thinking) and emotional sequelae (Goldsmith and Plunkett 2004). Children may be assumed to be unintelligent, but in reality have difficulties with executive functions (including basic attention and orientation, and working memory) (Middleton 2001). Executive functions allow individuals to adapt; therefore impairments to these functions cause children to perform poorly on tasks that require switching between cognitive strategies (Aaro Jonsson et al. 2004). Ewing-Cobbs et al. (1999) showed that 14.6 months after injury approximately 50% of infants and young children did not achieve average scores for emotional regulation and motor quality. Long-term deficits in executive functions and behaviour are interconnected with psychosocial and adaptive functioning. For instance, children with moderate to severe injuries are not socially advanced and have less developed problem-solving skills because these skills involve adaptation between academic and social functioning (Middleton 2001).

PSYCHOSOCIAL OUTCOMES

Psychosocial symptoms (see Table 7.1) are often observed during the early recovery phase, even in patients with no previous psychiatric history. Many children with MTBI will have favourable functional recoveries, but daily challenges and/or setbacks may still occur (temper outbursts, mood swings, memory problems, learning difficulties) (Hawley et al. 2004).

Personality/emotional outcomes

Profound personality changes are common and can lead to anger, aggression, violence and inappropriate sexual behaviour (Poggi et al. 2003). After a few months, a majority of patients will recover from these symptoms but some will experience persisting behavioural disturbance (Poggi et al. 2003); 28.1% of families have reported personality changes in their children after head injury, across all groups from mild to severe (Hawley et al. 2004).

Disordered personality following TBI has been observed by a number of clinicians and researchers. Most commonly observed has been the pseudo-depressed personality characterized by apathy and limited emotional response. Dorsomedial frontal lobe lesions have been associated with this type of personality. The pseudo-psychopathic personality on the other hand is characterized by disinhibition, egocentricity and sexual inappropriateness, and is reportedly associated with orbital frontal lobe lesions (Poggi et al. 2003).

Behaviour and development
Studies conducted to quantify the behavioural disturbance profile of TBI patients during the sub-acute phase of recovery found that the most common behavioural sequelae were disorganization, inaccurate self-appraisal, poor insight, unrealistic goals, poor planning, memory deficits, disorientation, depression, expressive speech deficits, blunted affect, fatigue and somatic concerns (McKinlay et al. 2002). Comparing children with mild, moderate and severe head injuries, researchers found that the severity of the injury was related to disordered cognition and deficits in insight, goals and planning (Anderson et al. 2004). However, they found that the extent of somatic concern was inversely proportional to the severity of the injury (McKinlay et al. 2002).

The original effects of early TBI may manifest if they interact with developmental processes and prevent emergence of new skills (McKinlay et al. 2002). It is also possible that the intensity, duration and frequency of premorbid behavioural issues may be exacerbated after injury (Middleton 2001). Visual impairment and blindness caused by cortical injury (occipital lobe injury, occipital lobe atrophy, optic atrophy, retinal fibrosis, and retinal shearing) can lead to developmental problems hindering learning and social attainment (Makaroff and Putnam 2003). Developmental delays and learning disability are frequent sequelae especially in severe TBI populations (Makaroff and Putnam 2003). The late onset of skills controlled by the prefrontal cortex is a critical factor in deviant psychosocial behaviour following brain insult (McKinlay et al. 2002). Psychosocial outcomes were examined among a group of 10- to 13-year-olds with mild head injury accompanied by a temporary hospital stay (less than 10 days), and significant hyperactive conduct was observed (McKinlay et al. 2002). Conversely, socially challenged children are more likely to experience behavioural disruptions and deficits in cognitive and educational processes (Anderson et al. 2004).

Social environments (school and employment outcomes)
Although it is encouraging that 90.6% of children return to regular school after injury, the outcome of this may become problematic. Research showed that, after

the injury, 18.3% of post-trauma children were disciplined at school for their behaviour, while a further 5.1% were excluded entirely from day school. It has been shown that 18.7% of children with TBI have problems with school work, but only 7.6% are evaluated as students with special education needs, the majority of them having been severely injured. One study reported that only 26 out of 40 special needs children received the special attention or assistance in school they required. Teachers were aware of the brain injury in only 39.8% of the cases. Clearly, education for children post-head injury is severely lacking (Hawley et al. 2004).

The school environment is an important tool in assessing social outcomes for children after injury. Children may have difficulty in trying to enter peer groups and in expressing their affirmative answers in wanting to do so. This can result in loneliness or isolation for the affected child. Alternatively, the child with TBI, living up to their social 'outcast' status, may seek and become friends with people parents feel are 'unsuitable' (Middleton 2001).

For the most part, children and adolescents suffering from severe TBI must cope with a diminished capacity for an independent life and inadequate assimilation into society. The earlier the child's stage of development when the injury occurred, the worse the long-term outcome. For example, for young children with TBI who were also unconscious for a short period of time, only 50% will remain in academic settings and 25% will hold full-time jobs as adults. The literature describing the life situation for many of these individuals over time reports early retirement or withdrawal from the workforce for those who fail to adjust in school. This relation between the lack of adjustment in school and eventual early retirement suggests that the conditions in the educational environment are not supportive ultimately of a good life situation for TBI individuals (Aaro Jonsson et al. 2004).

Family outcomes
When confronted with the realities of the injury, family members often become defensive. Denial is very commonly observed. Family members believe that their child will recover from the injury despite all the evidence to the contrary. Health care professionals may be disbelieved and distrusted when conveying a grim but realistic picture (Anderson et al. 2005).

Family members of head-injured children suffer deterioration in social as well as psychological functioning. A recent study found that relatives of TBI patients reach clinical levels of mental distress three months post-injury (Taylor et al. 2002). The deterioration in mental health of family members can also be long-term and progressive. Parents caring for TBI patients gradually over the years lose most or all of their social contacts. Divorce rates are high among those who were married at the time of the injury. Those who remain married frequently experience a shift in family roles of either one or both partners, from spouse and parent to primary caretaker. An educational and supportive approach to families and caregivers should be adopted as the psychological burden on them is enormous (Middleton 2001, Anderson et al. 2005).

COMORBIDITIES

Individuals with only mild brain injury have been shown to have good recovery, spanning a few weeks to three months (Mooney and Speed 2001). The question of why some cases deviate from the expected path of recovery then arises. Apparently, there are numerous components that interact to determine an individual's prognosis (Anderson et al. 2004). By pooling the results of several studies, it is clear that functional outcome is dictated not only by physical factors (injury severity, age), but also by psychological comorbidities (pre-existing personality characteristics, pre-morbid psychiatric conditions, new psychiatric conditions) and environmental factors (social and demographic aspects, family functioning) (Mooney and Speed 2001, Anderson et al. 2004).

Physical factors

It is possible that an individual suffering from TBI may not be making the expected gains simply because the initial injury severity was underestimated (Mooney and Speed 2001).

Of greater significance is the effect of a child's age on their post-injury outcome. There is research that predicts favourable outcomes in very young children with focal or unilateral cerebral pathologies. This finding is explained by the controversial theory of neuroplasticity. Younger children are neurologically more 'plastic', allowing for accelerated recovery post-injury (McKinlay et al. 2002, Anderson et al. 2004).

Conflicting evidence exists among severe TBI groups indicating that those sustaining injury later on in childhood have a better prognosis than younger children (Aaro Jonsson et al. 2004, Anderson et al. 2004). This is qualified by the fact that neuronal plasticity does not necessarily translate into functional plasticity, given the presence of residual neurobehavioural impairments in some patients (Aaro Jonsson et al. 2004). Hawley et al. assert that comparable minor residual deficits are more detrimental in children than in adults, possibly because impairments that are not observed initially may emerge later when other regions of the brain completely mature (Middleton 2001, Anderson et al. 2004, Hawley et al. 2004). Younger, preschool-aged children are vulnerable because they frequently sustain diffuse brain injuries, which obstruct cerebral development (Anderson et al. 2004). This is critical as neuronal myelination and frontal lobe maturation occur rapidly in the first five years of life, and are precursors to information processing and development of executive skills (Anderson et al. 2004). Consequently, children below the age of 5 years are more often affected in their motor and cognitive skills because these are less established, while older children and adolescents commonly have attention, behavioural, and adaptation deficits (Middleton 2001). The less these skills are established, the more deleterious and persistent are the subsequent outcomes after injury (Anderson et al. 2004).

Psychological factors

There are mixed opinions on behavioural and psychiatric sequelae, suggesting that premorbid personality not only increases the likelihood of sustaining an injury but also influences the outcome of the neurological effects of the injury (Middleton 2001, Thompson and Irby 2003, Massagli et al. 2004). Children with TBI appear to be a self-selecting group in that an elevated incidence of premorbid behavioural difficulties has frequently been documented (Middleton 2001). Children with pre-existing learning problems were identified as risk groups for moderate to severe head injury (Middleton 2001). Some researchers have suggested that disinhibition is the sole factor involved in pathological behaviour after TBI. This means that there are actually no personality changes after the injury; rather it is the emergence of maladaptive tendencies that were present premorbidly but were sensibly restrained during social interaction. This is, however, controversial (Middleton 2001, Thompson and Irby 2003, Massagli et al. 2004).

Personality characteristics that are common in head injury include over-achievement, perfectionism and dependency (Mooney and Speed 2001). There is also evidence of increased incidence of premorbid hyperactivity, impulsivity and antisocial personality (Middleton 2001). Many injuries are alcohol-related (MVAs) and those suffering have a high degree of alcoholism, which can be linked to dependent personalities (Greenwald et al. 2003). A similar situation can manifest with substance abuse.

Psychiatric comorbidities

Studies show that children and adults with mild TBI suffer greater disability when there is post-injury psychiatric illness than when there are no psychiatric sequelae (Thompson and Irby 2003, Massagli et al. 2004). A two- to threefold increase in the prevalence of psychiatric conditions (largely depression and anxiety disorders) was noted in one study. Also, it was shown that twice as many of those who developed psychiatric illness post-injury compared with those who did not had poor recoveries, implying that good recoveries are predicted by the absence of psychiatric comorbidities (Mooney and Speed 2001).

Mild TBI has been correlated with high rates of emotional disorders, including adjustment disorder, phobic disorder, panic disorder, post-traumatic stress disorder, major depressive disorder and somatoform disorders, as outlined in Table 7.1 (Middleton 2001, Thompson and Irby 2003, Massagli et al. 2004). Depressed and emotionally disturbed children are more liable to engage in self-destructive activities such as driving at excessive speed – the automobile often representing an ideal means for the direct expression of suicidal ideation (Middleton 2001, Thompson and Irby 2003, Massagli et al. 2004). Emotional disorders combined with cognitive loss and neuropsychological symptoms result in the inability of the individual to adapt. Consequently, a biphasic clinical course occurs whereby the effects of the initial mild TBI are heightened by post-injury mental health conditions that impede normal recovery (Mooney and Speed 2001).

The development of depression due to TBI is a common feature – more so in people with previous personality and family psychiatric history. Recent studies have been able to distinguish acute post-traumatic depression from depression developing months after the injury. Acute post-traumatic depression is typically characterized by vegetative symptoms whereas later onset of depression is characterized by psychological symptoms. It has been proposed that acute post-traumatic depression is secondary to neurophysiological or neurochemical changes to the brain after injury. Later onset of depression may be secondary to psychosocial factors and psychological reactions to the consequences of the injury. Depressive mood disorder secondary to TBI has been associated with frontal lobe lesions (Poggi et al. 2003).

ENVIRONMENTAL FACTORS

Several researchers have addressed the question of whether there exist familial characteristics which predispose to acquired brain injury (McKinlay et al. 2002, Taylor et al. 2002, Anderson et al. 2004, Hawley et al. 2004). History of psychiatric disorder in the immediate family or dysfunctional family dynamics would increase the probability of psychiatric sequelae (Taylor et al. 2002).

Family disruption/dysfunction

The concept that children suffering from brain injury are more dependent on a positive and supportive family environment also raises the point that those with severe TBI are then even more vulnerable to family adversity than children without injury. Anderson et al. found that a smaller number of children with severe TBI had intact family units compared with children without injury (Anderson et al. 2004). Taylor et al. report that abnormal behaviour is frequent among disadvantaged groups due to family dysfunction, ineffective child management, and negative parent–child interactions. In addition, detrimental effects of TBI on child behaviour and development of social skills are exacerbated by adverse family situations. Low-stress environments actually promote recovery, as exemplified by short-term gains in mathematics skills in severe TBI groups (Taylor et al. 2002).

It is important to note that underreporting symptoms can cause injury severity to be underestimated and the prognosis miscalculated. Whether this is mainly the result of lack of family response and caring or a case of denial remains to be seen. It has been demonstrated that parents frequently fail to report sequelae, and that teachers more than mothers will note hyperactivity, inattention and conduct disorders in the same child (Anderson et al. 2004).

Socio-economic status

Hospital surveys show links between children from deprived regions and poor recoveries after brain insult, suggesting that parent social economic status (SES) influences outcomes (Hawley et al. 2004). This is substantiated by the fact that children with TBI commonly represent a disadvantaged subset of the population, and that risk factors include decreased levels of maternal education and low SES (Anderson et al. 2004). Disadvantaged backgrounds have been correlated with long-term declines in academic performance, as well as increases in behavioural sequelae such as slower advances in short-term social skills (Taylor et al. 2002).

The reasons why SES has a negative impact on TBI recovery can be considered from two perspectives: the restrictions of low SES, and the benefits of high SES. First, parents may have limited financial and supportive resources to invest in educational programs, evaluations and therapies. This limits a child's access to special interventions. There may be distraction by other life stressors (including unemployment, single-parent homes, working in more than one job, or the demands of other children), and therefore less time to spend on remedial tasks with the injured child. Second, the advantage of having an affluent background is that children have more opportunities to augment behavioural adjustment and learn compensatory skills. Greater stimulation coupled with more appropriate encouragement from parents and other team workers significantly improves recovery. As long as access to care for children with TBI is based upon financial ability, socio-economic status will remain a factor in child outcomes (Taylor et al. 2002).

TIME OF ASSESSMENT

Due to the circumstantial and sometimes inconsistent nature of recovery in TBI patients, time since insult is a critical factor when assessing outcome after injury in childhood and adolescence (Aaro Jonsson et al. 2004). Final assessment should not be carried out before the child reaches adulthood, even in cases of mild TBI (Aaro Jonsson et al. 2004). Children with mild TBI should be required to have follow-up assessments as this type of injury has been found to have numerous persisting sequelae many years later (Hawley et al. 2004). Late changes in or late emergence of sequelae may regress a child's recovery causing additional burden on families, communities, and health care systems.

MANAGEMENT

The management of traumatic brain injuries is complex and time consuming. There is no one treatment that is effective for all. This is especially so in children. The sequelae of brain injury are numerous and are often dependent on the characteristics and qualities of the individual. In children, not only the child who has had the head injury suffers, but also the family and environment from which the child has originated. In terms of management, each strategy has to be individualized for that particular patient and/or family. It is beyond the scope of this chapter to fully describe all of the various treatment modalities available. This is especially so with psychopharmacological treatments where a multitude of medications could be tried.

Broadly, programs to rehabilitate children with traumatic brain injuries have medical, cognitive, behavioural and supportive subsets. Prior to initiating any of these treatments, a full neuropsychiatric assessment needs to be conducted, which should evaluate a child's cognitive ability, behavioural issues, family and social relationships, academic achievement and/or employment abilities or interests, daily living skills, financial status, social skills, and recreational activities. The assessment may include not only direct evaluation of the child and his/her family, but also requires interviews with the child's school and/or place of employment, friends, and social outlets. For those individuals who may have a therapeutic team already working with the child, the various members of the team may have different opinions as to the child's abilities and status.

Following this initial assessment, a strategy is developed for each individual to deal effectively with the kinds of problems that they may be facing. Psychiatric problems are complicated by an inability to integrate and cope with environmental and community stressors. This includes academic stressors as well. Management strategies for these individuals would include:

1 Psychopharmacological intervention
2 Cognitive therapies
3 Behavioural strategies
4 Family therapy
5 Financial and housing support
6 Academic support

PSYCHOPHARMACOLOGICAL INTERVENTION

This section covers broad generalities in psychopharmacological treatment. Many neuropsychiatric sequelae are possible. These include premorbid, immediate post-injury, and long-term sequelae. In children, premorbid deficits often involve attention and concentration, personality development including issues of judgement and insight, oppositional behaviour, and in some instances even aggression. Immediate post-injury difficulties usually include emotional overactiveness, disinhibition, inappropriate behaviour, and again anger and aggression. Longer-term difficulties could include maladaptive personality, specifically within the cluster B group, which includes borderline, narcissistic and antisocial personality disorders.

There may also be substance abuse and dependence even in relatively young individuals, which could worsen the behaviour that often brings the child to a physician. There may be significant apathy, impulsivity, and even the development of formalized psychiatric syndromes such as anxiety disorder, depressive disorder, or even a psychotic disorder.

Psychopharmacological treatment often has to play a significant role in treating these individuals. Numerous medications have been tried with some efficacy. Identification of the problem behaviour forms the key to its treatment. The problem behaviour has to be understood in terms of the environmental and familial impact so that the psychopharmacological treatment can be structured to enhance community and familial functioning.

Various types of medication are available (Yudofsky et al. 1994). They include:

1 Antidepressants
2 Antipsychotics
3 Mood stabilizers
4 Stimulants
5 Anxiolytics
6 Hypnotics
7 Memory enhancers
8 Other miscellaneous pharmacological treatments

Antidepressants
The most commonly used antidepressants are the newer selective serotonin reuptake inhibitors (SSRIs) and the serotonin norepinephrine reuptake inhibitors (SNRIs). The classical triad of the SSRIs is fluoxetine, sertraline and paroxetine. There are newer SSRIs, specifically citalopram, escitalopram and mirtazepine. The standard SNRI is venlafaxine (Effexor). The usual form of venlafaxine is the slow release form, which is marketed as Effexor XR. The dosing of these various medications needs to be titrated to the age and size of the child. Other antidepressants that could be tried include buproprion, which is also considered an anxiolytic and is quite effective in relieving anxiety in some instances, especially if there is a panic disorder present.

Antipsychotics
Antipsychotics fall within the major tranquillizer group of medications and the classical usage includes medications such as haloperidol. It is extremely uncommon for any traditional neuroleptics to be used. Most use is essentially of the atypical antipsychotics of which risperidone is the oldest and, in children, often the most widely used. This is followed by olanzapine and quetiapine. These antipsychotics or neuroleptics can be useful as antipsychotics addressing an individual's psychotic features, but are also used as anxiolytics in patients with severe panic disorders or

even generalized anxiety and/or obsessive-compulsive disorders, and in the management of difficult behaviour. Patients with oppositional behaviour or even violent tendencies often respond well to the judicious use of neuroleptics in combination with other medications. Patients with significant cognitive deficits, especially frontal lobe deficits with impulsivity and poor judgement, also benefit from the use of antipsychotics even if no psychotic features are in fact present.

Antipsychotics have also recently been shown to augment the effectiveness of antidepressants in treating patients with refractory depression (in adults, however – research in children is sparse to non-existent). Patients with bipolar affective disorders which occur post-acquired brain injury also often respond well to the use of antipsychotics.

Mood stabilizers

Patients may require treatment with an antipsychotic prior to the initiation of mood stabilizers, especially when a child (especially an older child or teenager) has a manic phase of a bipolar affective disorder which may occur following an acquired brain injury. Various mood stabilizers are available, including carbamazepine and valproic acid. These medications are also used as an augmentation of antidepressant treatment in refractory depression, as well as for stabilizing behaviour in individuals who may have frontal lobe dysexecutive syndromes. Aggression is also at times alleviated by use of mood stabilizers, often in combination with other medications.

Stimulants

The most typical stimulant used is methylphenidate. These medications have been used for a number of years in the treatment of attention-deficit hyperactivity disorder (ADHD), which often manifests in childhood and is identified in school-age children. Considering that the majority of post-injury children have difficulties with attention and concentration, as well as suffering from apathy (poor interest and difficulty initiating tasks), stimulants are often helpful in enabling these children to return to some form of functioning, either in the community or at school. Methylphenidate is used – usually a morning dose – to try to improve daytime functioning. Caution has to be exercised in its use during the latter part of the day as methylphenidate can often lead to problems with insomnia. A new form of methylphenidate – Concerta – may alleviate this particular difficulty. These newer forms also make it easier for once a day dosing, as opposed to methylphenidate which has to be given at intervals during the day to maintain functioning for a number of hours.

Other stimulants that have been known to be effective include dextro-amphetamine and modafinil, a non-controlled substance which was initially marketed for the treatment of narcolepsy. In some individuals, especially children, modafinil in smaller doses has been noted to improve daytime functioning, specifically interest and ability to initiate and perform activities. Atomoxetine has been used for selected patients with ADHD symptoms post-head injury (Ripley 2006) with some success although there remains concern about the potential for liver toxicity. Stimulant medications, however, are considered first choice.

Anxiolytics

Bupropion, both the regular as well as the slow-release form, is often classified as an anxiolytic and can be used in the treatment of a significant anxiety disorder following a brain injury, especially in older children and certainly in adults. These medications are used to treat conditions such as panic disorder with or without agoraphobia, generalized anxiety disorder, obsessive-compulsive disorder, and even somatoform disorders, which often manifest in older individuals. Other anxiolytics which are often used in the shorter term include benzodiazepines, especially clonazepam or lorazepam. The latter two medications are often used as adjuncts for relatively short periods of time to try to effect a decrement in acute agitation or anxiety. Clonazepam is often used for longer periods of time in the treatment of specific sleep disorders, such as periodic leg movements in sleep, which may occur in individuals following a brain injury. This symptom is more commonly seen in older individuals and adults. Anxiolytics can be taken alone or in combination.

Hypnotics

Sleep disorders often play a large role in post-injury rehabilitation. In adults, difficulties with sleep are often the presenting complaint to neuropsychiatrists and sleep specialists following a brain injury. There has been no one particular sleep disorder that has been identified as pathognomic in individuals with head injuries. Disrupted sleep with fragmentation is often clinically evident. Hypnotics can play a role in the treatment of children and adults post-traumatic brain injury.

The two common hypnotics that are used are the non-addictive, non-habituating hypnotics such as zopiclone and zaleplon. Zopiclone tends to be somewhat longer acting than zaleplon, with zaleplon often aiding in initiation of sleep as well as maintenance. Zopiclone more specifically improves the quality of sleep, with very little effect in initiating sleep. These medications are often prescribed for a short time, or in some instances for long periods of time, to try to improve an individual's sleep and thus daytime functioning, and even treat some of the other psychiatric syndromes.

Memory enhancers

There is no research on the use of memory enhancers in children. There have been anecdotal clinical trials of memory enhancers in adults with inconclusive results as to whether there was stabilization or improvement in memory.

Other miscellaneous pharmacological treatments

Infrequently, there have been attempts to use other medications, such as gabapentin, amantidine, levadopa, and other dopamine-enhancing medications such as prami-paxole, following a brain injury to treat very specific syndromes. These medications have been used in adults, with little or no research in children. Use in children has to be extremely cautious and is often to an extent experimental. The medication strategies described above should be attempted prior to initiation of these medications.

A component of any of the treatment modalities is the expert assessment and follow-up by an experienced neuropsychiatrist who also has extensive knowledge and experience of psychopharmacological management of post-TBI neuropsychiatric sequelae, especially in children. It is a given that patients with neuropsychiatric sequelae are not static. This is true of children who have varying stressors during development. Following initial stabilization, possibly with psychopharmacological management in addition to other treatment modalities, patients do not necessarily remain static and well managed. They may decompensate for no apparent reason. In these situations, treatment plans need to be revamped quite extensively. It is absolutely essential that long-term follow-up be maintained.

It is also clear that in the treatment of patients with traumatic brain injuries one modality is generally inadequate. This also applies to psychopharmacological management in that often one medication may be similarly inadequate. Thus, various medications from different classes, as described, need to be titrated for individual response.

COGNITIVE THERAPIES

Psychopharmacological management is only one part of the treatment. It does and should play a prominent role. The 'therapies' that are often employed in children and adults with post-TBI difficulties are often ineffective unless patients are to an extent amenable to the time and effort required for these therapies to be successful. If a child or adult is extremely aggressive, severely anxious or depressed, these 'therapies' or community manipulations will often fail.

The cognitive behavioural therapy that is used in adults and children with acquired brain injuries needs to be context-sensitive, support-oriented, and multi-component. The therapy needs to be long-term and solution-focused, breaking down each task into simple steps that are then repeated on numerous occasions to try to take into account an individual's memory deficits (which may be quite prominent following an acquired brain injury). Repetition is often a key to the cognitive behavioural therapy being internalized. The therapy is often more behavioural in the earlier stages then becomes cognitive in the latter stages, when patients are more stable and have had a chance to integrate some of the behavioural strategies that have been taught. There also has to be an age component, with behavioural therapy being more useful in younger children, whereas cognitive treatments may be possible in teenagers and adults.

The therapy has to be individualized for each patient. There is no standard treatment that is universally effective. Often the therapy needs to be modified to fit each situation on an ongoing basis. Initial assessments and the beginnings of therapy often do not indicate long-term response. If the therapy is malleable enough to be modified, even extensively, part way through treatment, there is a higher chance of a more successful outcome.

Cognitive behavioural training may include simple strategies such as use of a daily planner, and electronic devices such as palm pilots which act as memory aids. They help with simple tasks, both in activities of daily living, including cooking, cleaning, and independent skills. More extensive treatment of the neuropsychiatric syndromes may be required.

OTHER TYPES OF THERAPY AND SUPPORT

Other types of 'therapies' include supportive individual therapy, as well as family therapy. Families of individuals with TBI, especially children, have a variety of emotions including guilt, shame and anger. These all have to be addressed and the families need to be helped to work through these feelings. A family therapist with experience in treating patients and families with TBI is often an invaluable member of the team.

Patients require case management services which can coordinate the various treatment modalities. Families are in total disarray following a brain injury to a child, and cannot coordinate the care required. Children often need not only manipulation of their pharmacological state, but also of their school, social and recreational environments, and indeed their family structure. Without coordination, there is a likelihood that the treatment modalities that may be suggested from extensive neuropsychiatric or neuropsychological assessment may not be instituted appropriately. It should also be kept in mind that delayed treatment often leads to poorer response as behaviour and family dysfunction, as well as delays in academic development and social skills, often become entrenched and difficult to change with time. An advocate who can coordinate the treatments is essential.

Patients with TBI require help reintegrating into their community, their social and recreational structure, as well as back into school. An educational liaison worker who can interact with the child's school and smooth the path of learning can be very beneficial. Children will need special accommodation in how they learn, as well as how long it takes them to learn. Schools are often unaware of the extent of the difficulty in children with TBI as in many instances there is no external evidence of disability. Frank discussion with school administration and individual teachers as to the cognitive difficulties that a particular child may have and their possible solutions (e.g. extra time for assignments, projects or tests, review sheets, and open-book testing) may prove invaluable to school performance. Success in school often translates into improved self-image and self-esteem for the patient with TBI, which may then also lead to better functioning in many other neuropsychiatric aspects. This may even include improvement in specific neuropsychiatric syndromes. The same holds true for successes in social and recreational domains. Within these domains, case management or rehabilitation coaches, such as child/youth workers, may be able to help reintegrate some of these children into their own social and recreational fields – not only within the community but also within the school setting.

Patients with TBI, especially if they are children, and/or their families often have difficulties not specifically of a neuropsychiatric nature but more in the nature of community support. They have difficulties with housing, finances, and the basic obtainment of the necessities of life. These can, understandably, act as severe stressors to the support structure of a child and lead to exacerbation of neuropsychiatric syndromes. Advocacy and support in obtaining appropriate housing, financial help and/or social skills training have to play a large role in the overall rehabilitation and management.

Children, teenagers and adults with TBI often exhibit poor judgement, are impulsive, and at times aggressive. This combination leads to increased contact with the legal system. Education of crown attorneys and the judicial system often aids in preventing unduly harsh sentences for individuals who may not necessarily have been able to help themselves. A diversion program through treatment rather than through the penal system is often beneficial and leads to more effective rehabilitation of post-TBI complications.

The management of TBI patients requires a multi-modal approach which has to be tailored to each individual, their family, and their environment. It needs to be broad in terms of assessment, and long in terms of the duration of treatment and follow-up.

CONCLUSION

Neuropsychiatric difficulties following an acquired brain injury can be numerous, difficult to manage, and disabling, not only to the individual but also to his or her family, environment and community, with many of these difficulties being lifelong. It should also be kept in mind that children with brain injuries grow up to be adults with brain injuries. Thus, ineffective management of these children, especially if they have maladaptive personalities, often leads to difficult individuals as adults who are much more resistant to receiving or responding to treatment. Better understanding and treatment often lead to better outcomes at all ages and all levels.

REFERENCES

Aaro Jonsson C, Horneman G, Emanuelson I (2004) Neuropsychological progress during 14 years after severe traumatic brain injury in childhood and adolescence. *Brain Inj* 18(9): 921–934.

American Psychiatric Association (1994) *Diagnostic and Statistical Manual of Mental Disorders, 4th edn.* Washington, DC: American Psychiatric Association.

Anderson VA, Morse SA, Catroppa C, Haritou F, Rosenfeld JV (2004) Thirty month outcome from early childhood head injury: a prospective analysis of neurobehavioural recovery. *Brain* 127(12): 2608–2620.

Anderson VA, Catroppa C, Haritou F, Morse S, Rosenfeld JV (2005) Identifying factors contributing to child and family outcome 30 months after traumatic brain injury in children. *J Neurol Neurosurg Psychiatry* 76: 401–408.

Campbell CGN, Kuohn SM, Richards PMP, Ventureyra E, Hutchison JS (2004) Medical and cognitive outcome in children with traumatic brain injury. *Can J Neurol Sci* 31: 213–219.

Canadian Institute for Health Information. National Trauma Registry (2004) *Report: Injury Hospitalizations* (includes 2001/2002 data). Ottawa: Canadian Institute for Health Information, 21.

Carroll LJ, Cassidy JD, Peloso PM, Borg J, Von Holst H, Holm L, Paniak C, Pepin M (2004) Prognosis for mild traumatic brain injury: results of the WHO collaborating center task force on mild traumatic brain injury. *J Rehabil Med* Suppl 43: 84–105.

Ewing-Cobbs L, Prasad M, Kramar L, Landry S (1999) Inflicted traumatic brain injury: relationship of developmental outcome to severity of injury. *Pediatr Neurosurg* 31: 251–258.

Fraser Health Authority. Health Planning and Systems Development (2003) *Fraser Health Strategic Plan for Acquired Brain Injury Services: 2004–2006.* British Columbia: Fraser Health Authority.

Goldsmith W, Plunkett J (2004) A biomechanical analysis of the causes of traumatic brain injury in infants and children. *Am J Forensic Med Pathol* 25(2): 89–100.

Greenwald BD, Burnett DM, Miller MA (2003) Congenital and acquired brain injury. 1. Brain injury: epidemiology and pathophysiology. *Arch Phys Med Rehabil* 84(Suppl 1): S3–S7.

Hanten G, Chapman SB, Gamino JF, Zhang L, Benton SB, Stallings-Roberson G, Hunter JV, Levin HS (2004) Verbal selective learning after traumatic brain injury in children. *Annals of Neurology* 56(6): 847–853.

Hawley CA, Ward AB, Magnay AR, Long J (2004) Outcomes following childhood head injury: a population study. *J Neurol Neurosurg Psychiatry* 75: 737–742.

Kushner D (1998) Mild traumatic brain injury: toward understanding manifestations and treatment. *Arch Intern Med* 158: 1617–1624.

Limond J, Leeke R (2005). Practitioner review: Cognitive rehabilitation for children with acquired brain injury. *J Child Psychol Psychiatry* 46(4): 319–352.

Makaroff K, Putnam FW (2003) Outcomes of infants and children with inflicted traumatic brain injury. *Dev Med Child Neurol* 45: 497–502.

McKinlay A, Dalrymple-Alford JC, Horwood LJ, Fergusson DM (2002) Long term psychosocial outcomes after mild head injury in early childhood. *J Neurol Neurosurg Psychiatry* 73: 281–288.

Massagli TL, Fann JR, Burington BE, Jaffe KM, Katon WJ, Thompson RS (2004) Psychiatric illness after mild traumatic brain injury in children. *Arch Phys Med Rehabil* 85: 1428–1434.

Middleton JA (2001) Practitioner review: Psychological sequelae of head injury in children and adolescents. *J Child Psychol Psychiatry* 42(2): 165–180.

Mooney G, Speed J (2001) The association between mild traumatic brain injury and psychiatric conditions. *Brain Inj* 15(10): 865–877.

Muszynski CA, Yoganandan N, Pintur FA, Gennarelli TA (2005) Risk of pediatric head injury after motor vehicle accidents. *J Neurosurg* 102(4 Suppl): 374–379.

Poggi G, Liscio M, Adduci A, Galbiati S, Sommovigo M, Degrate A, Strazzer S, Castelli E (2003) Neuropsychiatric sequelae in TBI: a comparison across different age groups. *Brain Inj* 17(10): 835–846.

Provincial Acquired Brain Injury Advisory Committee (1999) *Provincial Review of Services for Children and Youth Living with the Effects of an Acquired Brain Injury.* Final Report. Ontario.

Ripley DL (2006) Atomoxetine for individuals with traumatic brain injury. *J Head Trauma Rehabil* 21(1): 85–88.

Taylor HG, Yeates KO, Wade SL, Drotar D, Stancin T, Minich N (2002) A prospective study of short- and long-term outcomes after traumatic brain injury in children: behavior and achievement. *Neuropsychology* 16(1): 15–27.

Thompson MD, Irby JW Jr (2003) Recovery from mild head injury in pediatric populations. *Sem Pediatr Neurol* 10(2): 130–139.

Walker J, Williams JI, Chipman M, Cusimano M, McLellan B, Simson H, Tator C, Verrier M (2002) *An Analysis and Dissemination of Current Neurotrauma Incidence and Causal Data in Ontario.* Ontario: Ontario Neurotrauma Foundation.

Yudofsky SC, Silver JM, Hales RE (1994) Neuropsychiatric aspects of traumatic brain injury. In: *American Psychiatric Press Textbook of Neuropsychiatry.* Washington, DC: American Psychiatric Press, pp 521–560.

8

SLEEP AND METABOLISM

Rajesh RamachandranNair, Shelly K Weiss and
Daune L MacGregor

PART 1: SLEEP

INTRODUCTION

Sleep disturbance in patients following traumatic brain injury (TBI) can have a significant impact on outcome and recovery. It is well recognized that disordered sleep can cause behavioural and cognitive consequences (Thaxton and Myers 2002). Therefore individuals with cognitive sequelae from TBI can be further compromised in recovery by problems resulting in non-restorative sleep.

The presence of sleep disturbance following traumatic brain injury (TBI) is a well recognized problem in the adult population but has been inadequately evaluated in pediatric patients. Studies of adult patients include adolescents over 15 years of age, as young people, particularly men between the ages of 15 and 24, are the most common individuals involved in accidents resulting in TBI (Lee et al. 2003). In these studies the reported rates of disturbed sleep following recent TBI range from 36% to as high as 59 and 70% (Keshavan et al. 1981). In a prospective study of post-acute TBI patients, 30% of 50 consecutive patients were diagnosed with insomnia based upon DSM-IV criteria (Fichtenberg et al. 2002).

Studies of adults report that subjective evaluation of individuals after minor head injury revealed complaints of difficulties in initiating and maintaining sleep, early morning awakenings, decreased ability to function and a generally decreased sleep quality (Parsons and Ver Beek 1981, Perlis et al. 1997). These effects were reported to be potentially long-term. Among 145 patients with a history of head injury, 50% had difficulty sleeping: 64% described waking up early, 25% described sleeping more than usual, and 45% described problems falling asleep. Eighty percent of individuals reporting sleep problems also reported problems with fatigue. In this study, the more severe the brain injury, the less likely the subject was to suffer from sleep disturbance (Clinchot et al. 1998).

Disorders in initiating or maintaining sleep (DIMS) occur more often in patients with recent injury, and disorders of excessive somnolence (DOES) occur more often in those patients with injuries sustained two to three years previously (Cohen et al. 1992). Other sleep disturbances have been reported in adults who have sustained significant head trauma, including hypersomnia, narcolepsy, central and obstructive sleep apnea and insomnia (Castriotta and Lai 2001).

A study of adolescents with mild brain injuries has found similar rates of sleep disturbance to those in the adult studies. Prevalence and risk factors of long-term sleep disturbance were studied in 98 adolescents who experienced mild closed head injury (CHI) 0.5–6 years before the study, and were compared with 80 controls. The prevalence of sleep disturbance was significantly greater in the adolescents who had mild CHI than in the age-matched controls (28% vs. 11%). Bruxism (teeth grinding or clenching) was also more common in the study group. In this study, sleep walking and enuresis were not increased in the individuals with mild CHI (Pillar et al. 2003).

CLASSIFICATION OF SLEEP DISORDERS

An extensive review of the classification of sleep disorders is beyond the scope of this chapter. Pediatric and adult sleep disorders are classified according to the International Classification of Sleep Disorders into four groups of disorders: (1) dysomnias or disorders that result in insomnia or excessive sleepiness; (2) parasomnias or disorders resulting in unusual nocturnal behaviour, disorders of arousal, partial arousal, or sleep stage transition; (3) sleep disorders associated with medical or psychiatric disorders; and (4) proposed sleep disorders (ICSD 2001).

ETIOLOGY AND MECHANISMS OF PATHOPHYSIOLOGY OF SLEEP DISTURBANCE FOLLOWING TBI

The etiology of sleep disturbance following TBI may be multifactorial. Some of the factors include disruption of normal neurologic function required for sleep initiation and maintenance, comorbidity caused by the TBI (such as depression), psychosocial factors relating to changes in individual and family dynamics, effect of chronic pain on sleep, and side effects of medication used to treat other problems encountered as a result of the TBI. In addition, there may be pre-existing diagnosed or undiagnosed sleep disturbance exacerbated by the TBI.

During the acute stage of recovery following TBI, dysregulation of sleep appears to be a function of the diffuse disruption of cerebral functioning due to both direct physical damage to the brain and secondary neuropathological events. Sleep abnormalities are more likely to occur in patients with lesions in the pontine tegmentum in the midpontine region (Markand and Dyken 1976). As brain functioning becomes reorganized and some degree of neurological stability is re-established, sleep can be expected to normalize in the absence of damage to neural sleep structures (Ron et al. 1980).

This theory of pathophysiology is consistent with clinical studies reporting adolescents who develop sleep disturbance within the acute stage of mild CHI (Casey et al. 1986, Hefez et al. 1987). Although the acute sleep disturbances commonly improve, adolescents may develop emotionally derived insomnia (Dagan et al. 1991). In this disorder it is postulated that the acute stress that leads to insomnia, instead of resolving with time, leads to substantial concern and distress which focuses on sleep itself. Ultimately, a vicious cycle of poor sleep leading to further anxiety regarding insomnia is created.

A further example of sleep disturbance related to the timing of the injury concerns insomnia and depression. The determinants of insomnia and depression may differ from the acute to the post-acute stage. Neurological factors may play a role in the early recovery process, and psychosocial factors may contribute later (Fichtenberg et al. 2000).

Another explanation for sleep disturbance following TBI may be a premorbid personality or character, which results in sleep disturbance after a relatively minor trauma (Pillar et al. 2003). Hypersomnolence after TBI may result from a pre-existing sleep disorder. Motor vehicle crashes have been reported to occur more frequently in people with sleep apnea (Young et al. 1997).

It may be difficult to separate the relative contribution of the neurologic injury from that of the emotional distress caused by the TBI, in relation to the development of sleep disturbance. It is reported that there is an increased incidence of sleep disturbance in children and adolescents who have undergone trauma, including road traffic accidents, child abuse and severe burns without neurologic injury (Kramer and Kinney 1988, Glod et al. 1997, Ellis et al. 1998).

Finally, the high prevalence of hypersomnia among children and adolescents in many studies could be influenced by the possibility that persons with a sleep disorder would be more likely to agree to participate in a sleep research study. Subjective versus objective complaints in adolescents with sleep disturbance after mild CHI were recently compared. The subjective complaints were largely confirmed by objective sleep measurements in the patients' homes and in the laboratory (Kaufman et al. 2001). Short-term memory disturbances are extremely common in brain-injured persons and may affect the validity of questionnaire-based data.

CHANGE IN SLEEP ARCHITECTURE FOLLOWING TBI

Sleep is divided into two distinct stages: rapid eye movement (REM) and non-rapid eye movement (NREM). NREM sleep is divided into four stages with stages 1 and 2 considered light sleep and stages 3 and 4 considered deep or slow wave sleep. The studies are inconsistent in the changes detected after TBI. In the acute phase of recovery after head injury in children, it has been reported that there is an increase in stage 2 and a decrease in stages 3-4 sleep, with no consistent changes in percentages of REM sleep. In the same analysis it was found that the children had increased spindle activity in stages 2–3 NREM sleep and increased REM density (Lenard and Pennigstorff 1970). In contrast, another study in 105 individuals reported a decrease in spindles and K complexes during NREM sleep and decreased REM activity (Harada et al. 1976).

LIMITATIONS TO EVALUATION OF INDIVIDUALS FOLLOWING TBI

It is important to be alert to the limitations of the studies which are based on questionnaires and self-reports. Individuals with TBI may have poor awareness of hypersomnolence and sleep quality, limiting the reliability of self-reporting questionnaires and interviews for the evaluation of sleep disturbance and post-traumatic hypersomnolence (Masel et al. 2001). The scales which are commonly used in adult sleep research (for example, the Epworth and Pittsburgh Sleep Quality Index questionnaire) include questions relating to activities, such as driving, that these individuals may not perform. This limits the validity of these data (Masel et al. 2001). In addition, individuals with TBI and cognitive compromise in addition to possible depression may have difficulty with accurate reporting of sleep and other disturbances due to poor self-awareness of their impairment and disability. These limitations may not be applicable to pediatric studies if the parent or adult caregiver reports symptoms of sleep disturbance.

RISK FACTORS FOR SLEEP DISTURBANCE AFTER HEAD INJURY

In a study of 184 patients with a history of head injury, post-traumatic somnolence was associated with variable degrees of impaired daytime functioning in more than 98% of patients. Patients who were in coma for more than 24 hours, who had a head fracture, or who had immediate neurosurgical interventions were likely to have scores > 16 points on the Epworth Sleepiness Scale (ESS) and sleep onset <= 5 minutes on a multiple sleep latency test – both indicators of hypersomnolence. Pain at night was an important factor in nocturnal sleep disruption and daytime sleepiness (Guilleminault et al. 2000). Sleep complaints of patients with brain injury are found to correlate with presence of fatigue, higher Glasgow Coma Scale scores, better immediate memory, a positive substance abuse history, and female gender (Clinchot et al. 1998). In a study of 87 patients with mild to severe TBI admitted to a comprehensive outpatient neurorehabilitation program, persons with mild head injury severity met the criteria for sleep disorders more frequently than persons with moderate or severe injury. It is not likely that these findings reflected a general response bias toward over-reporting of symptoms by persons with mild injury, because these patients did not report more symptoms of depression or pain, and they were not more likely to be pursuing litigation than were persons with moderate or severe injuries. These results suggest that reports of sleep disturbance are associated with intact executive functioning in the presence of some deficits in primary cognitive abilities (Mahmood et al. 2004).

INVESTIGATIONS AND TREATMENT

Any sleep disturbance which continues without evaluation and treatment can impact cognitive recovery and function. Undiagnosed hypersomnia may impair the rehabilitative process. Excessive sleepiness of any cause may be an obstacle to learning (Castriotta and Lai 2001). Cohen et al. suggest that problems with insomnia when untreated become more chronic and lead to disorders of excessive somnolence (Cohen et al. 1992). Sleep disturbance could significantly exacerbate neuropsychological deficits in patients with a history of head injury (Mahmood et al. 2004). Patients with TBI may also be placed on medications that have a deleterious impact on their sleep patterns, which needs to be considered in their evaluation and treatment (Zafonte et al. 1996).

The evaluation and treatment of sleep disorders are dependent on the specific disorder, as outlined in the sleep literature. The treatment of pediatric sleep disorders is not well researched and further studies in the area of these disorders in general and in sleep disturbance following TBI are warranted.

In some of the adult and pediatric sleep disorders pharmacotherapy for sleep disturbance is usually the last option after non-pharmacological interventions in sleep hygiene and environment have been exhausted. In TBI patients, pharmacotherapy may be warranted to treat comorbidity (including chronic pain). In adult patients, various sedative/hypnotic medications can be prescribed in conjunction with non-pharmacotherapeutic interventions to aid insomnia in TBI patients on a short-term basis. Sedative/hypnotic medications may produce negative cognitive effects. Disturbances in memory and new learning have also been reported from these medications (Zafonte et al. 1996). The role of pharmacotherapy in pediatrics is not well understood.

Melatonin has been studied in circadian rhythm sleep disorders but there is no evidence for its efficacy in patients with TBI. Melatonin is a hormone secreted by the pineal gland and has sleep-inducing properties. The rationale for therapeutic use of melatonin is based on its ability to shift circadian rhythms and to induce sleep (American Sleep Disorders Association 1995). There are data to support the use of melatonin in treating disorders of the sleep–wake cycle; however, there is little published evidence on the efficacy of melatonin in treating post-TBI sleep disturbances. In a randomized double-blind controlled cross-over trial to compare melatonin (5 mg) and a tricyclic antidepressant, amitriptyline (25 mg), in a small sample of seven adults with TBI, no differences in sleep latency, duration or quality or daytime alertness were found for either drug compared to baseline (Kemp et al. 2004).

PART II: METABOLISM

There is now significant evidence available documenting the effects of traumatic brain injury on the pituitary end organ axis (Cernak et al. 1999, Bondanelli et al. 2005). In order of frequency of observation, these are as follows:

1 Gonadotropin and somatotropin deficiency
2 Altered cortisol levels (corticotropin deficiency)

3 Impaired thyroid function (low triiodothyroxine (T3) and thyroid stimulating hormone), described as the 'low T3 syndrome'

Clinical effects can be caused by inappropriate anti-diuretic hormone secretion (SIADH) with hyponatremia and more rarely diabetes insipidus (DI) (Agha et al. 2005) and hypopituitarism. Most cases with neurohypophyseal dysfunction (DI and SIADH) recover completely; however, there is evidence supporting occurrence of long-term diabetes insipidus. The pathophysiology of hypothalamic and pituitary dysfunction in acquired brain injury includes areas of petechial hemorrhage in the anterior hypothalamus and hemorrhage and infarction in the pituitary gland (Kaufman et al. 1993).

Hormonal function should be assessed in trauma patients in the acute stages after the head injury and in the longer term. Undiagnosed abnormalities may have an effect on treatment and rehabilitation outcomes. A study evaluating patients with severe traumatic brain injury in a rehabilitation setting, with an effect on growth hormone (GH) and insulin-like growth factor–1 (IGF–1), showed no significant alteration in GH secretion – with normal central regulation of the GH–IGF–1 axis (Bondanelli et al. 2002).

Insatiable appetite in hyperphagia is recognized clinically in some patients after head injury, although considered rare (Shinoda et al. 1993). Hyperphagia can occur with lesions in the dorsomedian hypothalamic nucleus. Obesity after head injury is thought to be caused by lesions of the ventromedial hypothalamic and paraventricular nuclei, disorders of the limbic system or hypercortisolism (Cushing syndrome).

Hyperphagia as a symptom of limbic system disorders occurs and is recognized in Kluver–Bucy syndrome (KBS) – characterized by emotional changes, aberrant sexual behaviour, excessive oral tendencies and increased appetite. Cases of KBS are described after mild and severe head trauma (Salim et al. 2002, Yoneoka et al. 2004). The pathophysiology may relate to either bilateral orbitofrontal lesions or direct or indirect bilateral temporal lobe lesions (hypoperfusion or contusion).

Respiridol has been used successfully to attempt control of insatiable appetite after traumatic hypothalamic lesions (Bates 1997).

SUMMARY

Patients with acquired brain injuries, including mild and severe injuries, should be thoroughly evaluated for the presence of disturbances of sleep and/or metabolic dysfunction. The etiology and diagnosis of the sleep disturbance should be identified to allow appropriate remediation and/or pharmacotherapy. This is an important area where further research is warranted to identify the incidence, the type of sleep disturbance, the efficacy of treatment, and the potential impact on neurocognitive recovery by amelioration of comorbid sleep problems.

REFERENCES

Agha A, Sherlock M, Phillips J, Tormey W, Thompson CJ (2005) The natural history of post-traumatic neurohypophysial dysfunction. *Eur J Endocrinol* 152(3): 371–377.

American Sleep Disorders Association: Diagnostic Classification Steering Committee (1990) *International Classification of Sleep Disorders*. Lawrence, KS: Allen Press.

American Sleep Disorders Association: Standards of Practice Committee (1995) Practice parameters for the use of polysomnography in the evaluation of insomnia. *Sleep* 18(1): 55–57.

Bates JB (1997) Effectiveness of respiridone in insatiable appetite following hypothalamic injury. *J Neuropsychiatry Clin Neurosci* 9(4): 626.

Bondanelli M, Ambroscio MR, Margutti A, Boldrini P, Basaglia N, Franchetti P, Zatelli MC, Degli Uberti EC (2002) Evidence for integrity of the growth hormone/insulin-like growth factor-1 axis in patients with severe head trauma during rehabilitation. *Metab Clin Exp* 51(10): 1363–1369.

Bondanelli M, Ambroscio MR, Zatelli MC, De Marinis L, Degli Umberti EC (2005) Hypopituitarism after traumatic brain injury. *Eur J Endocrinol* 152(5): 679–691.

Casey R, Ludwig S, McCormick MC (1986) Morbidity following minor head trauma in children. *Pediatrics* 78(3): 497–502.

Castriotta RJ, Lai JM (2001) Sleep disorders associated with traumatic brain injury. *Arch Phys Med Rehabil* 82(10): 1403–1406.

Cernak I, Savic VJ, Lazarov A, Joksimovic M, Markovic S (1999) Neuroendocrine responses following graded traumatic brain injury in male adults. *Brain Inj* 13(12): 1005–1015.

Clinchot DM, Bogner J, Mysiw WJ, Fugate L, Corrigan J (1998) Defining sleep disturbance after brain injury. *Am J Phys Med Rehabil* 77(4): 291–295.

Cohen M, Oksenberg A, Snir D, Stern MJ, Groswasser Z (1992) Temporally related changes of sleep complaints in traumatic brain injured patients. *J Neurol Neurosurg Psychiatry* 55(4): 313–315.

Dagan Y, Lavie P, Bleich A (1991) Elevated awakening thresholds in sleep stage 3–4 in war-related post-traumatic stress disorder. *Biol Psychiatry* 30(6): 618–622.

Ellis A, Stores G, Mayou R (1998) Psychological consequences of road traffic accidents in children. *Eur Child Adolesc Psychiatry* 7(2): 61–68.

Fichtenberg NL, Millis SR, Mann NR, Zafonte RD, Millard AE (2000) Factors associated with insomnia among post-acute traumatic brain injury survivors. *Brain Inj* 14: 659–667.

Fichtenberg NL, Zafonte RD, Putnam S et al. (2002) Insomnia in a post-acute brain injury sample. *Brain Injury* 16(3): 197–206.

Glod CA, Teicher MH, Hartman CR, Harakal T (1997) Increased nocturnal activity and impaired sleep maintenance in abused children. *J Am Acad Child Adolesc Psychiatry* 36(9): 1236–1243.

Guilleminault C, Yuen KM, Gulevich MG, Karadeniz D, Leger D, Philip P (2000) Hypersomnia after head-neck trauma: a medicolegal dilemma. *Neurology* 54(3): 653–659.

Harada M, Minami R, Hattori E, Nakamura K, Kabashima K (1976) Sleep in brain-damaged patients. An all night sleep study of 105 cases. *Kumamoto Med J* 29(3): 110–127.

Hefez A, Metz L, Lavie P (1987) Long-term effects of extreme situational stress on sleep and dreaming. *Am J Psychiatry* 144(3): 344–347.

ICSD (International Classification of Sleep Disorders revised) (2001) *Diagnostic and Coding Manual*. Chicago, IL: American Academy of Sleep Medicine.

Kaufman HH, Timberlake G, Voelker J, Pait TG (1993) Medical complications of head injury. *Med Clin North Am* 77(1): 43–60.

Kaufman Y, Tzischinsky O, Epstein R, Etzioni A, Lavie P, Pillar G (2001) Long-term sleep disturbances in adolescents after minor head injury. *Pediatr Neurol* 24(2): 129–134.

Kemp S, Biswas R, Neumann V, Coughlan A (2004) The value of melatonin for sleep disorders occurring post-head injury: a pilot RCT. *Brain Inj* 18(9): 911–919.

Keshavan MS, Channabasavanna SM, Reddy GN (1981) Post-traumatic psychiatric disturbances: patterns and predictors of outcome. *Br J Psychiatry* 138: 157–160.

Kramer M, Kinney L (1988) Sleep patterns in trauma victims with disturbed dreaming. *Psychiatr J Univ Ottawa* 13: 12–16.

Lee HB, Lyketsos G, Rao V (2003) Pharmacological management of the psychiatric aspects of traumatic brain injury. *Int Rev Psychiatry* 15: 359–370.

Lenard HG, Pennigstorff H (1970) Alterations in the sleep patterns of infants and young children following acute head injuries. *Acta Pediatr Scand* 59: 565–571.

Mahmood O, Rapport LJ, Hanks RA, Fichtenberg NL (2004) Neuropsychological performance and sleep disturbance following traumatic brain injury. *J Head Trauma Rehabil* 19(5): 378–390.

Mann NR, Fichtenberg NL (1997) Sleep disturbance among TBI survivors: a comparison study. *Arch Phys Med Rehabil* 78: 1055.

Markand ON, Dyken ML (1976) Sleep abnormalities in patients with brain stem lesions. *Neurology* 26(8): 769–776.

Masel BE, Scheibel RS, Kimbark T, Kuna ST (2001) Excessive daytime sleepiness in adults with brain injuries. *Arch Phys Med Rehabil* 82(11): 1526–1532.

Parsons LC, Ver Beek D (1981) Sleep-wake patterns following cerebral concussion. *Nurs Res* 31: 260–264.

Perlis ML, Artiola L, Giles DE (1997) Sleep complaints in chronic post-concussion syndrome. *Percept Mot Skills* 84(2): 595–599.

Pillar G, Averbooch E, Katz N et al. (2003) Prevalence and risk of sleep disturbances in adolescents after minor head injury. *Pediatr Neurol* 29: 131–135.

Ron S, Algom D, Hary D, Cohen M (1980) Time-related changes in the distribution of sleep stages in brain injured patients. *Electroencephalogr Clin Neurophysiol* 48(4): 432–441.

Salim A, Kim KA, Kimbrell BJ, Petrone P, Roldan G, Asensio JA (2002) Kluver-Bucy syndrome as a result of minor head trauma. *South Med J* 95(8): 929–931.

Shinoda M, Tsugu A, Oda S, Masuko A, Yamaguchi T, Yamaguchi T, Tsugane R, Sato O (1993) Development of akinetic mutism and hyperphagia after left thalamic and right hypothalamic lesions. *Childs Nerv Syst* 9(4): 2430–2435.

Thaxton L, Myers MA (2002) Sleep disturbances and their management in patients with brain injury. *J Head Trauma Rehabil* 17(4): 335–348.

Yoneoka Y, Takeda N, Inoue A, Ibuchi Y, Kumagai T, Sugai T, Takeda KI, Ueda K (2004) Human Kluver-Bucy syndrome following acute subdural haematoma. *Acta Neurochirurgica* 146(11): 1267–1270.

Young T, Blustein J, Finn L, Palta M (1997) Sleep-disordered breathing and motor vehicle accidents in a population-based sample of employed adults. *Sleep* 20(8): 608–613.

Zafonte RD, Mann NR, Fichtenberg NL (1996) Sleep disturbance in traumatic brain injury: pharmacological options. *NeuroRehabilitation* 7: 189–195.

9

NEUROPSYCHOLOGICAL CONSEQUENCES

Erin M Picard and Mary L Stewart

PART I: NEUROPSYCHOLOGICAL CONSEQUENCES OF PEDIATRIC TRAUMATIC BRAIN INJURIES

Within the last decade, the amount of research devoted to the topic of pediatric brain injury has increased substantially, as has our understanding of the factors determining outcome. Our past reliance on adult research and testing paradigms to guide assessment and intervention in children has given way to a focus on approaches based in childhood development – approaches that recognize that there are indeed fundamental differences between adults and children.

In this chapter we will summarize the literature related to pediatric brain injury outcome in the areas of cognitive, behavioural and psychosocial functioning. The contribution of the neuropsychological assessment to the rehabilitation process will be discussed, as will our clinical experience related to the content and timing of assessments.

TRAUMATIC BRAIN INJURY AS A SUBSET OF ACQUIRED BRAIN INJURY

The majority of research in the area of childhood acquired brain injury (ABI) focuses on children who have sustained traumatic brain injuries (TBI) (Ewing-Cobbs et al. 2003), a specific subset of children with ABI. For the purpose of this discussion, we define ABI as all brain injuries sustained postnatally. Our definition of TBI includes those injuries sustained more specifically as a result of an acceleration or deceleration impact (for example, from a motor vehicle crash, a fall or an assault). The literature on TBI in childhood provides a useful model for understanding the impact of diffuse, early injury on the brain. The nature of medical conditions affecting the developing brain (including bacterial meningitis, encephalitis, stroke, and tumours) is such that they tend to have a more widespread or diffuse effect. Even when the effects of the primary injury/illness mechanism are more circumscribed, secondary medical complications often result in a more diffuse pattern of damage (Dennis 2000).

In the case of TBI in children, there are several factors that predispose to more diffuse injury. Incomplete fusion of the skull results in the forces of impact being more likely to be absorbed by the brain. As a child has a disproportionately large head, the risk of diffuse axonal injury is greater. The architecture of the brain is such that the convolutions are shallow, again leading to a greater likelihood of diffuse axonal injury (Anderson 2006).

IS EARLIER BETTER?

For many years, a child's brain was thought to be more flexible or plastic than that of an adult and, therefore, less susceptible to permanent impairment following an injury or illness affecting the brain. Kennard has been repeatedly cited as the originator of the notion that earlier is better when it comes to brain damage, likely to be the result of her emphasis on resiliency over delayed effects in her work with monkeys (Kennard 1936, 1938, 1940, 1942). While it is true that Kennard extended her findings to human infants based on clinical case studies, her findings were always specifically related to *motor* recovery. She did not generalize her findings to resiliency in cognitive recovery. In fact, the results of Kennard's early studies have been more enduring and do support a widely held belief that, in some instances, it may well be to one's advantage to have been injured at a young age. Recovery from early focal lesions is a case in point here. Although the 'earlier is better' theory may hold true for focal lesions incurred in childhood, recovery from prenatal injury, early diffuse injury, or early injury to particular brain regions (that is, prefrontal) may have very profound and long-lasting effects.

Further support for the notion of 'earlier is better' came from a set of studies documenting children's recovery of language skills following fairly localized or circumscribed lesions (Lenneberg 1967), in a group of children initially believed to have a very good recovery. As pointed out by Taylor and Alden (1997), children with early left hemisphere disease may go on to acquire many age-appropriate language abilities. Language-related impairments become evident, however, as they mature.

As we now know, individuals at both ends of the age spectrum (children and older adults) are more susceptible to the deleterious effects of a brain injury. The end of the spectrum we are concerned with here – children – presented as a puzzle in the early research in this area. While it is true that damage occurring to a developing system may not appear to be particularly severe at an early age (Anderson 2003), these children remain at risk of falling further behind peers as they develop and of demonstrating late effects related to the injury. This interaction between development and brain injury can produce a phenomenon known colloquially as 'growing into deficit'. The child may present well on initial assessment, but later demonstrate impairments in specific cognitive or behavioural areas. Given the protracted maturation of prefrontal regions of the brain, executive dysfunction with resultant impact on future success and productivity in social and occupational realms remain a concern when we see a child for assessment. In terms of adult outcome, those sustaining severe injuries are highly unlikely to go on to university, up to 40%

are unemployed, and 60% are poorly adjusted or have frank psychiatric disturbance (Anderson 2006).

In 1949, Hebb postulated that brain injury early in life could, under some circumstances, result in more severe behavioural disruption than similar damage in later life. In the case of traumatic brain injury (TBI) in childhood, the evidence does suggest that the youngest children are most vulnerable to adverse and persistent effects, regardless of the severity of the injury (Anderson et al. 2001). With diffuse, widespread, or bilateral injury, the same mechanisms for plasticity may not be available.

Not surprisingly, the factors determining outcome in a child with a brain injury are many and varied. Recovery occurs against a backdrop of brain growth (maturation) and cognitive development, with age at injury providing at best a rough estimate of a child's progress in these areas. Add to this the unique environmental context in which the child is embedded (educational opportunities, family functioning), and one begins to appreciate the complexity involved in predicting outcome for any given child. Outcome is not related directly to the extent or severity of the injury sustained, but is the result of a complex interplay between child-specific variables, medical variables and the environmental context.

FACTORS DETERMINING OUTCOME

It has long been identified that the severity of the brain injury plays an important role in the physical and cognitive outcomes after TBI (Carney and Gerring 1990). A similar relationship has been proposed between severity and psychosocial outcome. Important distinctions in outcome can be made using severity of injury as a method of grouping subjects.

Commonly used measures of severity include the duration of post-traumatic amnesia (PTA), the duration and depth of coma, the duration of impaired consciousness, neuroradiology findings, medical indicators (e.g. seizures, increased intracranial pressure), or some combination of these measures. While measures of severity such as the Glasgow Coma Scale (GCS) (McDonald and Jaffe 1992) score are useful in predicting long-term neurological and cognitive outcome for children and adolescents, duration of coma, impaired consciousness, and PTA have generally been found to be better predictors of outcome across studies (McDonald et al. 1994). As Yeates points out, 'the predictive utility of the duration measures might have been related to their utility as markers of recovery, rather than as measures of neurological status immediately after injury' (2000: 105).

The relationship between injury severity and neurobehavioural outcome (i.e. more severe injury suggests the likelihood of adverse outcome) has been well documented in the literature, beginning with the studies of Klonoff, Rutter and their colleagues (Klonoff 1971, Klonoff and Paris 1974, Klonoff et al. 1977, Brown et al. 1981, Chadwick et al. 1981a, 1981b, Rutter et al. 1983). Although injury severity is a reasonable predictor of poor outcome across a variety of neurocognitive and emotional/behavioural measures, it explains but a portion of the variance in outcome. Other factors implicated include age at injury, time since injury, and age at testing (Taylor and Alden 1997); premorbid ability and/or cognitive reserve (Dennis 2000, Stern 2002); family environment and perceived burden (Yeates et al. 1997, 2004); and reciprocal influences of family environment and injury characteristics (Taylor et al. 2001).

NEUROBEHAVIOURAL OUTCOME

As pointed out by Donders (2005), there is no 'signature' neurocognitive profile associated with childhood TBI. This reflects the uniqueness of the context in which the child is developing at any given point in time. The same can be said for all children with acquired brain injury. Although they are similar in some ways, there is always some 'twist' that makes each and every one of them different.

The most common difficulties with which these children present are in the areas of speeded information processing, attention, learning and memory, executive function, and behaviour. These impairments directly affect school performance, either by exacerbating pre-existing difficulties, altering their developmental trajectory, or by interfering with new learning.

MILD TRAUMATIC BRAIN INJURY

There continues to be some controversy regarding outcome at the mild end of the injury spectrum. According to the 'Best Evidence Synthesis on Mild Traumatic Brain Injury' (MTBI) (Carroll et al. 2004), which reviewed the available evidence regarding prognosis and outcome related to mild traumatic brain injury in childhood, there are no persistent cognitive changes associated with MTBI. The studies reviewed indicated that post-concussion symptoms appear to be largely resolved within two to three months of the injury. Carroll et al. (2004) found that the studies were remarkably consistent in their finding of no short- or long-term cognitive problems or behavioural deficits attributable to MTBI. With the exception of a single study which found more children with MTBI to be receiving remedial support (Wrightson et al. 1995), there were no other school-related deficits reported. Studies excluded from the Best Evidence review included those that did not report deficits specific to MTBI, that is, those that grouped mildly and moderately injured subjects together. In an addendum to the review, two recent studies were noted that raised a distinct possibility of an association between MTBI and later-onset behavioural disturbances (McKinlay et al. 2002, 2003). The association was greatest for those who were under 5 years of age and had been hospitalized as a result of their injury.

Whether or not there are persistent cognitive and behavioural deficits attributable to MTBI is still to be resolved. The results are mixed, with good recovery suggested by some among school-age children and those with no premorbid problems (Polissar et al. 1994, Asarnow et al. 1995), and no clear deficits identified by others (Ponsford et al. 1997) using MTBI and age-matched controls. Ponsford did make note of a subset of children exhibiting deficits, all of whom were later found to have had a pre-existing history of difficulties. Other research suggests that, while cognitive deficits may resolve, behavioural and psychosocial issues persist (McKinlay et al. 2002, 2003).

Beers summarized the concerns about the potential impact of MTBI in stating that 'although the effects seen after Mild Head Injury (MHI) are neither as common nor disabling as those associated with severe injury, they are important to address because the incidence of MHI is so much greater' (1992: 314).

DOMAIN-SPECIFIC OUTCOME

Early research in this area focused on determining whether there were any long-term sequelae associated with head injury (Klonoff 1971, Klonoff and Paris 1974, Klonoff et al. 1977). The prevailing view at that time was that outcome was more favourable following brain injury sustained in childhood, a notion that has since been well refuted in the literature (Taylor and Alden 1997). It has now been demonstrated that an injury sustained at a young age – regardless of injury severity – can have more deleterious effects on outcome than one sustained in later childhood, adolescence, or adulthood (Ewing-Cobbs et al. 2003). According to Taylor and Alden, 'current findings suggest that the sequelae of childhood brain lesions remain relatively constant over time since insult, or worsen' (1997: 562).

INTELLIGENCE

Early studies in the area, mainly those of Klonoff and colleagues (Klonoff 1971, Klonoff and Paris 1974, Klonoff et al. 1977), documented a relationship between TBI and impairment, however grossly. Just how complex the relationship between injury severity and outcome would prove to be is seen in the initial work of Rutter's group (Brown et al. 1981, Chadwick 1981a, 1981b, Rutter et al. 1983) who noted that although intelligence scores improved over time, psychiatric symptomatology worsened. Initially depressed intelligence (IQ) scores improved to within normal limits in all groups studied. Psychiatric symptoms increased, particularly within the severely affected group. The Rutter studies are also notorious for suggesting that children sustaining TBIs are not representative of the normal population; instead, this early research indicated that those with TBI include a disproportionate number of individuals with pre-existing pathology.

More recent research has documented impairments in a range of areas, with those sustaining the most severe injuries experiencing a significant and persisting pattern of deficits. Intelligence scores have been found to be depressed follow-ing moderate to severe TBI, with maximum recovery noted within six months (Anderson et al. 2001, Ewing-Cobbs et al. 2003), following which scores level off for up to two years. Persisting deficits are nevertheless observed among the most severely injured and among those who sustained their injuries at a young age (Ewing-Cobbs et al. 1997, Donders 2005). In the case of mild injuries, although the literature seems to indicate that IQ remains unaffected, this does not rule out the presence of more subtle deficits that IQ measures lack the sensitivity to detect.

There are many intelligence tests currently in use, most of which are based on hierarchical theories of intelligence, which presume that there is at least a general, overall factor and a set of specific abilities. As Sattler points out, 'The IQ should be viewed as a somewhat arbitrary summary index of many abilities' (2001: 152). Composite scores (Full Scale IQ) can more generally be problematic as they may mask important variations in abilities.

Our clinical experience is consistent with the research that used earlier versions of intelligence tests which placed a premium on speed and fine motor skills. When visual-perceptual and spatial abilities are confounded by time pressure, scores on the Performance IQ scale are likely to be affected. A recent revision of the Wechsler Intelligence Scale for Children (WISC-IV) assesses perceptual reasoning without relying on speed and fine motor ability to the extent of the earlier versions of this test. As a result of this change, we are now finding that children and adolescents who are tested three to six months post-injury may do well on both the Verbal Comprehension and Perceptual Reasoning Indices, likely a reflection of intact previously acquired skills. Decrements are most likely to be seen on the subtests that load on the Processing Speed and Working Memory Indices of the WISC-IV.

MOTOR, VISUAL-MOTOR, AND VISUAL-PERCEPTUAL SKILLS

Visual-perceptual skills involve the ability to interpret and organize visually perceived material. Visual-spatial ability, in contrast, is the processing of visual orientation or location in space. Many of these tasks also have a constructional component and require the individual to either draw or assemble objects. With most severe injuries, there are persisting motor deficits, which tend not to be as apparent at the milder end of the injury spectrum. Subtle deficits, such as motor slowness and reduced eye–hand coordination, may occur even following relatively mild injury (Anderson et al. 2001). Donders' (2005) recent work supports our clinical impressions that the deficits noted on visual-motor and visual-perceptual tasks are the result of a primary impairment in processing speed. By processing speed we mean the child's ability to quickly and efficiently take in information and act upon it. Consequently, these children seldom get bonus points awarded for completing tasks quickly and do poorly under time pressure.

Donders (2005) has highlighted the need for careful consideration of the impact of deficits in speeded processing across several areas typically assessed as part of a neuropsychological evaluation. In addition to the obvious impact on visual-perceptual tasks with timed components, processing speed limitations can affect performance on any timed task or any task in which a lot of information is presented at a specific rate (e.g. list learning tasks).

LANGUAGE

Early studies were limited by their reliance on Verbal IQ as a measure of language ability. It has been our experience that children with obvious difficulties with language formulation and expression can, and do, do well on the verbal subtests of the commonly used measures of intelligence. These are not scored based on the structure of the language used; instead, reliance is upon the content of the information they are able to convey regardless of how difficult it is for them to do so.

A dose-response relationship between language outcome and injury severity holds, with both expressive and receptive language skills being susceptible to impairment. Included among the types of language difficulties identified in the literature are dysnomia (Levin and Eisenberg 1979), reduced verbal fluency (Chadwick et al. 1981a, 1981b), problems in writing to dictation and copying sentences (Ewing-Cobbs et al. 1987), reduced speed and comprehensiveness of written expression (Yorkston et al. 1997), and object naming latency and confrontation naming impairments (Chadwick et al. 1981a, 1981b). Again, controversy remains regarding the impact of a mild injury on language outcome. Children injured at a young age seem to be at a greater risk for language difficulties, regardless of injury severity.

More recently, the research has focused on discourse deficits following TBI and has included evaluating the maintenance of overall coherence and organization of information, as well as the amount and complexity of the language used (Brookshire et al. 2000).

ATTENTION

Overall, the findings in this area are mixed, which could well relate to the fact that components of attention and their developmental trajectories have not always been considered. Nevertheless, a dose-response relationship has again been found to hold, with difficulties reported on measures of sustained attention, vigilance, and selective attention (Timmermans and Christensen 1991, Dennis et al. 1995, Anderson and Pentland 1998, Robin et al. 1999, Catroppa and Anderson 2003).

More recent investigations have been devoted to understanding the impact of injury on different components of attention. In a prospective study of the recovery of attention in the two years following a TBI, Catroppa and Anderson (2005) found that children with severe TBI generally performed the most poorly overall, with deficits most evident on the complex and timed tasks. Although there was recovery noted in some areas, deficits persisted over 24 months, particularly with respect to sustained attention. Children with severe TBI achieved fewest correct responses, had problems maintaining attention and working efficiently over time, showed a gradual increase in errors with time on task, and presented with a vigilance decrement.

LEARNING AND MEMORY

Memory has been identified as the most frequently disrupted ability following severe brain injury in children (Levin and Eisenberg 1979). Slower rates of learning have been reported, as have difficulties acquiring information over trials. Furthermore, persistent deficits in memory encoding, storage, and retrieval have been described among children sustaining severe traumatic injuries. At the milder end of the injury spectrum, memory retrieval difficulties have been reported (Jaffe et al. 1992, 1993, Levin et al. 1993, 1994, Jaffe et al. 1995, Yeates et al. 1995). Donders and Minnema (2004) found susceptibility to proactive interference to be more common in children with TBI when compared to a normative sample. In Donders' most recent research on list-learning paradigms, reduced processing speed was suggested as contributing to poor overall performance across repeated trials.

ACADEMIC ACHIEVEMENT

In most studies, academic issues are addressed in a perfunctory manner with little consideration given to assessing these skills beyond a single-word level (single-word recognition, spelling tests). The sparing of acquired skills post-injury may lead one to believe that a child is doing well when there should be cause for concern. Clinically, we have noted that difficulties with written expression mirror difficulties with oral expression: namely, many of the children we see have difficulties with form, fluency, and organization in both areas. Impairments in speeded processing and working memory often translate into reduced reading fluency, which in turn undermines comprehension of text.

These skills need to be more comprehensively assessed early post-injury and monitored at specific intervals (i.e. Grade 4, Grade 8, mid-to-late high school) through to late adolescence/early adulthood. Educational outcome studies have moved away from evaluating specific test performance to a focus on special education placements. It has been found that many more children who sustain injuries at a young age are receiving remedial support five years post-injury. Across a number of studies, these children have been more apt to experience school-related difficulties (Donders 1994, Kinsella et al. 1995, 1997).

Within the literature it has been noted that reading skills tend to be more resilient, provided the injury occurs after decoding skills have been learned (Barnes et al.1999). Nevertheless, efficient word recognition may be affected during the primary grades, leading to impaired fluency and comprehension.

EXECUTIVE FUNCTION

Among those children and adolescents sustaining severe brain injuries, impairments in several aspects of executive functioning have been described. These include poor planning and problem solving, reduced capacity for abstract thought, and slowed speed of response (Garth et al. 1997, Levin et al. 1997, Anderson et al. 2001). Gioia and Isquith (2004) report a linear trend across TBI groups, with the greatest deficits in executive function in those who sustained the most severe injuries. Injury severity was associated with everyday manifestations of executive dysfunction, which in turn was associated with poor neuropsychological test performance. Both test-based performance and behavioural ratings seem to account for a unique portion of variance in outcome, suggesting both are required to more fully appreciate the impact of executive dysfunction on everyday skills.

RECOVERY AND REHABILITATION

It would seem that the children at the mild end of the injury spectrum experience a relatively rapid and uncomplicated recovery. Certainly, they are in need of further study, given the mixed findings to date within the literature. Having had the opportunity to follow these children for many years, psychosocial and academic difficulties are the most common reason for referral for reassessment.

With respect to moderate to severe impairment, the recovery process is a longer one and often involves acute care hospitalization and rehabilitation. Over the years, we have come across some children and adolescents who have been severely injured but have recovered rapidly with few adverse sequelae. Moderate to severe injury is, nevertheless, more often associated with ongoing impairment.

Following discharge from active rehabilitation, these children require long-term follow-up at key transition periods during development and schooling (Anderson et al. 2001). The need for support and the types of support provided have to be revisited frequently, as we have found that these can and do change in the years following the injury. There is often a need to educate the community-based professionals with whom the child is involved. Key transition points include beginning school, participating in a full school day, Grade 4 (age 9/10 years), Grade 8 (age 13/14 years), and mid-to-late high school for post-secondary planning.

THE ROLE OF THE NEUROPSYCHOLOGIST

The notion that the primary purpose of the neuropsychological evaluation is to identify an underlying lesion or process is *not* widely accepted by child neuropsychologists (Fletcher and Taylor 1984). As Fletcher and Taylor note, 'it is important to recognize that the cause of brain injury (etiology) and the effects on the brain (pathophysiology) are not directly linked, but are related to a variety of other factors, such as the severity of the injury and how it is treated' (1997: 454–455). While it is true that neuropsychology is the study of brain–behaviour relationships, there may not be a direct relationship between test performance (a behavioural response) and 'lesion' location (a disruption of neuroanatomical functioning). The extent of damage does not bear a direct relationship to cognitive outcome. Where children are concerned, the neuropsychological assessment may in fact be more sensitive in determining the functional impact of more diffuse injuries to interrelated systems within the brain: that is, those skills that are more widely distributed and, therefore, more susceptible to damage. Taylor describes this notion well with his comment that 'in essence, the neuropsychologist's task is to isolate the "signal" produced by ABI from background "noise", examine reasons for variations in signal characteristics, and integrate this information to formulate probable causes and recommend treatment' (2004: 201). This applies more generally to TBI as well.

THE NEUROPSYCHOLOGICAL ASSESSMENT

An important aspect of neuropsychological rehabilitation of the child or adolescent with brain injury is the neuropsychological assessment. The determination of cognitive strengths and weaknesses is key to understanding what 'cognitive reserve' (Stern 2002) is available to the child or adolescent in the recovery process. The development of appropriate recommendations that assist with deficit reduction and the implementation of compensatory strategies are key to ensuring the success of the child or adolescent in their school programs. With respect to neuropsychological assessment of the child who has sustained a brain injury, our focus early post-injury has been to monitor their progress, consult with interdisciplinary team members, provide behavioural support and management, and determine the timing of the neuropsychological assessment.

In the acute rehabilitation phase, the most appropriate timing of a neuropsychological assessment is often at the point of discharge from the rehabilitation facility to the home community. The involvement of other disciplines (occupational and physical therapy and speech-language pathology) who complete their own baseline and discharge cognitive assessments is most helpful in setting specific short-term and longer-term therapy goals. In contrast, many of the tests used in the neuropsychological assessment are not intended to be administered too frequently, otherwise significant test–retest issues (practice effects leading to improved performance as an artifact of serial assessments) arise. The clinically recommended retest period would be at least nine months to one year after completion of the initial assessment, precluding the ability to reassess during most inpatient admissions.

In terms of when a client is ready to be seen for assessment, this decision is made for each client individually and is based on such factors as their stage of cognitive and physical recovery, ability to sustain focus and concentrate, and level of fatigue. Feedback from team members and family, as well as observations in group therapy or school settings, helps to determine readiness for assessment. Typically, the neuropsychological assessment is completed towards the end of the rehabilitation stay, unless there are indications of good recovery and ability to tolerate testing earlier.

It has been our experience that there is a significant demand from school board personnel and community professionals for the results of a neuropsychological assessment to assist with school placement, school program planning, and community intervention. A critical feature of the neuropsychological assessment is to identify impairments related to the injury, as well as the diagnosis of any coexisting childhood disorders (including learning disabilities, attention deficit disorders, and developmental disabilities). In contrast to the United States, in Canada (Ontario), the existence of a brain injury, in and of itself, is insufficient to meet the threshold for identification by the school system, unless there are significant physical impairments present. A child or adolescent with a brain injury may meet the threshold for diagnosis of a Learning Disability, under the Communication exceptionality, only if there exists an ability–achievement discrepancy. It is sometimes the case that students with brain injuries will meet the definition of Language Impairment, and this exceptionality may be supported by the assessment completed by either a neuropsychologist or a speech and language pathologist.

APPROACHES TO NEUROPSYCHOLOGICAL ASSESSMENT IN CHILDREN

There are a number of different approaches to neuropsychological assessment, the most common of which are the fixed test battery approach (the use of a specific set of tests for each client), an individually tailored approach (the tests are picked based on the presenting problems), or a combination of the two. The combination approach has merit in providing the flexibility to add or subtract test measures as appropriate while also allowing for the collection of systematic data which is useful for clinical tracking or research purposes. It also appears that many neuropsychologists, especially those working with children, have moved away from the use of traditional neuropsychological measures (for example, Reitan tests) in favour of those with a broader standardization sample and better norms.

Whatever the assessment approach used, neuropsychologists are also concerned with other factors that may affect the child's performance on the test battery (including level of fatigue, behavioural presentation, test environment, family functioning, and school history). It is important for the neuropsychologist to interpret test findings within the context of the unique circumstances of the child or adolescent. More important than the type of testing model used, is the degree to which the neuropsychological assessment is able to identify the strengths and weaknesses of the child and generate specific intervention strategies. As such, the neuropsychological assessment is a means to an end.

THE TESTING ENVIRONMENT

There are factors unique to the testing environment that may influence the child's test performance. It is absolutely essential that the testing is undertaken with minimal disruption. As a rule, no one other than the examiner and the child should be in the room during testing (Wechsler 2003). Our experience has been that the presence of an observer (other professional or parent) in the room during testing has an adverse impact on the child's performance and has, on occasion, invalidated the test results. Furthermore, there are legal issues in that psychological 'test materials are proprietary, copyrighted, confidential commercial information, analogous to trade secrets', and must be treated accordingly (MHS 2006). Recent legislation in Canada is restricting access to these materials, and making it the user's responsibility to ensure test security, even when the court subpoenas this information.

When testing a child, we are interested in securing their best performance: that is, what they are capable of under optimal circumstances. Nevertheless, we recognize that the testing environment is artificial – purposefully so. We structure the evaluation for the client, cue them to initiate, monitor their performance, and help them to stay on track. In addition to allowing frequent breaks (if needed), we redirect them and give them feedback. In the end, what we have done is to compensate for executive dysfunction, allowing them to demonstrate their potential in discrete skill areas. Consequently, it is within the realm of possibility that the results of the neuropsychological assessment may be incongruent with reports of actual behaviour in other settings. Working within the context of a multidisciplinary team enables the neuropsychologist to gather additional information about the client's functional status and allows for more meaningful interpretation of the test data. As will be discussed later, there are other measures that can be used to get a sense of the impact of executive dysfunction on everyday skills. Our personal bias is that the information can be found if one chooses to look for it.

WHY NEUROPSYCHOLOGICAL ASSESSMENT?

School board psychologists usually conduct psychoeducational assessments to determine the presence of learning or behavioural difficulties in their students. In contrast, a neuropsychological assessment addresses more comprehensively the underlying cognitive deficits that affect academic achievement. As many students with brain injuries perform at similar levels on tests of intellectual ability and academic achievement early post-injury, a typical psychoeducational assessment may fail to identify the attention, learning and memory, and speeded processing issues that place the child at risk for academic failure. Children and adolescents with acquired brain injury require systematic domain-by-domain assessment of skills. A comprehensive and systematic neuropsychological assessment more readily addresses the considerable variation in outcome seen in clients with acquired brain injuries.

COMPONENTS OF A NEUROPSYCHOLOGICAL ASSESSMENT

A comprehensive neuropsychological assessment includes a wide range of measures of specific neurocognitive skills, as well as the evaluation of emotional/behavioural and personality functioning. The timing of the assessment during a client's inpatient or day-patient rehabilitation stay is crucial. An assessment completed too early may result in an estimate of cognitive functioning confounded by fatigue and decreased endurance.

Ideally, the assessment should be completed prior to the client's discharge to their home community to assist with school placement decisions and program planning. The timing of *outpatient* neuropsychological assessments is usually planned around transition periods (for example, beginning a high school program), when there is suspected deterioration in cognitive skills or behavioural functioning, or when the school or community agencies require updated information to further refine the program plan for the client. The key areas assessed include the child or adolescent's intellectual ability; language-related skills; sensorimotor, visual-motor, visual-perceptual, and visual-organizational abilities; attention; verbal and visual memory and learning abilities; academic achievement; executive functions; and behaviour and personality. The majority of these tests are paper and pencil measures, with some fine motor testing completed with the use of a finger tapper, pegboard, and dynamometer. Some assessment measures are timed, either having a time limit or performance based on the speed as well as quality of performance. Many tasks require language output, ranging from single words to formulating sentences. The following is a summary of the skills and abilities typically assessed during a neuro-psychological assessment.

Intellectual ability

One of the fundamental components of a neuropsychological assessment is to determine the child or adolescent's ability level post-brain injury. It is sometimes the case that a client's ability level remains very similar to the level the client was at prior to their injury when seen for assessment in the post-acute recovery phase. This finding is particularly true with the advent of revised assessment tools that remove the timed component from several of the visual-perceptual tests. The speed and time demands of earlier versions of the Wechsler scales typically translated into reduced scores on the subtests of the Performance Intelligence Quotient (PIQ). The removal of speed and time demands has allowed for a clearer delineation of the impact of injury on perceptual-organizational as opposed to visual-motor processing speed abilities, the latter of which are particularly susceptible to the effects of a brain injury.

Tests of ability are varied but most include tests of verbal comprehension/ expression (vocabulary, comprehension, general knowledge, verbal reasoning abilities), perceptual-organizational abilities (nonverbal problem solving, understanding picture concepts), working memory (recall of digit series, letter/number sequencing, mental arithmetic), and processing speed (coding, search, and cancellation tasks).

Traditionally, intelligence tests have been considered instrumental in determining whether an ability–achievement discrepancy exists, for the purpose of diagnosing a learning disability; however, the validity of this approach to diagnosis has been questioned (Fletcher et al. 1992, Stuebing et al. 2002). Despite this, many school boards rigidly adhere to this diagnostic approach. With respect to the child with a brain injury, this discrepancy may not be evident as the injury may serve to lower – although not necessarily permanently – performance scores due to reduced visual-motor processing speed. When it comes to brain injury, an overall estimate of intellectual ability may not adequately represent the variability in scores across subtests and indices.

Using intelligence tests in isolation is problematic. Intelligence testing, while an important component of the neuropsychological assessment, should never be interpreted without reference to performance in other areas when it comes to the child with a brain injury. Composite scores, such as Full Scale IQ, can be meaningless as they may mask important variations in test performance. For example, in the case of significant variations across Index scores, the Full Scale IQ becomes a poor indication of overall cognitive ability. The intelligence test is perhaps most useful to obtain data on specific abilities. Although it can be sensitive to the effects of a brain injury, it does not sample memory, attention, or problem-solving skills directly.

Interpreting the results from intelligence tests without reference to assessment of other skills may result in a failure to determine the presence of significant deficits that could impact on a child's learning and behaviour. In turn, this could result in an inability to access much-needed educational and community resources.

Motor, visual-motor, and visual-perceptual skills
The nonverbal domain is assessed with a combination of perceptual reasoning measures as well as additional measures of fine motor skills (strength, speed, and coordination), visual scanning, visual-motor integration, visual-motor processing speed, and visual-organization skills. Given that the child with a brain injury may have reduced processing speed and fine motor impairments, it is critical that untimed and motor-free tests of visual-perceptual skills be administered.

Language skills
Both the neuropsychologist and the speech-language pathologist complete language assessments within the rehabilitation context. While the child is undergoing active rehabilitation it is typically the speech-language pathologist who completes a detailed language assessment to determine basic expressive and receptive abilities, as well as more complex or higher-order language skills.

There are a number of test measures that may be used to assess a child's language skills. In addition to assessing verbal comprehension/expression abilities broadly on intelligence testing, a language assessment is likely to include specific tests of receptive and expressive language (at the single word, sentence, and paragraph levels), word generation, verbal fluency and oral expression, pragmatics and discourse, screening for aphasic symptoms, verbal problem solving and reasoning, ability to express and interpret intents, inferencing, and understanding of figurative language. A child's ability to understand and use language is assessed informally by means of their ability to follow instructions and to respond to the examiner's questions. These assessment measures may be used in conjunction with those administered by the team speech language pathologist, if available. As stated earlier, the assessment of language skills may be critical to determine whether the client meets criteria for a Language Impairment exceptionality within the special education system.

When a comprehensive neuropsychological assessment is completed in isolation from other team members, as is often the case in the outpatient setting, a more detailed language assessment is undertaken by the neuropsychologist. We have found these extended language assessments to be particularly helpful in identifying the more subtle deficits associated with the mild end of the injury spectrum, deficits often overlooked when the child is seen for assessment within the school system.

Attention

Early during the course of recovery from a brain injury, attentional skills are compromised, making assessment of cognitive abilities difficult. These difficulties are often compounded by fatigue. When compared to adults, children tend to experience more global attention difficulties that persist beyond the acute recovery phase (Anderson 2003). Attention difficulties may affect a child's performance across a number of skill areas, particularly on measures of learning and memory. Identifying the nature and severity of the attention difficulties is important, given the potential for these to interfere with testing more generally.

Formal assessment may be initiated once the client is able to tolerate at least an hour-long block of testing. Currently, we have at our disposal tests that are designed to assess different components of attention, including selective attention, sustained attention, divided attention, and attentional control/switching. Selective attention (also called focused attention) is the ability to resist distraction, to sort through information, and to discriminate elements that are important to the task at hand. Sustained attention is the ability to keep one's mind on a task despite the task being repetitive or boring. Divided attention is the ability to do more than one thing at a time; and attentional switching is the ability to switch the focus of attention smoothly between one thing and another (Manly et al. 1999).

The use of rating scales and inventories is also helpful in evaluating parents' perceptions of the child's ability to attend, and whether this represents a problem relative to the child's peers. Teachers can complete these same questionnaires, providing an indication of the severity of difficulties the child is experiencing at school.

Learning and memory skills

A major emphasis is placed on the assessment of learning and memory skills when working with children with brain injuries, given the prevalence of these types of disorders in this population (Fletcher and Taylor 1997). Understanding the nature of the memory impairment is important given the potentially devastating impact on school performance. When difficulties on memory testing are identified, poor attention needs to be ruled out as the driving mechanism.

Memory disorders in children with TBI are diverse. The assessment process examines the impact on modality (verbal vs. visual), method of presentation (repeated vs. heard only once), context (meaningful vs. unrelated information), duration of delay (immediate vs. delayed), and the way memory is tested (spontaneous recall vs. cueing vs. recognition). Our clinical experience with children who have had severe injuries is that they perform most poorly with lengthy and/or complex information presented just once, particularly after a delay period.

Academic achievement

Our approach to assessing academic achievement in children with TBI has extended beyond the more traditional screening assessments of skills at the single-word level (word recognition, spelling) to a broader assessment of the impact of cognitive impairment on reading comprehension, written expression, and reading fluency. In terms of assessing skills in mathematics, reasoning skills are evaluated in addition to a child's knowledge of mathematical facts and procedures.

Even among the most severely injured of our clients, academic performance on initial assessment early post-injury tends to be unremarkable, unless the child has a history of learning difficulties. These acquired skills tend to remain intact, providing an indication of premorbid levels of functioning. An exception to this is when there is a timed component or speed is involved.

Skills acquired formally through learning tend to be spared early on, with academic impairments evolving over the course of the first few years post-injury. These intact academic skills that are dependent on old learning are frequently misinterpreted as indicating that the child is doing reasonably well. Incorporating fluency measures into the academic assessment is necessary to demonstrate the potential impact of the injury on academic performance and to highlight to those in the community the need for close monitoring over time.

Executive functions

The executive functions are a collection of control processes that are responsible for guiding, directing, and managing cognitive, emotional, and behavioural functions (Gioia et al. 2000). Executive dysfunction is a common outcome in children who have sustained traumatic brain injuries (Gioia and Isquith 2004), but is not only associated with prefrontal pathology directly (Anderson 2002). A range of brain injury syndromes may disrupt pathways connecting to prefrontal areas, hence the need for a thorough assessment of skills in this area.

As noted previously, the inherent structure of the testing situation can offset the effects of executive dysfunction. This is part of our overall strategy so that we may directly assess underlying cognitive skills (memory functioning) that may have been affected as a result of the injury. Specific aspects of executive function that are assessed include a child's fundamental self-regulatory abilities as well as their cognitive self-management skills. In addition to formal testing, these are assessed by means of ratings of their everyday behaviours and skills.

Contrary to what Ylvisaker et al. (2005) would have us believe, it is the exception rather than the rule that executive dysfunction is not directly observable on formal assessment. The tests used in assessment have become increasingly sophisticated, as has our understanding of early manifestations of executive dysfunction. In those rare cases in which executive dysfunction is not apparent upon formal testing, these concerns emerge from informal observations of behaviour in the child's daily environment – a standard practice in the rehabilitation context. This includes the collection of information from family members, teachers, and other involved team members.

It has been our experience that children and adolescents admitted for rehabilitation during the acute stages of recovery may not exhibit executive impairments due to the inherent structure of the rehabilitation program and associated supports built in (for example, cueing). Furthermore, family members frequently do not identify executive deficits as primary concerns, as their focus tends to be upon the child's physical recovery. Following discharge to their home community, the executive deficits may become more pronounced, particularly if the appropriate supports have not been anticipated and put into place. Routine follow-up clinic visits are necessary to ensure that the child is well supported and that his/her needs are understood.

Behaviour and personality

Difficulties with coping and adjustment may be present during the rehabilitation admission as a reaction to physical and cognitive changes. Behaviour changes post-injury are common and occur most frequently among children and adolescents who have sustained severe traumatic brain injuries. They present a significant barrier to successful community reintegration, given the adverse impact on social adaptation.

Our approach to assessing behavioural and emotional disorders in children and adolescents with TBI involves the administration of a core set of questionnaires and inventories, with the use of semi-structured screening interviews and diagnosis-specific scales (for depression and anxiety) as necessary. Psychosocial outcome has been found to be the result of a complex interaction between injury characteristics and other variables, with pre-injury family environment being in some cases a significant moderator of the effect of a traumatic brain injury (Yeates et al. 1997, 2004). Difficulties with coping and adjustment have been documented even among those at the mild end of the injury spectrum.

Among those whose injuries are milder, a lack of needed supports within their home communities has frequently been identified as the source of difficulties with coping and adjustment in the long term. Their injuries are not obvious, and their actions and behaviours may be misinterpreted as being intentional when they do indeed relate to the injury sustained. Lack of support at school more specifically has been identified as the catalyst for emotional difficulties experienced by those who are seen for long-term follow-up. Increasing demands made of students, as well as delayed cognitive effects of the injury, may lead to periodic emotional/behavioural difficulties – hence the need to monitor their progress over a number of years.

In addition to having scales that help to identify difficulties with coping and adjustment, we now have at our disposal measures that tap into the neurobehavioural manifestations of brain disease. These have helped us to anticipate difficulties that may arise following discharge, as well as to document the nature and severity of the behaviour problems exhibited.

PART II: PSYCHOSOCIAL FUNCTIONING FOLLOWING PEDIATRIC TRAUMATIC BRAIN INJURY

INTRODUCTION

Psychosocial is an umbrella term that encompasses a child's emotional, behavioural, social, and family functioning. TBI can affect all these areas, either as a direct consequence of the injury sustained or as a result of secondary complications related to family functioning and perceived burden, available resources and supports in the home community, or difficulties coming to terms with the injuries sustained. Further, these injury-related effects may be exacerbated by pre-existing personality, behavioural, and/or family difficulties. Taken together, predicting outcome in any individual case can be complex. This review will focus on the problems of children and adolescents during their rehabilitation admissions, as they prepare to make the transition to their home communities, and in the years that follow.

Whether one considers the psychosocial sequelae of TBI to fall under the rubric 'emotional', or 'behavioural', or 'social' is more a matter of perspective than of actual difference. Considerable overlap between these terms exists, with researchers often using them interchangeably. To further complicate matters, there are references to neurobehavioural and social outcomes (Yeates et al. 2004, Yeates and Taylor 2005), personality change disorder (Max et al. 2000, 2001, 2005), psychiatric disorders (Wassenberg et al. 2004), and disruptive behaviour disorders (Max et al. 1997). Presumably, these all fall under the broader term, psychosocial outcome.

BEHAVIOUR

Behaviour problems following TBI are common and come in a variety of forms. They are among the most troubling consequences of TBI to parents, families, and community professionals, with persistent problems occurring in approximately 40% of severe TBI cases. An additional 20% will experience transient behavioural changes (Max et al. 2000). In our experience, these changes can present a significant obstacle to successful community reintegration and participation in rehabilitation programming. When the behaviour problems emerge as a delayed consequence of an injury sustained at a young age, the effect on a child's coping and adjustment can be devastating. Moreover, the problems that develop as late effects are more often than not perceived negatively or misinterpreted outright.

TYPES OF BEHAVIOUR PROBLEMS OBSERVED FOLLOWING TBI

The behavioural difficulties observed following a TBI are many and varied. They have been classified in many different ways, ranging from the more general 'frontal lobe syndrome' (Alderman 2003), to distinct subtypes, such as the DSM-IV-based personality change disorder (Max et al. 2000). They are perhaps best characterized as behavioural excesses, behavioural deficits, or stimulus control disorders (Ylvisaker and Feeney 1998, Wilson et al. 2003). With respect to the first of these, disinhibition, agitation, aggression, behavioural outbursts, impulsivity, lability, reduced anger control, risk taking, perseveration, social inappropriateness, and euphoria have been reported (Feeney and Ylvisaker 1995, Persel and Persel 1995, Demellweek et al. 1998, Max et al. 2000, 2001, 2005). Behavioural deficits include reduced initiation, apathy, lack of drive, lack of interest, lethargy, slowness, inattentiveness, and reduced spontaneity (Stuss and Benson 1986, Feeney and Ylvisaker 1995, Persel and Persel 1995, Max et al. 2000, 2001, 2005). Stimulus control disorders refer to a behaviour that occurs in the wrong situation, such as hugging an unfamiliar person (Persel and Persel 1995).

As described by Sohlberg and Mateer (2001), different behaviours are seen at different stages of recovery and require different types of interventions. The early behavioural consequences of TBI include restlessness and agitation associated with confusion and disorientation. Crying, lashing out, moaning, and flailing are common, yet do not seem to be related to any external precipitant. Later on, the agitation is more clearly seen in response to environmental events and is thought to be related to confusion, fear, pain, and dyscontrol (Sohlberg and Mateer 2001). Thus, medical or therapeutic interventions may provoke these behaviours.

At this stage, the goals of behaviour management are to 'reduce the frequency and intensity of the behaviours, so as to reduce the likelihood of further injury to self or others; to support basic care and treatment goals; and to prevent the person from developing learned patterns of inappropriate behaviour through inadvertent reinforcement' (Sohlberg and Mateer 2001: 339). Due to a limited capacity for self-regulation and limited awareness, the most effective strategies emphasize factors external to the individual. Staff should be trained to maintain a calm and reassuring manner. They should reorient the patient by addressing the patient by name and identifying themselves and what they are going to do, and using clear and succinct explanations. Later still, as the individual becomes better oriented and begins to regain some degree of self-control, changes in their routine, higher levels of stimulation, and increased demands may lead to challenging behaviours. Management techniques at this point include increased rest time, keeping the environment and instructions simple, giving feedback and setting goals, being calm and redirecting to task, providing choices, increasing the opportunities for success, varying activities, and breaking down tasks (Persel and Persel 1995).

At later stages of the recovery process, behavioural problems may be worsened by fear and depression as the individual becomes increasingly aware of their limitations (Sohlberg and Mateer 2001). Unfortunately, by the time many children or adolescents reach this stage, they have been discharged from hospital to their home communities. It is at this stage that the emphasis of behavioural management changes to a focus on facilitating positive behavioural routines and emphasizing compensatory and self-regulatory strategies (Feeney and Ylvisaker 1995, Sohlberg and Mateer 2001). The latter of these are only effective once the individual has come to grips with changes in their abilities.

Contributors to Challenging Behaviour Following a TBI
There are many potential reasons why a child develops behaviour problems following TBI. These include the following: pre-injury behaviour problems or the psychosocial history of the individual; the direct physical, behavioural, or cognitive consequences of the injury; environmental factors such as the supports available, the expectations and demands made, and the appropriateness of the interventions implemented; reactive factors, such as the behavioural consequences of feelings of anger, loss, or frustration; late effects of the injury; and the backlog of successes and failures the individual has experienced in the aftermath of the injury (Sbordone 1990, Demellweek et al. 1998, Ylvisaker and Feeney 1998, Sohlberg and Mateer 2001).

Approaches to Working with Challenging Behaviours
There are many different approaches to managing challenging behaviours in children and adolescents. Historically, the field of behavioural modification and analysis can be traced to the writings of Thorndike who, in the latter part of the nineteenth century, articulated a fundamental principle of behavioural psychology known as the 'Law of Effect'. A revolutionary idea for its time, this law stated simply that the consequences of a behaviour could influence its future likelihood (Jacobs 1993). The principles of behavioural analysis were further developed by John B Watson, BF

Skinner, and Pavlov. In general, behaviour analysis focuses on the identification and manipulation of relationships between behaviours, their antecedents (i.e. what comes before them), and their consequences (i.e. what follows). Traditional approaches to behaviour management have placed a disproportionate emphasis on decreasing undesirable behaviours and manipulating consequences. Once perceived to be coercive and punitive, approaches to management have evolved to emphasize building positive behaviours and modifying antecedent events or circumstances. Moreover, antecedents, once restricted to events that immediately precede the behaviour, have, in the works of Ylvisaker (Ylvisaker and Feeney 1998), been broadened to encompass internal and external context variables (setting events).

Regardless of the techniques used, successful management of behaviour first requires careful analysis of the antecedents and consequences of that behaviour. Depending upon the stage of recovery and the degree of awareness or insight demonstrated by the child, different techniques may be used. Early on, the emphasis would be on environmental management therapies, such as changes in lighting, seating, or noise level. Due to a limited capacity for self-regulation and limited awareness, the most effective strategies emphasize factors external to the individual.

It is also important to teach parents and caregivers how to communicate effectively with the child or adolescent with a brain injury. This is especially true over the longer term, as the child returns to the community. Some parents unwittingly reinforce undesirable behaviours because they are anxious to see some type of response from their child. An example of this is a situation in which a nonverbal client is positively reinforced for any use of his hand, no matter how inappropriate (for example, hitting, pinching, grabbing). As pointed out by Sohlberg and Mateer (2001), there are many strategies that can be helpful in reducing disruptive behaviours, and parents require modelling, practice, and being supported to implement these effectively. They describe powerful behavioural techniques which include: (1) selectively ignoring behaviours, (2) distracting and redirecting, (3) providing choices, (4) reducing, but not eliminating, expectations, (5) backing off and trying again, (6) speaking quietly and maintaining a neutral stance, (7) identifying signs of a client's escalating distress, and (8) avoiding confrontation and power struggles. We have found that training staff in nonviolent crisis intervention has been an effective tool in managing a child's behavioural challenges.

While a behavioural management model can be effective in a rehabilitation setting, it is sometimes the case that a behavioural modification approach is necessary. There is a range of techniques available to target and decrease entrenched undesirable behaviours (e.g. verbal or physical aggression). At times, increasing the frequency of some behaviour (e.g. initiation, staying on task) is needed and can be accomplished by using prompting and shaping. It is essential to target a single behaviour and provide consistency across caregivers and environments.

COPING AND ADJUSTMENT

Emotional changes following brain injury have been documented, with specific mention made of decreased motivation, decreased self-esteem, depression, anger, over-arousal, irritability, apathy, lability, loss of self-reflective attitude, denial, low frustration tolerance, dependency, obsessive-compulsive behaviours, repression, euphoria, rapid mood swings, delusional thoughts, anxiety, and self-centredness. The most frequently reported emotional problems include irritability and apathy, followed by decrease in motivation, frustration, and obsessive traits (Demellweek et al. 1998). Again, decreasing lengths of stay in acute care and rehabilitation settings have translated into these consequences being more apt to occur after the child's discharge from hospital, when supports may no longer be readily available to them.

Both the emotional and behavioural sequelae of TBI have the potential to affect a child's coping and adjustment by undermining interpersonal relationships and social interactions. Executive impairments – in particular, difficulties with self-regulation – set the stage for difficulties with social adjustment. Specific impairments noted to affect a child's social adaptation include disinhibition, inappropriate social communication or judgement, decrease in compliance or oppositional behaviours, social withdrawal or isolation, and lack of social skills. Disinhibition, inappropriate social communication, and social withdrawal or isolation are the most commonly reported social interaction problems (Demellweek et al. 1998).

Given the potential of TBI to disrupt prefrontal areas and their associated networks and systems, cognitive, behavioural, and emotional outcomes are often inextricably interrelated. As Yeates et al. point out, 'childhood TBI leads to persistent problems in social functioning that are accounted for by multiple factors, including injury severity, specific neuropsychological and social information processing abilities known to be vulnerable to TBI, and the family environment' (2004: 423). Although there appears to be some controversy with respect to the role of the family environment in mediating psychosocial or behavioural outcome, this could well relate to the duration of follow-up (Yeates et al. 2004, Max et al. 2005).

PSYCHOLOGICAL STAGES OF RECOVERY

Following a traumatic event, the child and the family typically progress through a series of psychological stages of recovery. While these stages may parallel the physical and cognitive recovery of the child, they may also occur at a much later point in the recovery process. It is important for health care professionals to keep in mind that family members go through a very similar process of psychological recovery, but may be behind or ahead of their child's own recovery stage. The stages are not invariable, nor is it the case that all children and their families must go through all of these stages. Certainly, severity of injury and family support systems will play significant roles in the psychological recovery process (Yeates et al. 1997, 2004).

1 Denial

Once the TBI survivor has recovered from coma and is beginning to make physical and cognitive gains, the family may be very hopeful that all will be well and that their child will make a complete recovery. During the acute care hospitalization stage, families frequently hear rather pessimistic projections from physicians about the outcome expected for their child ('Your child may not live' . . . 'Your child may never walk or talk again'). When their child does survive the injury, wakes from coma, and does indeed begin to talk again, the parents become sceptical of the opinions of health care providers. In the rehabilitation setting, parents may have difficulty understanding that their son or daughter has serious cognitive deficits, especially if their child is making significant progress physically. The fact that cognitive deficits are sometimes 'hidden' makes it even harder for the rehabilitation team to convince family members that cognitive issues and goals are important. Further, the highly structured rehabilitation environment may mask important deficits, making it that much more difficult for families to come to terms with their child's situation.

Children who seem unaware of their physical or cognitive deficits and their implications are often considered to be in denial of their problems. This lack of insight into the effects of the brain injury may be a direct result of the injury sustained. It is interesting that family members who deny the presence of deficits in their children are considered to be in psychological denial while similar observations in the child with a TBI are attributed to the cognitive consequences of the injury.

2 Awareness of deficits/insight

The assessment process is often the launching point for the child to begin to become aware of their deficits. Insight occurs as the child realizes that certain skills and activities are not performed as easily as they once were. The family may also become more aware of their child's difficulties, especially if the child is unable to perform routine tasks, due to physical or cognitive limitations, when at home. The child's awareness of his/her deficits is crucial in terms of their motivation to work on the areas of difficulty or their acceptance of compensatory strategies designed to circumvent the problem area. In the rehabilitation setting, it is imperative to encourage families to take their child home for visits to enable them to more fully understand the neurobehavioural impact of their child's brain injury.

Although education about the brain injury is important, it is essential that this be delivered at a level accessible to the child. Too much information can be overwhelming, and can set the stage for the development of considerable anxiety. Alternatively, the child may use their newly acquired knowledge to try to avoid activities that are difficult for them. Emphasizing strengths and resilience in the child is important, particularly when the presenting issues are likely to cause lifelong difficulties.

3 Reactive depression

It is ironic that, as the child becomes increasingly aware of their limitations, there is the possibility that they may experience what appears to be a setback in their emotional coping. The more recent trend towards shortened hospital admissions has resulted in the likelihood of this consequence occurring in the community post-rehabilitation discharge, instead of during the rehabilitation stay. The development of a reactive depression in response to the realization that the person is not the same as they were before the injury can result in internalized distress causing decreased motivation to participate in the rehabilitation program. Left untreated, there is the potential risk of suicide among older children and in cases where the depression is severe. Difficulties with behaviour regulation may increase their risk of acting on impulse and without regard to consequences. As a result, they run a further risk of difficulties with noncompliance, substance abuse, and potential involvement with the criminal justice system.

The presence of depression in children with TBI is frequently stressful and uncomfortable for rehabilitation team members and families. This type of depression is also indicative of the child's progress through another stage of psychological recovery and may be viewed, therefore, as a positive and potentially necessary stage of recovery. Children with TBI may not experience depression while in active rehabilitation and it is important that children, families, and community team members be aware of the possibility that depression may occur. Supportive counselling may be needed to assist the child in identifying and expressing their feelings of sadness, anger, and frustration, as well as in developing ways of coping and dealing with their current life situation.

4 Adaptation and coping

It is thought that recovery from a brain injury is a lifelong process and it should be no surprise that the psychological adjustment to the injury may also be a long-term process. Children with TBI face the most significant challenges to their coping abilities when they return to their communities after their involvement in the rehabilitation facility. It is often at this point that children with TBI become fully aware of the extent to which their life has been altered as a result of their injury. One of the most significant concerns for children and adolescents is the loss of friends and the change in peer group, particularly if they have missed part or all of their school year. The difference in age of one or two years is of much greater significance for the child or adolescent than it is for the adult. The perception of being 'different' is very hard for the child or adolescent who is struggling to fit in with their peer group. Although necessary from a cognitive and academic support point of view, special education services such as teaching assistants and resource classes may have a stigmatizing effect on the child. Rehabilitation professionals working with the child with a TBI must be sensitive to these issues and attempt to provide needed supports in a manner that is acceptable and as least intrusive as possible for the child. This must be done, however, without compromising the need for support.

THE FAMILY
THE ROLE OF THE FAMILY IN PEDIATRIC REHABILITATION
1 The family as team members
The family is essential in the rehabilitation process for TBI survivors of all ages. The family provides the child with a support network that is critical to their eventual successful recovery, especially in terms of psychosocial outcome. It is important to remember that, no matter what the involvement of rehabilitation professionals, the child with a TBI will usually return to their home environment or at least to their home community. The success of community reintegration appears to be tied to the degree of family involvement in the rehabilitation process. Highly involved families have a greater understanding of their child's progress and are better equipped to provide for their child's needs before and after discharge home. This is particularly true if the child with a TBI presents with challenging behaviours that require the parents and siblings to develop new ways of interacting with them. The pre-injury family environment can be a significant moderator of TBI outcome, buffering its impact in high-functioning families and exacerbating it in low-functioning families (Yeates et al. 1997).

Many rehabilitation facilities are moving away from an 'expert' model to one in which the child's care is not only client-centred but goal-focused. Families are being encouraged to become more than passive recipients of professional recommen-dations. If the goal of rehabilitation is to help the child return to as normal a life as possible, the families can give valuable information about the child's previous life-style, and input into functional goals important to the child and the family. In this manner, families join the rehabilitation team as *collaborative* partners in developing the child's rehabilitation program.

Some common problems occur when parents experience guilt as a result of not having kept their child safe from injury. These feelings can often lead to parents' reluctance to hold their child accountable for their behaviour, and inability to effectively implement clear expectations, boundaries, and consequences. This may result in an escalation in the child's behaviour problems because the child is not receiving clear feedback about their behaviour. They may even feel unsafe in their environment. These feelings of guilt are not limited to situations in which the parents may feel responsible in some way for their child's injury. Many parents articulate being unable to hold their child accountable because of all they have been through. If not given sufficient guidance and support, parents with limited coping skills may eventually withdraw from a difficult situation, leaving the child at risk.

2 Involvement of the family in goal setting
Family members should be active participants along with the professional team members in the formulation of initial goals at the time of intake or admission prior to the formal assessment process. These initial goals may be quite global or general in nature and somewhat unrealistic but it is important to keep in mind that they are what the family view as relevant to the child and themselves. After the assessment period, the team should review the initial goals with the assessment results in mind so that more objective, short-term goals can be generated. For example, if the family have 'being able to walk' as a goal for their child, the team can suggest several subgoals such as 'improving balance' and 'standing with support' as necessary steps in order to achieve the ultimate goal of walking. An interdisciplinary care plan outlining the general and specific goals is very useful for both team and family members to keep track of the child's progress. The child, family members, and team should meet regularly to review the child's progress and to develop new rehabilitation goals. Parents often focus on physical problems and may need support to address psychosocial/cognitive issues, which often are more debilitating in the long term.

3 Bridging the gap between the institution and home
It is critical that the child's rehabilitation program be carried into the community as consistently as possible, and this is often achieved through the provision of case management services and rehabilitation therapists. The family plays an essential role in this process and the success of the child's community rehabilitation often hinges on the extent to which the family is prepared to support and cope with the child at home. The family must be comfortable with the prospect of having the child at home and any concerns about this should be dealt with before discharge. Often, there is disagreement between the child and the family members about when the child is ready for discharge. The child may not understand why they cannot go home when they feel they are ready, and the families may express discomfort or unwillingness to have the child home until they feel ready. Engaging children and families in the goal-setting and therapeutic aspects of the rehabilitation process may increase their comfort level in feeling capable of dealing with the issues at home. There may also be less distress felt at the time of discharge if the family feel more 'in control' of the child's program plan and are knowledgeable about intervention procedures.

In addition to ensuring that all necessary therapy and economic supports are in place in the community, it is also important that the family is supportive of and comfortable with all recommendations. The rehabilitative process in the community can be an intrusion on the privacy of the family and the team needs to realize that the family will have to adapt and change its way of operating to meet the needs of the child. Depending on the child's needs, demands on the family may range from having to take the child to various therapy appointments each day to having their home turned into a treatment centre. The role of the case manager with respect to this issue may be critical in bridging the gap between the institution and the community.

THE PSYCHOSOCIAL SEQUELAE OF TRAUMATIC BRAIN INJURY: A LONG-TERM CONCERN

Children and adolescents with TBI may experience a wide spectrum of behavioural, emotional, and social sequelae that may seriously interfere with their ability to recover from the injury. In addition to the direct effect (e.g. damage to frontal lobes and interrelated systems and networks) the brain injury may have on behavioural functioning, it is important to keep in mind that the TBI may have a significant impact on the emergence of skills at later developmental stages, particularly during the adolescent years.

Normal developmental stages of adolescence are significantly complicated by the presence of even minor brain injuries (Jacobson et al., cited in Sellars and Vegter 1993). McGuire and Rothenberg (1986) report that closed head injury presents a particular problem to adolescents who, prior to their injury, were moving towards a healthy separation from their families. This natural process may be reversed as the adolescent becomes more dependent as a result of their residual deficits. The stresses that accompany brain injury are multiplied by the naturally occurring developmental stresses of adolescence for both the family and the adolescent.

Brain injury during adolescence can occur at a time when even healthy teens are struggling with difficult developmental issues. Given the added distress related to increasing awareness of cognitive deficits and emergence of late effects, teens may feel isolated from their ever-judging peer group. Crosson (1987) reviewed literature that emphasized the consequences of adolescent brain injury in terms of contaminating dependence/independence issues between adolescents and their parents. He noted that those injured during their late teens and early twenties could find themselves involuntarily returned to a dependent relationship with their families. Slater (1989) describes a case study in which an 18-year-old felt that she was an outsider in her peer group subsequent to an acquired brain injury. This woman was concerned that she was not successfully addressing developmental tasks including identity and future career directions. Consequently, her level of distress increased as her feelings of self-efficacy and self-esteem decreased. An appropriate response to these difficulties may include group therapy, individual counselling, peer education, and supportive reintegration into social activities. The combination of increased complexity in their academic and social environments and the delayed or impaired development of executive functions (Sohlberg and Mateer 2001) leaves the adolescent vulnerable to considerable upheaval during the adolescent years.

The literature is just beginning to address the issue of long-term psychosocial outcome of those who sustained a TBI in childhood. The preliminary evidence is consistent with our clinical impressions suggesting that psychological adjustment issues outweigh physical and cognitive limitations over the long term (Anderson 2006). This is particularly true of those who sustained severe injuries, were injured at a young age, or sustained damage to prefrontal areas. Those who sustained their injuries at a young age are particularly vulnerable, given that they must go on to acquire many new skills to function in academic, social, and occupational realms. Difficulties with self-control and altered affect may significantly interfere with the ability of the child or adolescent to reintegrate successfully into academic and, eventually, vocational settings. Unless behavioural and emotional disturbances are treated promptly and efficiently, the psychosocial outcome of children with TBI will likely deteriorate over time.

CONCLUSION

The rehabilitation of the child or adolescent with TBI is a complex, multi-factor process that begins with the injury and continues for the rest of that individual's life. Children and adolescents are at particular risk in terms of compromised outcome because their injuries occur at a time when they are still developing cognitive and social skills. They lack the experience and learning previously acquired by adult TBI survivors and must continue to grow and develop with significant physical, cognitive, and psychosocial impairments. One of the most important indices of positive outcome would appear to be early comprehensive assessment and treatment, as well as a continuity of program planning and treatment into the home community. This is true for children from the mild to severe spectrum of the injury continuum.

Many children with mild brain injuries are sent home almost immediately and without support services; however, it is inappropriate to assume that all children will recover from TBI without some changes in their abilities. Health care professionals are becoming more aware of these issues and attempts are being made to follow children with mild TBI more comprehensively. Families and schools also benefit from increased monitoring of the child's recovery in terms of education and support that may be provided related to brain injury issues. The goal of future TBI rehabilitation efforts will be likely to focus on community intervention as the preferred means of service delivery and this will contribute substantially to the maintenance of the family unit.

REFERENCES

Alderman N (2003) Rehabilitation of behaviour disorders. In: Wilson BA (ed) *Neuropsychological Rehabilitation: Theory and Practice.* Lisse: Swets & Zeitlinger.

Anderson P (2002) Assessment and development of executive function (EF) during childhood. *Child Neuropsychol* 8(2): 71–82.

Anderson V (2003) Outcome and management of traumatic brain injury in childhood: the neuropsychologist's contribution. In: Wilson BA (ed) *Neuropsychological Rehabilitation: Theory and Practice.* Lisse: Swets & Zeitlinger.

Anderson V (2006) Do children really recover better than adults from brain damage? Presentation at the 16th Annual Nelson Butters' West Coast Neuropsychology Conference, *Advances in Pediatric Neuropsychology: From Toddlers Through School-Aged Children.* San Diego, CA.

Anderson V, Pentland L (1998) Residual attention deficits following childhood head injury. *Neuropsychol Rehabil* 8: 283–300.

Anderson V, Northam E, Hendy J, Wrennall J (2001) *Developmental Neuropsychology: A Clinical Approach.* Hove: Psychology Press.

Asarnow RF, Satz P, Light R, Zaucha K, Lewis R, McCleary C (1995) The UCLA study of mild head injury in children and adolescents. In: Broman SH, Michel ME (eds) *Traumatic Head Injury in Children.* New York: Oxford University Press, pp 117–146.

Barnes M, Dennis M, Wilkinson M (1999) Reading after closed head injury in childhood: effects on accuracy, fluency, and comprehension. *Dev Neuropsychol* 15: 1–24.

Beers S (1992) Cognitive effects of mild head injury in children and adolescents. *Neuropsychol Rev* 3: 281–319.

Bishop DV (1981) Plasticity and specificity of language localization in the developing brain. *Dev Med Child Neurol* 23: 251–255.

Brookshire BL, Chapman SB, Song J, Levin HS (2000) Cognitive and linguistic correlates of children's discourse after closed head injury: a three-year follow-up. *J Int Neuropsychol Soc* 6: 741–751.

Brown G, Chadwick O, Shaffer D, Rutter M, Traub M (1981) A prospective study of children with head injuries: II. Psychiatric sequelae. *Psychol Med* 11(1): 49–62.

Carney J, Gerring J (1990) Return to school following severe closed head injury: a critical phase in paediatric rehabilitation. *Pediatrician* 17(4): 222–229.

Carroll LJ, Cassidy JD, Peloso PM, Garritty C, Giles-Smith L (2004) Systematic search and review procedures: results of the WHO Collaborating Centre Task Force on Mild Traumatic Brain Injury. *J Rehabil Med* Suppl 43:11–14.

Catroppa C, Anderson V (2003) Children's attentional skills two years post-TBI. *Dev Neuropsychol* 23: 359-373.

Catroppa C, Anderson V (2005) A prospective study of the recovery of attention from acute to 2 years following pediatric traumatic brain injury. *J Int Neuropsychol Soc* 11: 84–98.

Chadwick O, Rutter M, Brown G, Shaffer D, Traub M (1981a) A prospective study of children with head injuries: II. Cognitive sequelae. *Psychol Med* 11: 49–61.

Chadwick O, Rutter M, Shaffer D, Shrout P (1981b) A prospective study of children with head injuries: IV. Specific cognitive deficits. *J Clin Neuropsychol* 2: 101–120.

Crosson B (1987) Treatment of interpersonal deficits for head-trauma patients in inpatient rehabilitation setting. *Clin Neuropsychol* 1(4): 335–363.

Demellweek C, O'Leary A, Baldwin T (1998) Emotional, behavioural, and social difficulties. In: Appleton R, Baldwin T (eds) *Management of Brain-injured Children.* New York: Oxford University Press.

Dennis M (1987) Using language to parse the young damaged brain. *J Clin Exp Neuropsychol* 9: 723–753.

Dennis M (2000) Childhood medical disorders and cognitive impairment: biological risk, time, development, and reserve. In: Yeates KO, Ris MD, Taylor HG (eds) *Pediatric Neuropsychology: Research, Theory, and Practice.* New York: Guilford Press, pp 3–22.

Dennis M, Wilkinson M, Koski L, Humphreys RP (1995) Attention deficits in the long-term after childhood head injury. In: Broman SH, Michel ME (eds) *Traumatic Head Injury in Children.* New York: Oxford University Press, pp 165–187.

Donders J (1994) Academic placement after traumatic brain injury. *J Sch Psychol* 32: 53–65.

Donders J (2005) Current issues in pediatric head trauma. Workshop presented at the annual meeting of the American Academy of Clinical Neuropsychology. Minneapolis.

Donders J, Minnema MT (2004) Performance discrepancies on the California Verbal Learning Test – Children's Version (CVLT-C) in children with traumatic brain injury. *J Int Neuropsychol Soc* 10: 482–488.

Ewing-Cobbs L, Levin H, Eisenberg H, Fletcher JM (1987) Language functions following closed head injury in children and adolescents. *J Clin Exp Neuropsychol* 9: 575–592.

Ewing-Cobbs L, Fletcher J, Levin H, Francis D, Davidson K, Miner M (1997) Longitudinal neuropsychological outcome in infants and preschoolers with traumatic brain injury. *J Int Neuropsychol Soc* 3: 581–591.

Ewing-Cobbs L, Barnes MA, Fletcher JM (2003) Early brain injury in children: development and reorganization of cognitive function. *Dev Neuropsychol* 24(2&3): 669–704.

Feeney TJ, Ylvisaker M (1995) Choice and routine: antecedent behavioral interventions for adolescents with severe traumatic brain injury. *J Head Trauma Rehabil* 10(3): 67–86.

Fletcher J, Taylor HG (1984) Neuropsychological approaches to children: towards a developmental neuropsychology. *J Clin Neuropsychol* 6: 24–27.

Fletcher JM, Taylor HG (1997) Children with brain injury. In: Mash EJ, Terdal LG (eds) *Assessment of Childhood Disorders, 3rd edn.* New York: Guilford Press.

Fletcher JM, Francis DM, Rourke BP, Shaywitz SE, Shaywitz BA (1992) The validity of discrepancy-based definitions of reading disabilities. *J Learn Disabil* 25(9): 555–561.

Garth J, Anderson V, Wrennall J (1997) Executive functions following moderate to severe frontal lobe injury. Impact of injury and age at injury. *Pediatr Rehabil* 1: 99–108.

Gioia GA, Isquith PK (2004) Ecological assessment of executive function in traumatic brain injury. *Dev Neuropsychol* 25 (1&2): 135–158.

Gioia GA, Isquith PK, Guy SC, Kenworthy L (2000) *Behavior Rating Inventory of Executive Dysfunction.* Odessa, FL: Psychological Assessment Resources.

Hebb DO (1949) *The Organization of Behaviour.* New York: McGraw-Hill.

Jacobs HE (1993) *Behavior Analysis Guidelines and Brain Injury Rehabilitation: People, Principles, and Programs.* Gaithersburg, MD: Aspen Publishers.

Jaffe KM, Fay GC, Polissar NL, Martin KM, Shurtlef HA, Rivara JB, Winn R (1992) Severity of pediatric traumatic brain injury and neurobehavioral outcome: a cohort study. *Arch Phys Med Rehabil* 73: 540–547.

Jaffe KM, Fay GC, Polissar NL, Martin KM, Shurtlef HA, Rivara JB, Winn R (1993) Severity of pediatric traumatic brain injury and neurobehavioral recovery at one year: a cohort study. *Arch Phys Med Rehabil* 74: 587–595.

Jaffe KM, Polissar NL, Fay GC, Liao S (1995) Recovery trends over three years following pediatric traumatic brain injury. *Arch Phys Med Rehabil* 76: 17–26.

Kennard MA (1936) Age and other factors in motor recovery from precentral lesions in monkeys. *Am J Physiol* 115: 138–146.

Kennard MA (1938) Reorganization of motor function in the cerebral cortex of monkeys deprived of motor and premotor areas in infancy. *J Neurophysiol* 1: 477–496.

Kennard MA (1940) Relation of age to motor impairment in man and in subhuman primates. *Arch Neurol Psychiatry* 44: 377–397.

Kennard MA (1942) Cortical reorganization of motor function: studies on series of monkeys of various ages from infancy to maturity. *Arch Neurol Psychiatry* 48: 227–240.

Kinsella G, Prior M, Sawyer M, Murtagh D, Eisenmajer R, Anderson V, Klug G (1995)

Neuropsychological deficit and academic performance in children and adolescents following traumatic brain injury. *J Pediatr Psychol* 20: 753–767.

Kinsella G, Prior M, Sawyer M, Ong B, Murtagh D, Eisenmajer R, Bryan D, Anderson V, Klug G (1997) Predictors and indicators of academic outcome in children 2 years following traumatic head injury. *J Int Neuropsychol Soc* 3: 608–616.

Klonoff H (1971) Head injuries in children: predisposing factors, accident conditions, accident proneness and sequelae. *Am J Public Health* 61: 2405–2417.

Klonoff H, Paris R (1974) Immediate, short-term and residual effects of acute head injuries in children: neuropsychological and neurological correlates. In: Reitan RM, Davison LA (eds) *Clinical Neuropsychology: Current Status and Applications.* New York: Wiley, pp 179–210.

Klonoff H, Low MD, Clark C (1977) Head injuries in children: a prospective five year follow-up. *J Neurol Neurosurg Psychiatry* 40: 1211–1219.

Lenneberg E (1967) *Biological Foundations of Language.* New York: Wiley.

Levin H, Eisenberg H (1979) Neuropsychological impairment after closed head injury in children and adolescents. *J Pediatr Psychol* 4: 389–402.

Levin H, Culhane K, Mendelsohn D, Lilly M, Bruce D, Fletcher J, Chapman S, Harward H, Eisenberg H (1993) Cognition in relation to magnetic reasonance imaging in head-injured children and adolescents. *Arch Neurol* 50: 897–905.

Levin H, Mendelsohn D, Lilly M, Fletcher J, Culhane K, Chapman S, Harward H, Kusnerick L, Bruce D, Eisenberg H (1994) Tower of London performance in relation to magnetic resonance imaging following closed head injury in children. *Neuropsychology* 8: 171–179.

Levin H, Song J, Scheibel R, Fletcher J, Harward H, Lilly M, Goldstein F (1997) Concept formation and problem solving following closed head injury in children. *J Int Neuropsychol Soc* 3: 598–607.

McDonald CM, Jaffe KM (1992) Neurobehavioral and family functioning following traumatic brain injury in children. *West J Med* 157(6): 664.

McDonald CM, Jaffe KM, Fay GC, Polissar NL, Martin KM, Lios S, Rivara JB (1994) Comparison of indices of traumatic brain injury severity as predictors of neurobehavioral outcomes in children. *Arch Phys Med Rehabil* 75: 328–337.

McGuire TL, Rothenberg MB (1986) Behavioral and psychosocial sequelae of pediatric head injury. *J Head Trauma Rehabil* 1(4): 1–6.

McKinlay A, Dalrymple-Alford JC, Horwood LJ, Fergusson DM (2002) Long-term psychosocial outcomes after mild head injury in early childhood. *J Neurol Neurosurg Psychiatry* 73: 281–288.

McKinlay A, Dalrymple-Alford JC, Horwood LJ, Fergusson DM (2003) Pre-injury and other non-specific factors do not explain adverse psychosocial development associated with childhood mild head injury. *Brain Injury* 17(Suppl 1): 39.

Manly T, Roberston IH, Anderson V, Nimmo-Smith I (1999) *The Test of Everyday Attention for Children (TEA-Ch): Manual.* Bury St Edmunds: Thames Valley Test Company Limited.

Max JE, Lindgren SD, Knutson C, Pearson CS, Ihrig D, Welborn A (1997) Child and adolescent traumatic brain injury: psychiatric findings from a paediatric outpatient specialty clinic. *Brain Injury* 11(10): 699–711.

Max JE, Koele SL, Castillo CC, Lindgren SD, Arndt S, Bokura H, Robin DA, Smith WA, Sato Y (2000) Personality change disorder in children and adolescents following traumatic brain injury. *J Int Neuropsychol Soc* 6: 279–289.

Max JE, Robertson AM, Lansing AE (2001) The phenomenology of personality change due to traumatic brain injury in children and adolescents. *J Neuropsychiatry Clin Neurosci* 13(2): 161–170.

Max JE, Levin HS, Landis J, Schachar R, Saunders A, Ewing-Cobbs L, Chapman S, Dennis M (2005) Predictors of personality change due to traumatic brain injury in children and adolescents in the first six months after injury. *J Am Acad Child Adolesc Psychiatry* 44(5): 434–442.

Multi-Health Systems Inc (MHS) (2006) Catalogue. Toronto: MHS, pp 184–185.

Persel CS, Persel CH (1995) The use of applied behavior analysis in traumatic brain injury rehabilitation. In: Ashley MJ, Krych DK (eds) *Traumatic Brain Injury Rehabilitation.* New York: CRC Press, pp. 231–273.

Polissar N, Fay G, Jaffe K, Liao S, Martin K, Shurtleff H, Rivara J, Winn H (1994) Mild pediatric traumatic brain injury: adjusting significance levels for multiple comparisons. *Brain Injury* 8: 249–264.

Ponsford J, Wilmott C, Rothwell A, Cameron P, Kelly A, Ayton G, Curran C, Nelms R (1997) Cognitive and behavioural outcome following mild traumatic brain injury in children. *J Int Neuropsychol Soc* 3: 225.

Reitan RM (1969) *Manual for Administration of Neuropsychological Test Batteries for Adults and Children.* Indianapolis: Author.

Robin DA, Max JE, Stierwalt JAG, Guenzer LC, Lindgren SD (1999) Sustained attention in children and adolescents with traumatic brain injury. *Aphasiology* 13: 701–708.

Rutter M, Chadwick O, Shaffer D (1983) Head injury. In: Rutter M (ed) *Developmental Neuropsychiatry.* New York: Guilford Press, pp 83–111.

Sattler JM (2001) *Assessment of Children: Cognitive Applications, 4th edn.* San Diego: Jerome M Sattler.

Sbordone RJ (1990) Cognitive rehabilitation of the traumatic brain injured patient in the year 2000. *Psychother Priv Pract* 8(2):129–138.

Sellars CW, Vegter CH (1993) *Pediatric Brain Injury.* Tucson, AZ: Communication Skill Builders.

Slater EJ (1989) Does mild mean minor? Recovery after closed head injury. *J Adolesc Health Care* 10(3): 237–240.

Sohlberg MM, Mateer CA (2001) Children with acquired cognitive impairments. In: Sohlberg MM, Mateer CA (eds) *Cognitive Rehabilitation: An Integrative Neuropsychological Approach.* New York: Guilford Press, pp 429–452.

Stern Y (2002) What is cognitive reserve? Theory and research application of the reserve concept. *J Int Neuropsychol Soc* 8: 448–460.

Stuebing KK, Fletcher JM, LeDoux JM (2002) Validity of IQ-discrepancy classifications of reading disabilities: a meta-analysis. *Am Educ Res J* 39(2): 469–518.

Stuss DT, Benson FD (1986) *The Frontal Lobes.* New York: Raven Press.

Taylor HG (2004) Research on outcomes of pediatric traumatic brain injury: current advances and future directions. *Dev Neuropsychol* 25(1&2): 199–225.

Taylor HG, Alden J (1997) Age-related differences in outcomes following childhood brain insults: an introduction and overview. *J Int Neuropsychol Soc* 3: 555–567.

Taylor HG, Yeates KO, Wade SL, Drotar D, Stancin T, Burant C (2001) Bidirectional child–family influences on outcomes of traumatic brain injury in children. *J Int Neuropsychol Soc* 7: 755–767.

Teuber HL (1962) Behaviour after cerebral lesions in children. *Dev Med Child Neurol* 4: 3–20.

Timmermans SR, Christensen B (1991) The measurement of attention deficits in TBI children and adolescents. *Cogn Rehabil* 9: 26–31.

Wassenberg R, Max JE, Koele SL, Firme K (2004) Classifying psychiatric disorders after traumatic brain injury in children: adequacy of K-SADS versus CBCL. *Brain Injury* 18(4): 377–390.

Wechsler D (2003) *Wechsler Intelligence Scale for Children, 4th edn (WISC-IV)*. San Antonio, TX: The Psychological Corporation.

Wilson BA (2003) *Neuropsychological Rehabilitation: Theory and Practice*. Lisse: Swets & Zeitlinger.

Wilson BA, Herbert CM, Shiel A (2003) *Behavioural Approaches in Neuropsychological Rehabilitation: Optimising Rehabilitation Procedures*. New York: Psychology Press.

Wrightson P, McGinn V, Gronwall D (1995) Mild head injury in preschool children: evidence that it can be associated with persisting cognitive defect. *J Neurol Neurosurg Psychiatry* 59: 375–380.

Yeates KO (2000) Closed head injury. In: Yeates KO, Ris MD, Taylor HG (eds) *Pediatric Neuropsychology: Research, Theory, and Practice*. New York: Guilford Press.

Yeates KO, Taylor HG (2005) Neurobehavioral outcomes of mild head injury in children and adolescents. *Pediatr Rehabil* 8(1): 5–16.

Yeates KO, Enrile B, Loss N, Blumenstein E, Delis D (1995) Verbal learning and memory in children with myelomeningocele. *J Pediatr Psychol* 20: 801–815.

Yeates KO, Taylor HG, Drotar D, Wade SL, Klein S, Stancin T, Schatschneider C (1997) Preinjury family environment as a determinant of recovery from traumatic brain injuries in school-age children. *J Int Neuropsychol Soc* 3: 617–630.

Yeates KO, Swift E, Taylor HG, Wade SL, Drotar D, Stancin T, Minich N (2004) Short- and long-term social outcomes following pediatric traumatic brain injury. *J Int Neuropsychol Soc* 10: 412–426.

Ylvisaker M, Feeney T (1998) *An Integrated Approach to Brain Injury Rehabilitation: Positive Everyday Routines*. San Diego: Singular Publishers.

Ylvisaker M, Adelson D, Willandino B, Burnett SM, Glang A, Feeney T, Moore W, Rumney P, Todis B (2005) Rehabilitation and ongoing support after pediatric TBI: twenty years of progress. *J Head Trauma Rehabil* 20(1): 95–109.

Yorkston KM, Jaffe KM, Polissar NL, Liao S, Fay G (1997) Written language production and neuropsychological function in children with traumatic brain injury. *Arch Phys Med Rehabil* 78: 1096–1102.

10

COMMUNICATION REHABILITATION

Kim Bradley and Maya Kishida Rattray

INTRODUCTION

The purpose of this chapter is to define and catalogue an approach to the acute rehabilitation of communication in children with traumatic brain injury. An attempt has been made to reflect specialist research, the realities of clinical practice in a socialized medicine context, and the conceptual and theoretical underpinnings that define both the scope and the manner of the speech and language rehabilitation of children with acquired brain injury.

No attempt has been made to give a comprehensive survey of the theories and controversies that define the research questions as they are unfolding today. For 20 years research questions have been asked and answered that have assisted in understanding the anatomical and cognitive processing theories that underlie normal cognitive behaviour and the consistent and inconsistent changes that occur with an acquired brain injury. The reference list is not exhaustive but includes readings that have in some way informed clinical practice.

As recently as February 2005 Ronald Ruff commented when looking at the remediation of mild head injury that:

> it is essential that a range of treatment modalities be developed. There exist an abundance of reasonable techniques, but the science in support of their efficacy . . . is in its infancy. In contrast to the emphasis on diagnosis we are a very long way away from achieving a balance between diagnosis and treatment.
>
> (Ruff 2005: 16)

Research that clearly demonstrates the efficacy of much of the treatment discussed in these pages is not available. Often the treatment that is described is a logical extension of diagnostic research: an attempt to put into practice the one or two paragraphs at the end of a research article that address how the findings contained in the preceding lengthy discussion should inform rehabilitation practices. This chapter is a discussion of some of the 'reasonable techniques' that research, logic, intuition, and clinical experience have developed to treat the communication problems of children following an acquired brain injury.

Chapman et al. (1997) found that one-third of children with moderate to severe traumatic brain injury (TBI) exhibited language problems measurable by traditional developmental language testing. They further assert that a majority of children who sustain a severe brain injury show some form of communication difficulty, with a highly variable outcome. Pediatric inpatient rehabilitation by its very nature attracts the more severely head-injured and thus language difficulties that can be demonstrated with standardized language testing are the norm.

Several distinctions underlie assessment and therapeutic intervention with children with an acquired brain injury:

- a language disorder that is acquired versus a developmental language disorder
- a primary language disorder versus a cognitive communication disorder
- impairment-based versus functional therapy
- a developing language system versus an established language system

These distinctions are discussed below. The continuum of treatment in an acute rehabilitation centre is then described, followed by a short discussion of spontaneous recovery. The second part of the chapter looks at the presentation of communication problems in children who have suffered an acquired brain injury (ABI), most often a traumatic brain injury (TBI). Narrative discourse, word-finding, auditory processing, pragmatics and higher-level language are each discussed under the headings of presentation, assessment and therapy. Finally, two concluding sections look at communication and the preschool child with an ABI, and motor speech disorders in children following an ABI.

ACQUIRED LANGUAGE DISORDER AND DEVELOPMENTAL LANGUAGE DISORDER

Developmental language disorder or specific language impairment are terms used when a child does not acquire language in a manner and at a rate similar to their peers in the absence of hearing loss or emotional, environmental or intellectual disorder. Remediation of developmental language disorders is the focus of preschool language intervention programs and school-based speech language pathology services. An acquired language problem occurs as a result of accident or disease, when an acute event impacts the brain and changes previous language functioning or alters the developmental course of language acquisition. It is obvious that such events may occur to a person with or without previously existing language, learning and behavioural difficulties. After a head injury it is necessary to attempt to separate the effects of the acquired language problem, which are often remediable and changing in the short term, from pre-existing normal or abnormal language development, second language acquisition, and learning difficulties.

Developmental or specific language impairment affects phonology, syntax and morphology. Children with traumatic brain injury are often largely intact in these areas despite significant difficulties using language to communicate.

Primary Language and Cognitive Communication

The need for rehabilitation of communication occurs as a result of a wide range of aetiologies of brain injury. Lees in 1993 attempted to classify 34 children with acquired language disorder using Goodglass and Kaplan's (1972) traditional adult aphasia classification. Fifty-three per cent of children could not be classified. Almost half of the children who did not fit into aphasia classifications (8 of the 17) had closed head injuries. Closed head injury, then, can be consistently differentiated from aphasia. Aphasia is characterized by difficulty in the use of language, both receptive and/or expressive, whether by listening, reading, writing, speaking or gesturing, and this dysfunction is disproportional to dysfunction in other cognitive areas. It is commonly as a result of a focal lesion to language centres in the brain, as might happen with a stroke. Partial impairment may be referred to as dysphasia (Darley 1982).

Remediation of a focal lesion in the language centres of the brain has a different focus from remediation of the more usually diffuse injuries of a traumatic closed head injury. Clinical observation suggests that a child with a focal lesion, for example in Broca's area, after about the age of 8 shows clearly the agrammatism, word-finding and mild language processing difficulties and the intact social environmental astuteness of the similarly affected adult. In contrast, a child with a traumatic brain injury may have age-appropriate pre-existing grammatical skills but socially inappropriate behaviour, attention or organization issues that limit their ability to give a clear and understandable, age-appropriate, verbal description. Difficulties with expressive language are common to both but the nature of the difficulties is very different and, predictably, so are the resulting goals of therapy. The child with aphasia may be working on recognizing and choosing an appropriate pronoun; the child with TBI on how to use a rubric/graphic organizer to help them organize their explanations.

A child with TBI may also present with specific primary language deficits depending upon the site, nature and severity of the injury to the brain. Hartley and Levin (1990) note that the incidence of aphasia following TBI is consistently reported at 2 to 4 %. Admissions to rehabilitation centres, which by definition suggest a more severe injury, generate an incidence closer to 30% (Schwartz-Cowley and Stepanik 1969, Sarno et al. 1986). However, unless another disease function is occurring simultaneously, a child with aphasia as a result of stroke usually does not present with the other cognitive overlays that are so prevalent in traumatic brain injury.

The distinction is made between primary language difficulties and the impact of other cognitive processes, such as executive functions, attention, impulsivity or memory, on a child's ability to follow directions or to explain their thoughts and ideas. Understanding why a task is difficult for a child necessitates identifying the demands of the task and generating and testing hypotheses about why the child completed the task as they did. Fig. 10.1 conceptualizes this process.

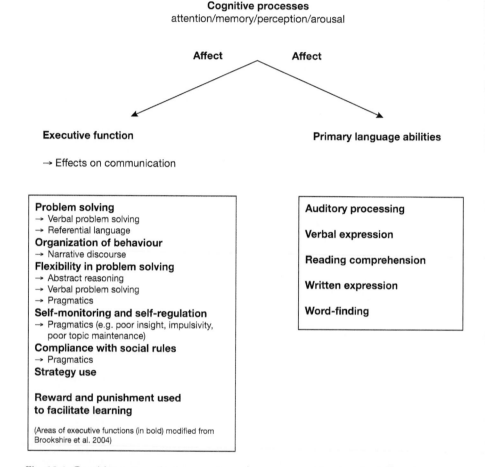

Fig. 10.1. Cognitive communication vs. primary language: cognitive domains influencing communication following ABI.

It is acknowledged that Fig. 10.1 is a simplistic view of the complex relationship between language and cognition. It is, however, a useful conceptualization of the assessment process and the cataloguing of the resources available to a child to counteract an identified deficit. How cognitive deficits are expressed in language and how a language disorder may present as behavioural or cognitive sequelae has to be clearly demarcated. It is only when the relative contributions of each are understood that a strategy for rehabilitation or compensation can be effectively generated. At times, these distinctions are obvious; at other times the separation of effects is difficult. For example, Turkstra and Holland (1998) adapted a syntax comprehension task so that it had a reduced load on working memory and storage, and adolescents with TBI did significantly better on the task. Control participants did not vary across the two tasks. The original comprehension task on its own might have yielded erroneous conclusions about the extent of the child's difficulty in understanding grammar. The improved performance yields both impairment level information about the child's memory and language processing abilities and strategies for improving comprehension in a functional setting.

IMPAIRMENT AND FUNCTIONAL THERAPY

Much of the approach towards pediatric cognitive communication rehabilitation in the last two decades has been influenced by the seminal work of Mark Ylvisaker (1985, 1993, 1998). One of the premises of his work is that a skill must be remediated in the context in which it will be used or generalization of that skill will not happen: cognitive skills are domain-specific. Ylvisakar's work challenges a style of speech therapy in which workbook-based drill work happens once a week, behind closed doors, and then the skills are expected to surface when needed in real life situations. His approach to therapy is from an information-processing model, which sees cognitive functioning as a functional integrative performance of a cognitive task, which in itself is made up of component processes and systems. His emphasis on the integrated nature of cognitive behaviour, and thus communication, led to the 'functional' emphasis of his therapy.

The focus of the Ylvisaker style of therapy is at the level of 'Activities and Participation' according to the World Health Organization's (WHO) 2001 International Classification of Functioning, Disability and Health (ICF). 'Activities' are the execution of a task or action by an individual, and 'participation' the individual's involvement in life. By focusing ABI intervention in functional situations, on activities and participation, solutions and compensatory strategies emerge in the environment in which they need to be used. This ultimately will lead to the most effective uptake and success of compensatory strategies.

'Impairments', conceived by WHO (2001) as problems in body function and structures (including psychological function), require remediation at the level of specifically affected components of cognitive or language behaviour. The evidence for the efficacy of this type of intervention comes largely from the traditional adult aphasia literature where remediation of specific aspects of linguistic functioning, both receptive and expressive, has been shown to be effective by various programs and techniques (for a summary see Cicerone et al. 2000). Similarly, therapy for developmental language problems is also largely impairment-based: the specific language structures that a child has and has not acquired are catalogued, and then remediation of those components is attempted. The generalization of these tasks into real world situations is presumed – once a concept is understood, the child starts to use it, as the situation requires. It is noted that both developmental language intervention through programs such as the Hanen Program (Watson 1995) which emphasize the communication relationships of the child, and aphasia therapy in the guise of 'supported conversation' styles of intervention (Kagan et al. 2001), have also moved towards therapy based at an activity or participation level. However, these therapies are also most often used in combination with traditional impairment level interventions as needed.

As was noted above, cognitive communication impairment is neither a developmental language nor a primary language impairment and thus remediation at the impairment level for cognitive communication deficits is less theoretically clear and certainly has a weaker published efficacy. With a child in the acute stage of rehabilitation following a brain injury, there is good justification for both impairment and functional/participation level tasks as the child is changing at both these levels. A clear picture of the component and process level of cognitive functioning is necessary to monitor or facilitate improving performance at the skill level. Strategies also need to be developed to circumvent or support difficult tasks. The continuum of treatment starts initially with more impairment-based diagnostic and therapeutic activities. What makes a task difficult is identified, practised and supported in component parts, building towards a more successful, integrated whole. At discharge this has evolved into functionally driven therapy, where knowledge of specific impairment drives environmentally based adaptive strategies and problem solving.

Therapy with children with an acute acquired brain injury and measurable language impact is most effective when it is both impairment-based in the history of traditional adult aphasia therapy and functional activity-based in the Ylvisaker mode. Children are admitted to acute rehabilitation typically one to six weeks post-traumatic event. This is the time of most significant spontaneous recovery and the time of maximum impairment. They will continue to change in terms of basic measurable abilities throughout the time they are in remediation. Specific cognitive and language skills need to function in the context of a child relearning to participate and function in an altered world. What that world will look like – what constellation of abilities and challenges the child will move back with into family, school and community – is still emerging.

The reality of intensive therapeutic intervention and emerging medical stability following a life-altering acquired brain injury often necessitates an inpatient hospital stay. Minimizing that stay by maximizing recovery and adaptation is the goal of rehabilitation. Ideally, all of that rehabilitation would take place in the environment in which the skills are eventually to be used. Barring that, intensive rehabilitation in an environment that is aware of its limitations is the next best alternative.

CONTINUUM OF INPATIENT MANAGEMENT

During acute rehabilitation initial baseline testing requires about 40 minutes spread across several sessions while talking with and getting to know the child. Isaki and Turkstra (2000) note that an aphasia test and auditory processing, speaking under pressure, discourse and verbal reasoning tasks were able to correctly classify 85% of

25 TBI adults as employed or unemployed. Impairment level tasks were able to provide functional and practical information. A similar array of baseline tasks sensitive to communication disability following TBI is used with children, including a test of vocabulary (which is often largely intact but is a positive starting point), a standardized test of auditory comprehension, and a replicable sample of discourse and problem-solving tasks to provide information for therapy. This is specifically discussed under the assessment headings in the communication topics below. Diagnostic language assessment batteries are not appropriate at the early stages of recovery.

Goals are set using Goal Attainment Scaling (e.g. Maloney et al. 1978, Joyce et al. 1994) and diagnostic therapy continues to explore the full picture of the child's functioning, with other children in the classroom, in group work, with their parents and siblings, and during recreation. Liaison with the child's classroom, parents and other therapists is facilitated by the inpatient/day-patient nature of the rehabilitation. Strategies to facilitate the child's communication success, such as the child asking for clarification or repetition, are practised individually and then cued for as needed in the environment. The actual words or action used to cue are shared among the adults dealing with the child so that the child's functioning is both facilitated and challenged to improve.

A battery of standardized tests (four to five hours of testing) is completed when the child's performance has stabilized, as close to discharge as possible, to facilitate the best and most accurate information for transition to school and to the community. This testing is used to advocate for community resources and to set a standard against which subsequent language functioning can be judged. Does the child continue to make the same developmental gains as their peers? Does their performance fall away from that of their peers over time? Does the child continue to narrow the gap between their own and the optimal age-appropriate function? For example, Jordan and Murdoch (1990) tested 8- to 17-year-olds at 12 months post-severe closed head injury with a standardized battery and showed they had significantly lower overall language performance. At 24 months post-injury, the children showed an improvement but still had a significantly lower performance than age-matched peers. That language batteries do not always reveal the communication challenges of children with mild to moderate TBI is well known. These tests were designed for children with developmental language disorders and therefore provide limited information if reported as standard scores on their own. Patterns of strengths and weaknesses, and additional cognitive information, as well as specific task analysis of why a child was or was not able to perform a task, are needed to make the test information valid and useful (Turkstra 1999).

The most usual exception to this continuum of management is in the case of a child who is to receive radiation therapy following surgery for a brain tumour, where standardized testing is completed as close to admission as possible so that potential deterioration as a result of radiation can be adequately monitored (e.g. Spiegler et al. 2004). The other exception is in the case of short admissions (up to six weeks) for mild head injuries, for assessment and recommendations only. Again, a full standardized and non-standardized language battery is completed immediately.

SPONTANEOUS RECOVERY

Would children recover to the same level without intervention? Certainly individualized Goal Attainment Scaling shows that most children have better communication skills, measured by improvement on their specific goals, when they leave the rehabilitation centre than when they were admitted. The question is whether this improvement is as a result of the intervention provided.

At the level of activity and participation the answer to that question is easy: adaptive strategies, graphic organizers, rubrics and cueing strategies are tools that would not have been available to the child had they not been designed and practised with him or her. However, at the impairment level, separating out spontaneous recovery from the effects of therapy is a more vexed question.

There is research on some impairment level therapy techniques. For example, Constantinidou et al. (2005) demonstrated that work with repetitive hierarchic categorization tasks improved performance and generalized to a functional decision-making task. The researchers interpreted this result as support for specific cognitive rehabilitation of moderate and severe TBI. Wiseman-Hakes et al. (1998) established the efficacy of specific pragmatic intervention techniques. There are other such impairment level studies but, as noted above, research on efficacy needs to be expanded across the multiplicity of rehabilitation tasks used with children with TBI.

Snow et al. (1998) assessed 26 severely impaired adults with TBI at three to six months and two years post-injury. Conversation abilities did not improve or became worse over time, except in a subgroup of eight who did improve. These eight were characterized by greater initial severity of symptoms and therefore longer speech language pathology involvement.

The Brain Injury Special Interest Group of the American Congress of Rehabilitation published the results of their evidence-based review of cognitive rehabilitation in 2000 (Cicerone et al. 2000). A 'practice standard' was set for an area if there was evidence of well-developed prospective randomized trials (Class I evidence), or overwhelming Class II evidence such as cohort studies, retrospective non-randomized clinical series, or case studies with well-designed controls. The following was recommended:

Cognitive-Linguistic Remediation
A. Practice Standards
1. Cognitive linguistic remediation is recommended for treatment of language deficits secondary to left hemisphere stroke during both the acute and post acute periods of rehabilitation.

2. Specific interventions for functional communication deficits, including pragmatic conversational skills, are recommended for persons with TBI.

B. Practice Guidelines
1. Cognitive remediation for specific areas of language impairment such as reading comprehension and language formulation is recommended after left hemisphere stroke and TBI.

(Malec 2001: 15)

Thus, speech language pathology intervention is generally endorsed because evidence is being amassed about efficacy of specific intervention techniques. However, there is a wide array of intervention strategies and facets of disability following a brain injury that still needs to be addressed, and efficacy for specific methodologies continues to need to be established and replicated.

COMMUNICATION PROFILE IN CHILDREN FOLLOWING TBI
Discourse
Presentation
It is a common observation that children usually generate grammatically and semantically correct sentences following a brain injury (Jordan et al. 1992, Chapman et al. 1997). Difficulties with language formulation emerge when ideas that are more complex need to be expressed coherently and efficiently in words. Impairment in discourse has been noted even in patients who perform normally on a standardized language battery (Groher 1977, Milton et al. 1984).

Difficulties with narrative speech following TBI do not reflect specific syntactic or morphologic challenges unless there is a more focal Broca's type lesion and then agrammatism similar to that seen in an adult emerges. Clinical observation suggests that agrammatism from a focal lesion in young children will reveal itself in the structures of grammar that the child has already acquired. Therapy needs to address both the specific deficits noted in the child's grammar and also the continued acquisition of developmentally appropriate grammar. Errors of grammar with the more diffuse TBI injuries generally occur during complicated explanations: pronoun referents or verb tenses become confused, not because the child cannot understand and use the grammar correctly, but because slow processing and organization issues confuse the idea that is being expressed and the language reflects this. However, as with the child with a focal lesion, in the child with more diffuse brain injury the acquisition of new and more complicated grammar appropriate to ongoing development will also need to be specifically addressed. While the child may have passively acquired language in a developmentally appropriate time frame previously, the impact of brain injury on cognitive functions means that continued development cannot be taken for granted.

That narrative speech is disorganized and impaired following a traumatic brain injury has been amply identified in both children and adults. Hartley and Jensen (1991) found that productivity was impaired on both procedural (giving directions) and narrative (telling a story) tasks, although narrative tasks were more compromised. Liles et al. (1989) found that story retelling tasks were incomplete, with fewer and less complex cohesive ties than occurred with typical speakers, as well as significantly fewer episodes from the original story. Mentis and Prutting (1987) found that story generation tasks were even more compromised than story retelling tasks. Chapman et al. (1997) made several observations about narration following TBI: narrative discourse was found to be more impaired than conversation; stories were fragmented and more difficult to follow; the organization of the narrative of children with TBI was as poor as that of children with specific language impairment despite the absence of the syntactic and morphologic impairments associated with the developmental language disorders. Ehrlich (1988) noted that adults with head injury gave lengthier explanations and were slower to generate information: it required more words and time to make the same point. Chapman et al. (1999) summarize the main difficulties that children with brain injury have with discourse as:

1   Retaining the most important information
2   Producing organized discourse
3   Making inferences and realizing meaning relations between adjacent ideas
4   Paraphrasing information contained in texts
5   Condensing and transforming the textual information in synthesized generalized statements

Different discourse tasks place different linguistic and cognitive demands on a child. The tasks used in the above studies varied considerably, as did the age, aetiology, severity of injury and time post-onset of the subjects. Hence, seemingly contra-dictory results, such as finding that individuals with TBI produce less information than controls (Liles et al. 1989) and more information than controls (Ehrlich 1988), are not inconsistent. A child who has not processed the information on a story retelling task will produce an impoverished version. A child who is disorganized and tangential will easily take more words than their peers to give a complete explanation. The literature is useful as an indicator of where to look for difficulties with higher-level expressive language in a child, but the pattern of difficulties is not consistent or predictable for a given child.

With traumatic brain injury, more difficult, higher-level tasks are more vulner-able to damage. For example, word-finding difficulties may be apparent in generative description or story telling which are not evident in conversation naming or sentence generation. Table 10.1 presents Chapman et al.'s (1999) analysis of the impact of executive function disturbance on discourse abilities, which is also part of the assessment schema of Fig. 10.1.

TABLE 10.1
Impact of cognitive disturbances of executive functions on discourse abilities

Impaired executive functions	Resulting discourse behaviours
Impaired global semantic representation	Unable to grasp the central meaning of discourse; or hold it in memory to use later for social or learning purposes
Unable to utilize organized memory systems	Impairment in episodic structure resulting in disorganization of information related to everyday happenings
Poor capacity for planning	Difficulty unfolding discourse coherently
Limited flexibility in problem solving	Difficulty conceiving of alternative interpretations, narrow or rigid interpretations of text, fluency of ideas reduced
Poor inhibitory control	Stream of consciousness in discourse producing intrusions of tangentially related information, unable to inhibit ideas that come to mind during talk or learning

Source: Chapman et al. 1999.

Assessment

As with the assessment of auditory comprehension, discussed below, the assessment of narration involves looking at the requirements of the task and the supports the child needs or uses to accomplish the task successfully. Therapy focuses on helping the child to recognize and use the compensations that are effective.

Assessment of narrative speech for research purposes is very different from narrative assessment in a therapeutic setting. Tasks used in clinical assessment must be replicable, quick to administer and easy to analyse. Often one of the best measures of a child's recovery is a comparison of expressive language generated on comparable tasks at successive points in time. Standardized narrative tasks that can be efficiently analysed in a clinical setting are not generally available, and therefore most tasks used are non-standardized.

A language sample of narrative tasks identified in the literature as sensitive to the discourse difficulties of ABI is collected. Tasks have progressively less inherent structure, with varying amounts of visual or auditory support. Thus, the first task is a story retelling task with pictures to help in the recall (e.g. 'The Bus Story Test': Renfrew 2001). Then there is a story retelling task without pictures. From the same story, the child is also required to condense the information into a central statement. Then there is a story generation task with sequenced pictures but no auditory model.

The next task is a picture description task with no auditory model (e.g. Boston Diagnostic Aphasia Exam, Cookie Theft picture). This is followed by a procedural discourse task (e.g. 'Tell me how to make a peanut butter sandwich') conceived within this framework as a generative task without an auditory or visual structure provided but with structure inherent in the task. The final tasks are a story generation task, a verbal problem-solving task, and an expressing opinion task with a verbal flexibility component where the opposite opinion must then be defended. These tasks have no inherent or provided structure.

Analysis of the speech sample identifies what level of support is needed for the child to produce a complete and meaningful piece of discourse. Does the child need external visual and/or auditory structures (i.e. pictures as well as having heard the story already) for their explanations to make sense, or is it only when they have to express an opinion, which they may be just forming, that coherence becomes a factor for their listener? If word-finding is a difficulty, with which task is this apparent? Are there grammatical errors? On which tasks? Is there a paucity of information or is there a lot of disorganized information? Is tangential information included? Does the child include the moral for the story they heard or the bare facts of the story? How fluent is the production? How complex is the syntax? Is story grammar apparent? Are the various components of the explanation linked to each other through devices such as conjunctions and personal pronouns?

Clinical experience is that an entire series of narrative tasks can be completed in about 15 minutes by children down to about the age of 6 years. Each task has a younger age task – 6 to about 9 years– and then another task suitable for an older child. The language sample is then transcribed and analysed. The same sample is repeated at a time closer to discharge. The tool gains power with repeated use as progression in abilities can be charted.

Therapy
Therapy for language formulation tasks consists of identifying situations, such as playing a game or discussing an episode of a TV program, where a coherent explanation might be needed. Rubrics of how to construct a complete and coherent explanation are developed and practised with the child, with particular attention to difficulties exposed by the speech sample described above. Analysis of previously tape-recorded exercises is one of the most powerful techniques for using an organizing rubric. When a child cannot later understand their own explanation and then hears the difference the rubric makes, further convincing of the necessity for structure is not needed. A rubric for a younger child may be as simple as including specific information about 'who' and 'what' is being talked about. With the older child, it usually involves the organization of information with planning, monitoring and revising of content. With sufficient cued practice, the structure can become internalized.

It is noted that discourse has been discussed in the context of an expressive language task although aspects of narration specifically rely on the ability to process information at a similarly complex level before it can be generated. If a child cannot paraphrase and condense information then they cannot hope to produce an effective, simple explanation. Some of these tasks require discourse processing at a global level, requiring the child to condense and transform information to produce summary statements and interpretations.

Discourse is not simply an expressive language task but a communication skill directly reliant upon executive function, cognitive processes such as attention and memory, and both receptive and expressive language abilities. Remediation of discourse is discussed again briefly in the section on higher-level language and cognitive communication below.

While oral discourse has been well studied in both children and adults, written discourse has not been as well analysed. Yorkston et al. (1997) found written language to be even more susceptible to the effects of a TBI than oral language. As with verbal expression, attention and organization issues most significantly affected performance. Children with severe TBI produced fewer sentences and generated less information than children without TBI. They also had significantly more capitalization, spelling and punctuation errors (Chapman and Lawyer 1997).

Language formulation difficulties following ABI occur in both oral and written modalities.

WORD-FINDING

Presentation

Word-retrieval or word-finding difficulty occurs when a person experiences difficulty retrieving a word despite his/her knowledge and comprehension of the word ('tip of the tongue' phenomenon).

Word-finding difficulties are noted with various types of brain injury, including left hemisphere stroke, hydrocephalus and TBI (Dennis 1992). The frequency of word-retrieval difficulties may be attributed to the widespread networks in the brain that underlie word meaning. Words are accessed by other words associated by, for example, definition, category, visual images and sound similarities. Damage to various parts of the brain interrupts these neural connections, interfering with the efficiency of word retrieval. Word-retrieval difficulties can also be attributed to poor organization of vocabulary, poor attention, lack of initiation, poor monitoring, or lack of compensatory strategies (Ylvisaker et al. 1998b).

Characteristics of word-finding difficulties in children include: (1) overuse of vague and non-specific words in conversation (e.g. 'thing', 'there', 'stuff'); (2) verbosity (i.e. using too many words to express ideas); (3) overuse of filler words (e.g. 'um . . .' and 'you know'); (4) hesitation and/or increased response time; (5) substitution of related words (e.g. 'cup' for 'glass'); (6) signs of word-searching behaviours (e.g. looking away, closing eyes to concentrate); (7) overuse of routine phrases (e.g. 'I'm gonna . . .'); (8) reduced content words (e.g. 'Get the thing from her'); and (9) circumlocution (i.e. talking around a topic).

Assessment

Word-finding difficulties have been found to be more readily apparent in timed tasks and/or in the context of discourse (Dennis 1992). Assessment therefore needs to be conducted systematically in various linguistic contexts, starting at the word level (e.g. confrontation naming) and advancing toward the level of narrative discourse. Linguistic and cognitive demands within a task need to be structured in order to determine the point of breakdown. When a child fails to name an object during a confrontation naming task, a speech language pathologist may provide a phonemic cue (first sound), a semantic cue (function and meaning), or sentence completion cue to evaluate if a child is then able to retrieve the intended word. If the child successfully retrieves the word with cueing, the difficulties are related to word-finding. In contrast, the inability to name an object in the presence of such cueing may simply suggest poor expressive vocabulary.

In addition to evaluating the word-finding difficulties in various linguistic contexts, it is important to evaluate them with imposed stress, fatigue, and time constraints, as these factors may exacerbate the problem. For example, classroom presentation and timed tests may impose a greater burden on a child with word-retrieval difficulties (Ylvisaker et al. 1998b).

Therapy

Word-finding difficulties are treated with a combination of skill building, compensation techniques and environmental modifications. To maximize generalization the intervention needs to be incorporated into practical and relevant activities such as preparing and rehearsing for a presentation while applying strategies.

Skill-building approach

In order to achieve optimal efficiency of word retrieval, words need to be organized with other words, concepts and images to establish effective storage and retrieval. Tools such as semantic webbing, concept exploration and visual organizers assist with organized word storage and retrieval. The goals of intervention in this approach are: (1) to establish a connected semantic knowledge base; (2) to build organized networks of concepts; and (3) to assist with deliberate use of such organization in moments of word-retrieval difficulty (Ylvisaker et al. 1998b).

Compensation approach

Based on the pattern analysis from the assessment, a speech language pathologist determines effective cueing strategies for the child. For example, if the child demonstrates the most successful word retrieval with phonetic cueing, the intervention focuses on establishing this strategy use. The ultimate goal is to help the child gain internal control of the most effective type of cueing to use as a self-cueing strategy. This may involve steps such as: (1) a speech language pathologist initially providing the phonetic cue; (2) the child using an alphabet board to cue him/herself; and (3) eventually the child mentally scanning the alphabet to cue him/herself for the intended word during conversation.

The child is encouraged to seek assistance and/or to provide specific attributes and descriptors for the intended word so that his/her communication partner can help figure out the intended word. A child may be explicitly taught phrases such as 'I am thinking' and 'I don't know what it's called' to welcome others to help before the child becomes frustrated. Use of gestures and pointing is also encouraged as a compensatory strategy to minimize frustration.

In addition, establishing an increased awareness of word-retrieval difficulties is addressed by encouraging the child to monitor and track incidences of vague word use and occasions of frustration, groping and self-correction. The child is also encouraged to pay attention to when others ask for clarifications. The child needs to become aware of when to use the strategies.

Environmental modifications and caregiver training

It is crucial to minimize the child's level of frustration as much as possible, hence environmental modifications and caregiver training for facilitating word retrieval are essential. Word-retrieval facilitation strategies include: (1) asking specific questions; (2) encouraging the child to show what he/she means; (c) encouraging the child to describe the association of words; and (d) encouraging the child to use cueing strategies that have been practised.

AUDITORY COMPREHENSION

Presentation

The ability to understand oral language, to comply with directions, understand stories or follow a conversation, is called auditory comprehension or auditory processing. Most children with a moderate to severe brain injury display difficulty with auditory processing, at least initially. After an ABI, progression through the Rancho Scale of cognitive levels includes the ability to respond promptly and appropriately to spoken language either by following a command or by responding to a question. Difficulties with comprehension of longer oral material have been shown to continue in the long term with even mild and moderate ABI (Brookshire et al. 2004).

Assessment

The speech language pathologist needs to analyse the child's understanding of and response to spoken language and establish the nature of any difficulty. There can be several reasons why a child does not appear to understand what is being said to them.

Fig. 10.1 (see p. 156) notes the impact of various cognitive functions on language. If a child does not attend to what somebody is saying then the information is not available to be processed. If through auditory perception difficulties the child does not perceive the information properly, then again the degraded signal cannot possibly be correctly interpreted. In both cases, the child may respond incorrectly but the difficulty is not with understanding the vocabulary or grammar of the statement. Similarly, if the information degrades very quickly in the working memory then it is unavailable for processing. In these cases, the child is not able to respond to auditory information but it is not an auditory processing difficulty. To be a true auditory processing difficulty the child must be able to attend to, perceive and retain the information but, when it comes to understanding, not be able to extract the complete meaning from the words. Distinguishing between these factors, all of which may result in an incorrect or incomplete understanding of oral information, is essential to optimizing auditory processing and developing appropriate compensatory strategies for the child.

Baseline testing of auditory comprehension skills is completed one-to-one in a quiet setting with conscious manipulation and observation of the need for redirection, refocusing, eye contact, and verbal cues for the child to attend to. A baseline test that gives a standardized score establishes whether the child comprehends language at an age-appropriate level. This is a short task completed in less than 15 minutes. Other auditory comprehension tasks may be used in a non-standardized way or in less optimal conditions to collect more information on the child's processing abilities.

A test such as the Revised Token Test/Token Test for Children (McNeil and Prescott 1978), originally developed to assess auditory comprehension in adult aphasia, generates very useful information that can be manipulated in therapy. Sarno et al. (1986) noted that 32% of adults with ABI had difficulty with the Token Test initially, with 25% continuing to have difficulty at six months. Because the test involves following directions with big/little squares/circles in five colours, vocabulary is limited and again a more controlled analysis of processing can occur. How much is too much information? A yellow square? A small yellow square? A yellow square and a red circle? A small yellow square and a big red circle? If it is known precisely when the information becomes too difficult then it is possible to direct activities in therapy at the point where comprehension is breaking down.

In addition, non-standardized interpretation of this quick task provides a wealth of other information. Does the child make most of their errors on the first part of the task or the second? Generally, a clear pattern emerges for each individual, of either understanding the initial information and then becoming overwhelmed, or of forgetting all of the early information and hearing only the most recent information.

If an adolescent understands this about him/herself, it allows for very specifically directed requests for repetition and knowledge of what it is they are likely to have missed. For the parent of the younger child this also provides valuable coping strategies as they too will become aware of when the child is most likely to be having difficulty. Also, how a child uses repetition will emerge during this task: does the child ask the speaker for repetition spontaneously? Does the child spontaneously rehearse the information while completing the task? Does, or can, the child repeat directions verbatim? Does the child spontaneously use strategies such as grabbing a token as soon as they hear it so they can move on to the next and keep up with the listener? What coping strategies the child has developed already and what other ones would appear to help them will all start to emerge during this short but very controlled task. When a child's coping mechanisms, or lack thereof, become apparent, then observation of the child within the classroom, playroom or with their family allows the therapist to see how both the difficulty and the strategies play out functionally.

The same analysis of how a child is coping with auditory information is carried over to looking at how a child is able to follow a short story or paragraph of information. The distinction between the two tasks is an important one. It is generally easier to process information if it is about a topic of which a child has pre-existing knowledge, or to which they are able to apply previously learned information. Thus while only able to process three pieces of unrelated information (i.e. Token Test type task) a child may be able to follow much more information if it fits into an existing schema. Another child may respond to paragraph/related information as if it were unrelated and simply be overwhelmed by the amount of information: the content and story do not help with the processing. This information is useful as a baseline and as part of the total picture of how the child is dealing with auditory information. Thus, response to paragraphs of increasing length is charted. Again, how much information is too much? Does the child retain detail but fail to synthesize what the main idea of the information was? Alternatively can the child identify the point of the information but not generate specific detail? Is the child aware of not processing? Can they identify when the point of too much is reached?

Tasks such as the Token Test or paragraph listening are not functional and are of limited use if they only generate a score of a child's performance in comparison to other children their age. When all of the information available from the performance of these tasks is analysed, it gives a strong direction to the investigation of how much information a child can manage and what strategies make it easier for the child. The practising of these strategies, in all of the contexts in which a child is having difficulty understanding, is the focus of the weeks and months of therapy that follow. The child needs to recognize when they are at a loss and to have internalized strategies of what to do when this happens.

Following acquired brain injury in a child, language processing difficulties are also often apparent with reading comprehension. While reading can compensate somewhat for memory and auditory perception difficulties, if a child is having difficulty extracting meaning from language it is most often apparent in both reading and listening. Because reading develops over years and involves many visual, phonological and cognitive processes, it is particularly vulnerable to the effects of TBI at any time in the process of the child acquiring reading competency. Children who sustain significant brain injury before the age of 8 years have significant reading disorders and those who are injured after this age are much less impaired (Chapman et al. 1999). There is little research as to the effect of ABI on reading abilities; however, clinical observation suggests that if the child demonstrates oral communication difficulties, reading usually requires support to develop appropriately.

Therapy

It is important to recognize that these tasks are used in an acute situation to establish baseline, measure change, and investigate compensatory techniques. Children are not trained to an assessment task: the goal is not to improve on the Token Test. Therapy for the younger child becomes an endless series of listening games which imitate real life . . . which teddy bear goes where in the doll's house, which dog is to be given which bone. The children are playing games but the strategies and demands of the task are controlled, specific and repetitive. Children learn through play and through practising the same base skill in an endless variety of presentations in the real world, at home and in the classroom. Speech and language therapy is a very concentrated and focused version of the same process. It is important that all the adults dealing with a child recognize when the child is having difficulty and use the same language to cue the child on what to do. Thus, generalization becomes less an issue because the understanding of language is approached in the same way in all situations.

Adolescent listening tasks may involve listening to a video of a TV court program where the picture of the judge and the plaintiff on the screen gives very little information as to the nature of the controversy being discussed and it is only by listening to their explanations that the teenager can understand the issue. Similarly, following directions to accomplish an age-appropriate task – origami or making a paper aeroplane, for instance – is a focused listening task which adolescents enjoy. Information is always given to them at the current limit of their ability. Therapy works at the impairment level in terms of the amount of information the child is processing but also practises strategies about what to do when difficulty occurs.

Listening tasks with the adolescent are almost always paired with a task of indicating how confident they are in their replies. The teenager needs to be able to interpret the signals that let them know that all is not well, before they know to use support strategies. Teens often very quickly become able to accurately assess if they followed a direction correctly. It is not unusual for a teen to assert that they are fine and there are no repercussions to an accident while concurrently being able to accurately identify probable errors in following directions. Metacognitive insight appears able to disconnect from specific experiences of difficulty.

At discharge, part of the complete standardized language assessment will be an impairment level evaluation of the child's receptive language in comparison to their peers. While this information is useful for school planning, it is only useful within the context of the interpretation of the demands of the task. The functional implications of the difficulty and the strategies the child either does or could use to overcome auditory processing difficulties must also be assessed and communicated.

HIGHER LEVEL LANGUAGE AND COGNITIVE COMMUNICATION
Presentation
Cognitive communication may be defined as how executive functions impact language and communication (see Fig. 10.1). This includes verbal planning and organization, making inferences, abstract reasoning, and verbal problem solving. Despite many children regaining competence in intelligence and primary language following an ABI (Levin et al. 1982, 1996), executive function deficits persist in problem solving, planning, and response modulation (Levin et al. 2001), as well as in oral and written narrative production (Dennis et al. 1998).

Following ABI, children may interpret proverbs and figurative language literally, presenting as concrete thinkers, lacking cognitive and linguistic flexibility. Difficulty understanding humour and sarcasm is also a result of concrete thinking. The inability to understand or generate alternative points of view may make the child look self-centred, rigid and concrete in their thinking.

Assessment
Informal assessment tasks using real life situations and less structured tasks are needed to assess higher-level language. Traditional assessment often compensates for difficulties with organization, planning, time management, initiation or sequencing because the testing items provided are already sequenced, clinician-driven, and have no time constraints. Thus, standardized language testing may mask the underlying deficits. Tasks such as planning for a picnic or delegating a task to others require the child to demonstrate the ability to attend to details, to plan for specific steps, to predict outcome, to demonstrate flexibility, and to adhere to imposed conditions.

The ability to make inferences, use abstract reasoning, understand humour and irony, predict outcome and identify emotions can be evaluated with the use of everyday materials, such as age-appropriate magazine advertisements and comics. The child's interpretation of what the advertisement is trying to sell, what is clever about it, why a certain image is used, how the person feels, and what could happen next provides insight into the child's cognitive communication/higher-level language skills.

Therapy

Intervention in the area of cognitive communication involves specific skill development as well as development of compensatory strategies. Explicit teaching of the steps of problem solving may include: (1) identifying if there is a problem; (2) stating what the problem is and why; (3) understanding the cause of the problem; (4) generating multiple solutions; (5) choosing the best option and stating why; (6) evaluating outcome and choosing a second option accordingly; and (7) generating prevention. Identifying which of these steps presents difficulty for a child allows focused intervention: one child may not be able to generate any solutions to a problem but may be very good at choosing the best solution when given options; another child may be able to generate solutions and judge them very well once they can clearly state what the problem is.

The speech language pathologist starts by asking a question for each step of solving an everyday problem, usually with written or symbolic support. When this has been modelled and practised, the child is encouraged to state each question and provide answers him/herself. Finally, the child goes through all the steps without stating the questions to provide a connected problem-solving sequence in a narrative format. This process assists not only with problem solving, but also with discourse organization and generation skills. This format is established initially with the speech language pathologist; the child and parents then use cueing when a problem presents that needs to be solved. With practice, it becomes an internalized problem-solving structure.

In order to assist with verbal organization (see the section on discourse above), a child may be introduced to various strategies such as semantic webbing, using charts and graphs of story grammar or usual sequence of an explanation, as well as assessing the content of an explanation using 5w-1h questions (i.e. who, what, when, where, why, and how). The strategies that work best for the child are developed with him/her, practised in isolation and in context and, eventually, internalized. Addressing figurative language and humour starts with recognizing environmental cues that indicate that something was meant to be funny, or that language was meant to be referential, and then analysing why it might be funny, or referential. In addition, modelling appropriate responses when the child realizes they have missed a joke or have misinterpreted a situation is important.

For higher-grade students, direct intervention in the areas of study skills, organization skills and note-taking skills must be addressed.

PRAGMATICS AND SOCIAL COMMUNICATION

Presentation

Pragmatics refers to knowledge of the social rules of language (Marsh 1999). These rules include knowledge and use of appropriate body language, tone of voice, turn taking, sharing, maintaining or switching conversation topics appropriately, and respecting personal space.

Ylvisaker and Gioia (1998) summarized common social communication deficits following a brain injury involving the frontal lobes, including disinhibition, socially inappropriate behaviour, and lack of initiation. The child may be overly friendly or present with difficulty reading social cues and interpreting social situations. Difficulty with organizing social responses, rigidity, and awkward behaviour are also common. An inability to respond to feedback in social situations may also be observed. These difficulties following a brain injury can be linked to underlying deficits of executive functions (Fig. 10.1).

Pragmatic difficulties are observed in how and with whom the child interacts. Parents and teachers may indicate that the child does not have many friends, or only likes to play with younger children, or, in contrast, with older children and adults. Children with pragmatic difficulties can be labelled as 'oppositional', 'behaviourally challenged' or 'antisocial', and consequently may be isolated, which further limits the child's opportunities to learn appropriate peer interaction.

Failure to learn social rules during play is seen in poor turn taking and sharing, which may make the child seem uncooperative or unfriendly. The inability to monitor the environment or the general tone of conversation may make the child seem to monopolize attention, appear uninterested or careless. Poor monitoring of own body language (e.g. facial expression, proximity, eye contact, tone of voice, volume) may give the impression of an awkward, overly friendly, inappropriately behaved, or sarcastic child. Poor initiation means the child may be seen as withdrawn and uninterested. The child may be inattentive, distracted, interrupting, and off-topic, with underlying deficits in attention or impulsivity.

Assessment

Marsh (1999) identifies three reasons for social incompetence associated with TBI: (1) skill deficit, resulting from lack of cognitive and social skill acquisition; (2) performance deficit, resulting from failure to perform the acquired social skills; and (3) impaired self-control, interfering with acquisition and performance of social skills. Identification of the child's specific difficulties, knowledge of executive function impact and Marsh's framework give a structure to the assessment of pragmatic skills.

While there are standardized assessment tools to evaluate social communication skills, interview is still the most commonly used assessment method (Marsh 1999). Through interviews with adults who are involved with the child in different settings (e.g. parents, teachers, soccer coaches), a speech language pathologist attempts to obtain a broad picture of the child's social communication skills. Teachers and educational assistants can provide input on the child's peer interaction. Primary caregivers can report on the child's interaction with siblings, neighbourhood friends, and relatives.

Further information may be obtained using a comprehensive social communication questionnaire. These types of questionnaires are also useful for pre- and post-intervention comparison. Older children are encouraged to be a part of this process by participating in an interview and completing a questionnaire. By comparing the completed questionnaires, it is possible to determine the commonly identified issues or discrepancies. For example, if there is a discrepancy between two adult reports, investigation of the environmental factors that may play a role in the child's social communication may be indicated. If a child self-evaluates a certain skill at a higher level than the adult informers, it might be an indication of poor insight. Similarly, a reverse situation may be an indication of a child's poor self-esteem or inadequate self-evaluation skills.

In addition, direct observation of the child's interaction within their natural environment and in real-life situations is essential. Monitoring of the child's preferred communication partners often indicates the developmental stages of the child's social communication skills.

Therapy

As, by its nature, social communication takes place in interaction with others, interventions are often provided most effectively in a group setting (Wiseman-Hakes et al. 1998). A speech language pathologist identifies individual and group goals based on the assessment and may facilitate the group in collaboration with other professionals, such as an occupational therapist to maximize functionality, or a child and youth worker to address behavioural needs.

The components of social skills training programs often include rehearsal, feedback, prompting, modelling, programming, and home assignment (Trower 1995). In social communication intervention with children with TBI, it is important to remember that social changes created in a training context do not generalize easily to everyday interactions with peers. Consequently, social communication intervention should be targeted in functional and naturalistic contexts (Ylvisaker and Szekeres 1998).

Ylvisaker (1998) proposes a project-based approach, where the group learns to set goals, plan, organize, initiate, predict outcome, solve problems and self-evaluate during natural interaction with peers. Children can target specific individual pragmatic skills (e.g. turn taking, not interrupting, sharing, being positive), as appropriate, during the course of the project. The target behaviour must be identified by the child, and a replacement skill learned, used consistently and generalized, for the behaviour to be considered consolidated. Goals are introduced one at a time, and facilitated throughout the project, while new goals are added when the child is ready. At the end of each session and at the end of the project, the participants are asked to evaluate their observations of their own and others' goals. Parents are encouraged to observe the sessions, for example through an observation mirror, and are part of the process of choosing target behaviours and establishing goals. Parents can then encourage the maintenance and generalization of targeted behaviours within the child's daily routine (e.g. planning what to take for a sleepover or having a successful play-date).

A project-based approach provides a context in which the child learns cognitive-communication and pragmatic skills while they collaboratively work on a personally relevant group project. This type of setting approximates the child's real demands at school, providing a context to make generalization of the learned skills and strategies more likely. The children in the group should be matched according to their chronological age, rather than their skill levels, as social communication demands as well as expectations for appropriate behaviour are mostly associated with chronological age.

Intervention may include the direct teaching of a communicative alternative that serves the same functions as the problem behaviour – 'functional communication training' (Durand 1991, Carr et al. 1994, Shirley et al. 1997). The target may be a decrease in the problem behaviour, for example interrupting, or an increase in a targeted behaviour, such as eye contact.

COGNITIVE COMMUNICATION AND PRESCHOOL CHILDREN
Despite the common belief that young children have advantageous brain plasticity, infants and toddlers are particularly vulnerable to the effects of TBI (Raimondi and Hirschauer 1984) and prefrontal injury seems to indicate negative outcomes in young children (Levin et al. 1993, Kolb 1995).

Executive function development and cognitive communication demands in preschool
Cognitive communication and executive function demands during the preschool years are basic compared to those for school-aged children and adolescents; however, executive functions such as working memory, flexibility and inhibition can be identified in preschool children (Espy et al. 1999a). In infancy, attention control, intentional problem solving and self-regulation start to emerge (Diamond 1985, Haith et al. 1988), and continue to develop into the preschool years (Espy et al. 1999a). In an attempt to investigate executive function development in preschoolers, Isquith et al. (2004) modified the Behaviour Rating Inventory of Executive Function (BRIEF) (Gioia et al. 2000). They concluded that while metacognitive aspects of executive function such as planning, organizing, initiating, monitoring and working

memory were less clearly discriminated, dimensions of inhibition, flexibility and emotional regulation were measurable and evident in preschoolers.

Despite this research showing that executive functions grow rapidly during preschool years and that TBI sustained during childhood disrupts working memory and inhibitory control (Ewing-Cobbs et al. 2004), preschoolers with TBI can present as age-appropriate among their peer group. The highly structured and concrete nature of preschoolers' activities may mask the underlying difficulties with executive function. For example, group instruction with preschoolers is usually accompanied by concrete visual information, demonstration and gestures. Instructions and concepts are repeated and adults often explicitly call for attention before instruction is provided. Routines are usually consistent and the children know what to expect during the course of a day or during a particular activity. In other words, demands for higher cognitive and executive function skills are relatively limited in the life of the preschool child.

Assessment and monitoring of cognitive communication: role of the speech language pathologist

Interviews and developmental checklists completed by parents and other caregivers give information about the child's pre-injury developmental status and the rate and pattern of new skill development in relation to the expected developmental milestones. The child's speech and language skills are assessed with the use of standardized tests. A preschool child may present with age-appropriate receptive and expressive language skills when tested following an ABI, and then fall away from their peers over time as their ability to continue to acquire language in a developmentally appropriate time frame is impacted by acquired language or cognitive impairments. Alternatively, an impact on primary language may be detected immediately.

Close observation of the preschool child is needed to detect preliminary deficits in the areas of executive functions during structured and unstructured play. Parents' and carers' reports of changes in behaviour or abilities following an ABI are particularly important as an indicator of what has become more difficult for the child. Areas to monitor include the ability to focus on a play task while ignoring distractions (e.g. attend to a task while peers are playing a different game); to shift from one activity to another (e.g. circle time to story time); to organize and categorize toys; to share and take turns with peers; to use age-appropriate social skills; to sequence and plan play activities; and to learn and apply new ideas in play. Monitoring of the development of symbolic and pretend play also provides insight into appropriate development of abstract thinking. A preschooler with ABI may present as a slow processor, as a follower rather than a leader in the context of a group activity. Monitoring whether the child typically follows instructions on their own initiative, or frequently relies on copying their peers' actions, provides insight not only into the child's basic auditory processing skills and learning of new information but also into initiation and self-regulation.

A speech language pathologist is involved in problem-solving the underlying reasons for reported behavioural issues. For example, lack of initiation, 'out of control' behaviours and/or temper tantrums, seen in typically developing preschoolers, are triggered more easily and may be prolonged and intensified in children with TBI (Ylvisaker et al. 1998c). From a cognitive-communication perspective, the speech language pathologist investigates the underlying reasons for such behaviour, keeping in mind a number of factors including: (1) executive function deficits such as difficulty shifting activity, rigidity, poor self-control, inability to take the other's perspective, and disinhibition; (2) difficulty understanding instructions and conversation (i.e. auditory processing); (3) difficulty expressing ideas (i.e. verbal expression and/or word-finding); and (4) difficulty understanding or complying with social routines or rules. A child may also be anxious due to lack of structure, organization and consistency within their environment. In such cases, collaborating with the neuropsychologist, occupational therapist and child and youth worker is imperative.

Facilitating the development of cognitive communication
Zelazo et al. (1997) reviewed the literature and concluded that there are dramatic changes within the domains of executive function between 2 and 5 years of age (i.e. flexible problem representation, planning, execution, and evaluation). While vocabulary associated with aspects of executive functions is abstract and not easily understood by preschoolers, adults are encouraged to use words such as 'think', 'remember', 'organize' and 'first – then' consistently to facilitate the child's organization and success (Ylvisaker et al. 1998c).

Ongoing and intensive collaboration with teachers, childcare workers and families, as well as education on normal language and cognitive development and brain injury and its common sequelae, is usually appropriate. This allows monitoring of the child's skill development in the long term and promotes early detection of difficulties associated with ABI.

Even when the preschool child seems to have recovered well from their brain injury, they need to be monitored over the longer term. Deficits may not become apparent until the child reaches the age where a particular skill should have developed but has not. An area of the brain may be appropriately functionally immature at the time of injury and the impact may not become apparent until the demand for the damaged region emerges (Sohlberg and Mateer 2001).

In preparation for grade 1, preschoolers who have sustained a brain injury should ideally be assessed for speech, language, cognitive communication and pragmatics, as well as phonological awareness and pre-reading skills, using standardized tests and informal tasks. A child with ABI may present with age-appropriate speech and language skills yet show signs of weaker cognitive-communication skills (e.g. generation of ideas in an organized manner or sequencing events). These are areas to be monitored and supported in the classroom setting in order to detect emerging signs of executive function/cognitive-communication difficulty. A reassessment at grade 3 or 4 to ensure readiness for higher learning is appropriate.

As it is not unusual for a child to have delayed developmental consequences following brain injury at an early age, long-term monitoring of infants and preschoolers is justified (Ylvisaker and Gioia 1998).

SPEECH FOLLOWING TBI

The prevalence of dysarthria following severe traumatic brain injury is consistently reported at between 30 and 40% (Sarno et al. 1986). This incidence is also reported at five years post-injury. Thompson et al. (1994) reported on the persistence of dysarthria in 15 individuals who had dysarthria acutely and continued to be dysarthric 10 to 15 years later. Ylvisaker (1993) reported that 8 to 10% of children were unintelligible following a severe head injury.

There are studies that show improved functional speech following intervention after a period of spontaneous recovery (Enderby and Crow 1990). Speech will still be dysarthric but speech control and intelligibility can be improved.

It is of note that the presentation of dysarthria in children who premorbidly had acquired fluent speech is similar to that following TBI in adults. Ataxic or spastic dysarthria in a child has the same perceptual correlates as dysarthria in an adult. Acquired apraxia presents with similar motor speech correlates to those seen in an adult and, as in adults, is a disorder distinct from developmental apraxia of speech.

Speech disorders following an acquired brain injury generally present as a mixed dysarthria. Yorkston et al. (1999) identify spastic, ataxic and flaccid dysarthria, and combinations of these, in patients following a TBI. Spastic and ataxic dysarthria are the most common presentations of a specific dysarthria and a combination of these two is the most common mixed dysarthria.

All possible combinations of spastic, ataxic, flaccid and, less commonly, hyperkinetic involvement at the levels of respiration, phonation, articulation and resonance are noted in speech following a TBI. Every child will present with different relative involvement of respiration, phonation, resonance and articulation. A clear description and diagnosis of the type and effect of dysarthria can be made from a complete motor speech examination, analysis of the perceptual characteristics of speech and a detailed history.

Therapy for dysarthria is chronicled in detail elsewhere (Dworkin 1991, Duffy 2005). The same techniques for therapeutic management of acquired dysarthria in adults have proved useful with children. Some techniques are observed to be consistently successful with children with TBI. With ataxic dysarthria, rate work with emphasis on final sound production and especially speaking 'one word at a time' is a technique that effectively slows speech and allows articulation targets to be reached without trying to get a child to gauge whether speech is too fast or too slow. If a child is speaking 'one word at a time', then rate takes care of itself. In addition, such techniques are often used with children as clarification tools – a pattern of speech to slip into when they are tired or someone is having difficulty understanding them. Compliance at this level is not a problem, whereas work on adoption of such a foreign way of speaking for habitual speech is resisted. If the emphasis is on clarification strategies, over time, especially with the adolescent, the rate and articulation control gradually takes over more and more of their speaking time.

Continuous positive airway pressure for work on hypernasality, usually in spastic dysarthria following ABI, has been reported recently in the literature (Cahill et al. 2004) and has been completed with several children. The youngest child to tolerate the entire protocol was aged 7, with emphasis on the 'Darth Vader' look of the equipment. Respiratory support is often the first level of intervention, with visual feedback from an inspiratory spirometer effective at improving exhalatory control.

Adaptation to the age and attention abilities of the child always needs to be made to keep the drill work, which is unavoidable in dysarthria therapy, fun and relevant to the child. Maxims for management of adult dysarthria are paramount when managing dysarthria in a child: speech therapy needs to be targeted at speech, and not non-speech, tasks, and visual biofeedback is essential for a child. Dysarthria work is rarely effective with a child without significant tactile, visual and auditory feedback. Remembering that for the child with an acquired brain injury sensory feedback is almost inevitably as impaired as oral motor control, all possible sensory support must be given to change or relearn a motor speech behaviour. While the basic techniques of speech rehabilitation are similar for children and adults, Love (2000) and Yorkston et al. (1999) look specifically at the challenges of their application to children.

Children must often be taught to recognize when somebody does not understand them and then to implement clarification strategies that have been practised and internalized. Some of these strategies will be oral ('over'-articulate, repeat using different words, spell), some behavioural (use a gesture, point) and some will involve the use of alternative or augmentative communication for part or all of the message (spell the message, point to the first letter of each word as you say it).

Therapy for acquired oral and verbal apraxia in children, as for dysarthria, follows similar strategies to therapeutic intervention with an adult. Rosenbek et al.'s (1973) hierarchy of facilitating articulatory accuracy with maximum verbal, visual and tactile cueing (integral stimulation) and then successively removing the support and increasing the complexity of the articulatory demands is readily adaptable to children (Yorkston et al. 1999). Prompts for Restructuring Oral Muscular Phonetic Targets (PROMPT) (Chumpelik 1984, Hayden 1994), which involves manipulation of the articulators by the therapist, can be used as a technique on its own or is effectively added as an extra source of support in the initial stages of Rosenbek et al.'s hierarchy. The amount of repetition and drill work necessary for successful rehabilitation of acquired apraxia in a child requires considerable creative energy from the speech language pathologist. The drill work must happen but often elaborate reward systems need to be negotiated.

CONCLUSION

The communication challenges of a child who has had a brain injury are complex and multifaceted. In addition to the potential for motor speech disorders, compromised cognitive processes can manifest themselves through language and language itself can be primarily affected. Speech language pathology management of these children in an acute rehabilitation setting focuses on the differential diagnosis of these difficulties and remediation through specific skill building, compensation and environmental modifications.

REFERENCES

Alderman N, Ward A (1991) Behavioural treatment of the dysexecutive syndrome: reduction of repetitive speech using response cost and cognitive overlearning. *Neuropsychol Rehabil* 1(1): 65–80.

Appleton RE, Baldwin T (1998) *Management of Brain-injured Children.* Oxford: Oxford University Press.

Bara GB, Cutica I, Tirassa M (2001) Neuropragmatics: extralinguistic communication after closed head injury. *Brain Lang* 77: 72–94.

Boston Diagnostic Aphasia Exam, see Goodglass and Kaplan (1972).

Brooks N (1991) The effectiveness of post acute rehabilitation. *Brain Injury* 5(2): 103–109.

Brookshire B, Levin HS, Song J, Zhang L (2004) Components of executive function in typically developing and head-injured children. *Dev Neuropsychol* 25(1&2): 61–83.

Cahill LM, Turner AB, Stabler PA, Addis PE, Theordoros DG, Murdoch BE (2004) An evaluation of continuous positive airway pressure (CPAP) therapy in the treatment of hypernasality following traumatic brain injury. *J Head Trauma Rehabil* 19(3): 241–253.

Carr EG, Levin HS, McConnachie G, Carlson JI, Kemp DC, Smith CE (1994) *Communication Based Intervention for Problem Behaviour.* Baltimore: Paul Brookes.

Chapman SB, Lawyer SL (1997) Recovery of written discourse abilities in children following closed head injury at three and twelve months post injury. Texas Speech-Language Hearing Association, Austin, Texas.

Chapman SB, Levin HS, Harward HN (1996) Long-term recovery of discourse, cognitive, and psychological abilities in pediatric head injury: a case illustration. In: Balejko A (ed) *Diagnoza i terapia os Harward HN (1996) Long-term recover.* Bialystok, Poland: Wydaniel.

Chapman SB, Watkins R, Gustafson C, Moore S, Levin HS, Kufera JA (1997) Narrative discourse in children with closed head injury, children with language impairment, and typically developing children. *Am J Speech-Lang Pathol* 6: 66–75.

Chapman SB, Levin HS, Wanek A, Weyrauch J, Kufera J (1998) Discourse after closed head injury in young children: relation of age to outcome. *Brain Lang* 61: 420–449.

Chapman SB, Levin HS, Lawyer SL (1999) Communication problems resulting from brain injury in children: special issues of assessment and management. In: McDonald F, Togher L, Code C (eds) *Communication Disorders Following TBI*. Hove, East Sussex: Psychology Press, pp 235–269.

Chapman S, Sparks G, Levin H, Dennis M, Roncadin C, Zhang L, Song J (2004) Discourse macrolevel processing after severe pediatric traumatic brain injury. *Dev Neuropsychol* 25(1&2): 37–60.

Chumpelik D (1984) The PROMPT system of therapy: theoretical framework and applications for developmental apraxia of speech. *Semin Speech Lang* 5: 139–156.

Cicerone KD, Dahlberg C, Kalmar K, Langenbahn DM, Malec JF, Bergquist TF, Felicetti T, Giacino JT, Harley JP, Harrington DE, Herzog J, Kneipp S, Laatsch L, Morse PA (2000) Evidence-based cognitive rehabilitation: recommendations for clinical practice. *Arch Phys Med Rehabil* 81: 1596–1615.

Constantinidou F, Thomas RD, Scharp L, Laske KM, Hammerly MD, Guitonde S (2005) Effects of categorization training in patients with TBI during post acute rehabilitation. *J Head Trauma Rehabil* 20(2): 143–157.

Darley F (1982) *Aphasia*. Philadelphia: WB Saunders Company.

Dennis M (1992) Word finding in children and adolescents with a history of brain injury. *Top Lang Disord* 13(1): 66–82.

Dennis M, Barnes MA, Wilkinson M, Humphreys RP (1998) How children with head injury represent real and deceptive emotion in short narratives. *Brain Lang* 61: 450–483.

Diamond A (1985) Development of the ability to use recall to guide action, as indicated by infants' performance on AB. *Child Dev* 56: 868–883.

Duffy JR (2005) *Motor Speech Disorders: Substrates, Differential Diagnosis and Management*. St Louis: Elsevier Publications.

Durand MV (1991) *Severe Behaviour Problems: A Functional Communication Training Approach*. New York: Guilford Press.

Dworkin JP (1991) *Motor Speech Disorders: A Treatment Guide*. St. Louis: Mosby Year Book.

Ehrlich JS (1988) Selective characteristics of narrative discourse in head injured and normal adults. *J Commun Disord* 21: 1–9.

Ehrlich J, Barry P (1989) Rating communication behaviours in the head injured adult. *Brain Injury* 3(2): 193–198.

Ehrlich JS, Sipes AL (1985) Group treatment of communication skills for head trauma patients. *Cogn Rehabil* 3: 32–37.

Enderby P, Crow E (1990) Long-term recovery patterns of severe dysarthria following head injury. *Br J Disord Commun* 25: 342–354.

Epsy KA, Kaufmann PM, McDiarmid M, Glisky ML (1999a) Executive functioning in preschool children: A-not-B and other delayed response format task performance. *Brain Cogn* 41: 178–199.

Epsy KA, Kaufmann PM, Glisky ML (1999b) Neuropsychologic outcome in toddlers exposed to cocaine in utero: a preliminary study. *Dev Neuropsychol* 15: 447–460.

Ewing-Cobbs L, Prasad MR, Kramer L, DeLeon R (2004) Executive functions following traumatic brain injury in young children: a preliminary analysis. *Dev Neuropsychol* 26(1): 487–512.

Friedland D, Miller N (1998) Conversation analysis of communication breakdown after closed head injury. *Brain Injury* 12(1): 1–14.

Freund J, Hayter C, MacDonald S, Neary M, Wiseman-Hakes C (1994) *Cognitive*

Communication Disorders Following Traumatic Brain Injury: A Practical Guide. Austin, TX: PRO-ED.

Giles GM, Fussey I, Burgess P (1988) The behavioural treatment of verbal interaction skills following severe head injury: a single case study. *Brain Injury* 2(1): 75–79.

Gillis RJ (1996) *Traumatic Brain Injury: Rehabilitation for Speech-Language Pathologists.* Boston: Butterworth-Heinemann.

Gioia GA, Isquith PK, Guy SC, Kenworthy L (2000) *The Behavior Rating Inventory of Executive Function.* Luts, FL: Psychological Assessment Resources.

Goodglass H, Kaplan E (1972) *The Assessment of Aphasia and Related Disorders.* Philadelphia: Lea & Febiger.

Groher M (1977) Language and memory disorders following closed head trauma. *J Speech Hearing Res* 20: 212–223.

Haith MM, Hazan C, Goodman GS (1988) Expectation and anticipation of dynamic visual events by 3.5-month-old babies. *Child Dev* 59: 467–479.

Hartley LL (1995) *Cognitive-Communicative Abilities Following Brain Injury.* San Diego: Singular Publishing.

Hartley LL, Jensen PJ (1991) Narrative and procedural discourse after closed head injury. *Brain Injury* 5(3): 267–285.

Hartley LL, Levin HS (1990) Linguistic deficits after closed head injury: a current appraisal. *Aphasiology* 4(4): 353–370.

Hayden D (1994) Differential diagnosis of motor speech dysfunction in children. *Clin Commun Disord* 4: 175–182.

Hebb DO (1942) The effect of early and late brain injury upon test scores and the nature of abnormal adult intelligence. *Proc Am Phil Soc* 1: 265–292.

Isaki E, Turkstra L (2000) Communication abilities and work re-entry following traumatic brain injury. *Brain Injury* 14(5): 441–453.

Isquith PK, Gioia GA, Espy KA (2004) Executive function in preschool children: examination through everyday behavior. *Dev Neuropsychol* 26(1): 403–422.

Jordan FM, Murdoch BF (1990) Linguistic status following closed head injury in children: a follow-up study. *Brain Injury* 4: 147–154.

Jordan FM, Cannon A, Murdoch BE (1992) Language abilities of mildly closed head injured children 10 years post injury. *Brain Injury* 6(1): 39–44.

Joyce BM, Rockwood KJ, Mate-Kole CCM (1994) Use of goal attainment scaling in brain injury in a rehabilitation hospital. *Am J Phys Med Rehabil* 73(1): 10–14.

Kagan A, Black SE, Duchan JF, Simmons-Mackie N, Square P (2001) Training volunteers as conversation partners using 'supported conversation for adults with aphasia' (SCA): a controlled trial. *J Speech Lang Hear Res* 44: 624–638.

Kolb B (1995) *Brain Plasticity and Behaviour.* Mahwah, NJ: Erlbaum.

Lees JA (1993) *Children with Acquired Aphasia.* London: Whurr Publishers.

Levin HS, Eisenberg HM, Wigg NR, Kobayashi K (1982) Memory and intellectual ability after head injury in children and adolescents. *Neurosurgery* 11: 668–673.

Levin HS, Culhane KA, Mendelsohn D, Lilly MA, Bruce D, Fletcher JM et al. (1993) Cognition in relation to magnetic resonance imaging in head-injured children and adolescents. *Arch Neurol* 50: 897–905.

Levin HS, Fletcher JM, Kusnerik L, Kufera J, Lilly MA, Duffy FF et al. (1996) Semantic memory following pediatric head injury: relationship to age, severity of injury and MRI. *Cortex* 32: 461–478.

Levin HS, Song J, Ewing-Cobbs L, Roberson G (2001) Porteus maze performance following traumatic brain injury in children. *Neuropsychology* 15: 557–567.

Liles BZ, Coelho CA, Duffy JJ, Zalagens MR (1989) Effects of elicitation procedures on the narratives of normal and closed head injured adults. *J Speech Hear Disord* 54: 356–366.

Lohman T, Ziggas D, Pierce RS (1989) Word fluency performance on common categories by subjects with closed head injuries. *Aphasiology* 3(8): 685–693.

Love RJ (2000) *Childhood Motor Speech Disability.* Needham Heights, MA: Allyn & Bacon.

McNeil M, Prescott T (1978) *The Revised Token Test.* Austin, TX: PRO-ED.

Malec JF (2001) *Evidence-Based Guidelines for Cognitive Rehabilitation.* Proceedings of Innovative Treatment Approaches for Acquired Brain Disorders. June 22, 2001. Mayo Clinic, Rochester, MN.

Maloney FP, Mirrett P, Brooks C, Johannes K (1978) Use of goal attainment scale in the treatment and ongoing evaluation of neurologically handicapped children. *Am J Occup Ther* 32(8): 505–510.

Marsh N (1999) Social skill deficits following traumatic brain injury: assessment and treatment. In: McDonald F, Togher L, Code C (eds) *Communication Disorders Following TBI.* Hove, East Sussex: Psychology Press, pp 175–210.

Mateer CA, Kerns KA, Eso KL (1997) Management of attention and memory disorders following traumatic brain injury. In: Bigler ED, Clark E, Farmer JE (eds) *Childhood Traumatic Brain Injury: Diagnosis, Assessment, and Intervention.* Austin, TX: PRO-ED, pp 153–175.

Matsuzawa J, Matsui M, Konishi T, Noguchi K, Ruben CG, Bilker W et al. (2001) Age-related volumetric changes of brain gray and white matter in healthy infants and children. *Cereb Cortex* 11: 335–342.

Mentis M, Prutting CA (1987) Cohesion in the discourse of normal and head injured adults. *J Speech Hear Res* 30: 88–98.

Milton SB (1988) Management of subtle cognitive communication deficits. *J Head Trauma Rehabil* 3(2): 1–11.

Milton S, Prutting C, Binder G (1984) Appraisal of communicative competence in head injured adults. In: Brookshire R (ed) *Clinical Aphasiology Conference Proceedings.* Minneapolis: BRK Publishers.

Murdoch BE (1995) *Acquired Speech and Language Disorders: A Neuroanatomical and Functional Neurological Approach.* London: Chapman and Hall.

Pondford J (1995) *Traumatic Brain Injury: Rehabilitation for Every Day Adaptive Living.* Hove, UK: Lawrence Erlbaum.

Raimondi AJ, Hirschauer J (1984) Head injury in the infant and toddler. Coma scoring and outcome scale. *Childs Brain* 11: 12–35.

Renfrew C (2001) *The Bus Story Test.* Bicester, UK: Speech Mark Publishing Ltd.

Rosenbek J, Lemme M, Ahem M, Harris E, Wertz R (1973) A treatment for apraxia of speech in adults. *J Speech Hear Disord* 38: 462–472.

Ruff R (2005) Two decades of advances in understanding of mild traumatic brain injury. *J Head Trauma Rehabil* 20(1): 5–18.

Sarno MT, Buonaguro A, Levita E (1986) Characteristics of verbal impairment in closed head injury. *Arch Phys Med Rehabil* 67: 400–405.

Schwartz-Cowley R, Stepanik MJ (1969) Communication disorders and treatment in the acute trauma center setting. *Top Lang Disord* 9: 1–14.

Shirley MJ, Iwata BA, Kahng SW, Mazaleski JL, Lerman DC (1997) Does functional communication training compete with ongoing contingencies of reinforcement? An analysis during response acquisition and maintenance. *J Appl Behav Anal* 30: 93–104.

Simmons N (1983) Acoustic analysis of ataxic dysarthria: an approach to monitoring treatment. In: Berry W (ed) *Clinical Dysarthria*. Austin, TX: PRO-ED.

Snow P, Douglas J, Ponsford J (1995) Discourse assessment following traumatic brain injury: a pilot study examining some demographic and methodological issues. *Aphasiology* 9(4): 365–380.

Snow P, Douglas J, Ponsford J (1998) Conversational discourse abilities following severe traumatic brain injury: a follow–up study. *Brain Injury* 12(11): 911–935.

Sohlberg MM, Mateer CA (2001) Rehabilitation of children with acquired cognitive impairments. In: *Cognitive Rehabilitation: An Integrative Neuropsychological Approach*. New York: Guilford Press, pp 429–452.

Spiegler BJ, Bouffet E, Greenberg ML, Rutka JT, Mabbot DJ (2004) Change in neurocognitive functioning after treatment with cranial radiation in childhood. *J Clin Oncol* 22(4): 706–713.

Thompson NM, Francis DJ, Stuebing KK, Fletcher JM, Ewing-Cobbs L, Miner ME, Levin HS, Eisenberg HM (1994) Motor, visual-spatial, and somatosensory skills after closed head injury in children and adolescents: a study of change. *Neuropsychology* 8(3): 333–342.

Trower P (1995) Adult social skills: state of the art and future directions. In: O'Donohue W, Krasner L (eds) *Handbook of Psychological Skills Training: Clinical Techniques and Applications*. Boston: Allyn & Bacon, pp 54–80.

Turkstra L (1999) Language testing in adolescents with brain injury: a consideration of the celf-3. *Lang Speech Hear Serv Sch* 30: 132–140.

Turkstra L (2000) Should my shirt be tucked in or left out? The communication context of adolescence. *Aphasiology* 14(4): 349–364.

Turkstra L, Holland AL (1998) Assessment of syntax after adolescent brain injury: effects of memory on test performance. *J Speech Lang Hear Res* 41: 137–149.

Turkstra LS, McDonald S, DePompei R (2001) Social information processing in adolescents: data from normally developing adolescents and preliminary data from their peers with traumatic injury. *J Head Trauma Rehabil* 16(5): 469–483.

Watson C (1995) *Making Hanen Happen – The Hanen Program for Parents*. Toronto: Hanen Centre Publications.

Webb SJ, Monk CS, Nelson CA (2001) Mechanisms of postnatal neurobiological development: implications for human development. *Dev Neuropsychol* 19: 147–171.

Wiseman-Hakes C, Stewart M, Wasserman R, Schuller R (1998) Peer group training of pragmatic skills in adolescents with acquired brain injury. *J Head Trauma Rehabil* 13(6): 23–28.

World Health Organization (2001) International Classification of Functioning, Disability and Health. www3.who.int\icf\icftemplate.cfm.

Ylvisaker M (1985) *Traumatic Brain Injury Rehabilitation: Children and Adolescents*. Boston: Butterworth-Heinemann. (*2nd edn*, 1998.)

Ylvisaker M (1993) Communication outcome in children and adolescents with traumatic brain injury. *Neuropsychol Rehabil* 3: 367–387.

Ylvisaker M (ed) (1998) *Traumatic Brain Injury Rehabilitation: Children and Adolescents, 2nd edn*. Boston: Butterworth-Heinemann.

Ylvisaker M, Gioia GA (1998) Cognitive assessment. In: Ylvisaker M (ed) *Traumatic Brain Injury Rehabilitation: Children and Adolescents, 2nd edn*. Boston: Butterworth-Heinemann, pp 159–179.

Ylvisaker M, Szekeres SF (1998) A framework for cognitive rehabilitation. In: Ylvisaker M (ed) *Traumatic Brain Injury Rehabilitation: Children and Adolescents, 2nd edn.* Boston: Butterworth-Heinemann, pp 125–158.

Ylvisaker M, Szekeres SF, Feeney T (1998a) Cognitive rehabilitation: executive functions. In: Ylvisaker M (ed) *Traumatic Brain Injury Rehabilitation: Children and Adolescents, 2nd edn.* Boston: Butterworth-Heinemann, pp 221–269.

Ylvisaker M, Szekeres SF, Haarbauer-Krupa J (1998b) Cognitive rehabilitation: organization, memory, and language. In: Ylvisaker M (ed) *Traumatic Brain Injury Rehabilitation: Children and Adolescents, 2nd edn.* Boston: Butterworth-Heinemann, pp 181–220.

Ylvisaker M, Sellars CW, Edelman L (1998c) Rehabilitation after traumatic brain injury in preschoolers. In: Ylvisaker M (ed) *Traumatic Brain Injury Rehabilitation: Children and Adolescents, 2nd edn.* Boston: Butterworth-Heinemann, pp 303–329.

Yorkston KM, Jaffe KM, Polissar NL, Liao S, Fay GC (1997) Written language production and neuropsychological function in children with traumatic brain injury. *Arch Phys Med Rehabil* 78(10): 1096–1102.

Yorkston KM, Beukelman DR, Strand E, Bell K (1999) *Management of Motor Speech Disorders in Children and Adults.* Austin, TX: PRO-ED.

Zelazo PD, Carter A, Reznick JS, Frye D (1997) Early development of executive function: a problem-solving framework. *Rev Gen Psychol* 1(2): 198–226.

11

REHABILITATION THERAPY

Janet Woodhouse and Trish Geisler

Occupation as defined by the Canadian Association of Occupational Therapists refers to 'a group of occupations and tasks of everyday life, named, organized, and given value and meaning by individuals and a culture' (Townsend 1997). Occupations are complex and vary according to environmental and personal factors, and change over an individual's lifespan. Through occupation, an individual will engage in meaningful activity, developing habits and roles.

Occupational performance is the dynamic relationship between individuals, their environment and their occupations (Townsend 1997). Chapparo and Ranka (1997) defined occupational performance as the ability to perceive, plan and carry out roles, routines, tasks and subtasks for the purpose of self-maintenance, productivity, leisure and rest in response to demands of the internal and/or external environment.

The World Health Organization's Model of International Classification of Functioning, Disability and Health (ICF) (2001), comprised of Body Function (*impairment*), Activities (activity *limitation*), and Participation (participation restriction), provides a useful framework for pediatric rehabilitation (see Fig. 11.1). Functioning and disability are conceived as a dynamic interaction between health conditions and contextual factors. Participation is defined as involvement in a life situation or, within an occupational therapy framework, occupational performance. The process of rehabilitation of children with an acquired brain injury, and their families, involves the identification and understanding of the nature of their impairments in order to develop interventions that promote participation in daily occupations.

The philosophy of occupational therapy is based on key concepts such as the occupational nature of human beings, their capacity for adaptation, and their ability to influence their own health (Ferland 2005). Enabling participation in the occupations of childhood is the major focus of paediatric occupational therapy.

EFFECTS OF BRAIN INJURY ON DAILY ACTIVITIES

The effects of a brain injury on a child's occupational performance are all-encompassing. Occupational performance can be impacted by sensory-motor, cognitive and social-behavioural impairments sustained as a result of the injury. The effects of a traumatic brain injury (TBI) grow more complex as a child matures and

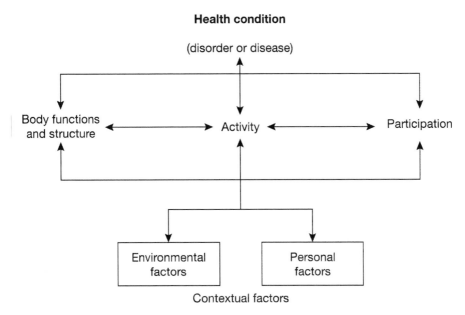

Fig. 11.1. The World Health Organization's Model of International Classification of Functioning, Disability and Health (ICF) (2001).

faces new challenges (Cronin 2001). Deficits can emerge as the child develops and persistent deficits can affect skill acquisition. As children are naturally supervised, problem areas may present in a subtle manner and are often difficult to identify. However, as expectations of occupational performance increase with maturation, these deficits become more apparent and have greater impact on the child's participation in daily occupations.

SENSORY-MOTOR IMPAIRMENTS
Children with severe brain injuries are more likely to exhibit motor impairments including spasticity, ataxia, contractures, paralysis and speech impairments. Blaskey and Jennings (1999) found that the incidence and severity of motor disorders increase with the length of coma following head trauma (Cronin 2001). Long-term motor impairments include altered joint mobility and stability, muscle weakness and reduced endurance (Winkler 1995). Sensory impairments reported following a brain injury include impaired postural awareness and orientation, and tactile hyper-sensitivity. Carney and Gerring (1990) found that children might demonstrate impaired motor planning, tactile sensory dysfunction and spatial disorientation. Porr (1999) found that these impairments could lead to specific problems in the area of swallowing and eating. Visual system impairments that occur as the result of a brain

injury include diplopia, hemianopsia and changes in visual acuity (Massagili et al. 1996, Cronin 2001, Warren 1991).

Cognitive Impairments

Cognitive impairments limit occupational performance for children of all ages. Deficits in cognition cause some of the most severe sequelae of traumatic brain injury (Cronin 2001). Common areas of impairment in children with acquired brain injury include: attention, concentration, judgement, initiation, task orientation, and impulse control. Difficulties with memory and decreased speed of information processing are more long-term impairments. These cognitive problems in isolation or in combination will influence occupational performance.

The principal cause of impaired activities of daily living (ADL) independence in TBI is the range of complex behavioural and cognitive disturbances associated with executive functions (Stuss and Benson 1986, Toglia 1991, Cicerone et al. 2000). Executive functions have been defined as a set of interrelated skills necessary to maintain an appropriate problem-solving set for attainment of a future goal (Anderson and Catroppa 2005). The sub-components of executive functions include: attentional control, strategic planning or problem solving, cognitive flexibility of thought and action, and concept formation.

Psychosocial and Behavioural Impairments

Walleck and Mooney (1994) report that post-concussion syndrome is seen after any type of brain injury and may involve personality changes, mood lability, loss of self-confidence, impaired short-term memory, headaches and other subtle cognitive impairments. Functionally these impairments may present as a lack of goal direction and initiative, social withdrawal, depression, denial of disabilities, immature behaviour, apathy, self-centredness, disinhibition, and aggression (Miller 1991).

More difficult and long-lasting effects are loss of friends, decreased involvement in social activities and lack of social support (Willer et al. 1993, Glang et al. 1997). Students with TBI exhibit maladaptive behaviours including: disinhibition, impulsiveness, decreased frustration tolerance, reduced anger control, poor judgement, decreased motivation and insensitivity to others.

Physical, cognitive and behavioural impairments may restrict the child's participation in daily occupations, impacting on their development of autonomy and self-reliance. A traumatic brain injury does not always occur in isolation. Many children and adolescents also experience other complications including orthopedic injuries and multi-system involvement – for example, spinal cord injuries that impact upon occupational performance. Factors such as fatigue, medical stability and psychological status influence interventions and outcomes.

In addition, pre-existing conditions such as ADD, ADHD, PDD/autism, high-level risk-taking behaviours, and drug and alcohol involvement further compound the situation. These conditions need to be taken into consideration in working through the process of rehabilitation with the child and family.

ENVIRONMENT

The child is part of a larger family system and it is vital to involve the entire system in the rehabilitation process. Daily occupations occur within the context of a family system. The family's understanding of the child and their environment is essential to family-centred practice. Family-centred practice refers to 'the attitudes and behaviours of a therapist that facilitate and esteem the family's role as lead negotiator in assessment, treatment and discharge'. Evidence suggests that family-centred practice is linked to efficient attainment of meaningful goals, greater carry-over of program recommendations and increased consumer satisfaction (Van Benthem 2004).

Research has demonstrated that physical, cognitive, behavioural and academic skills are embedded in an environmental context (Ylvisaker et al. 2005). The following environmental considerations are important factors to consider when working with children with acquired brain injuries:

- Parents/families are part of the child's rehabilitation program.
- The hospital/rehabilitation centre is not home.
- Physical environments must be age-appropriate.
- Physical environments must be accessible/safe and barrier free.
- Interventions need to be developed around the child's routines and schedules.
- The child's and adolescent's environment includes their peers, school and community.
- Rehabilitation goals and interventions need to reflect the entire range of the child's/adolescent's occupations and the environments in which they occur.

ASSESSMENT OF DAILY OCCUPATIONS

Assessment is core to the delivery of occupational therapy services and serves as the foundation for all subsequent clinical decisions, professional opinions, interventions and recommendations. The completion of an occupational therapy assessment involves a comprehensive and consistent process, whether it is condensed into one visit or continued over several sessions (COTO 2005).

Function is often applied narrowly in the field of rehabilitation. It is typically interpreted as encompassing basic self-care activities such as bathing, feeding and dressing. These activities are frequently viewed from a physical performance perspective. The assessment of daily occupations requires a broader perspective involving an understanding of the roles, tasks, activities and skills required by the individual to perform meaningful occupations in a specific context (Nelson 1988, Ponsford et al. 1995, Trombly 1995). The focus on daily occupations necessitates an understanding of individuals in the context of their previous lifestyle, relationships, abilities, values, personality and behavioural patterns, life goals and roles in the community. A child with a traumatic brain injury needs to be assessed within the context of their previous developmental stage and behaviour patterns (Ponsford et al. 1995, Coster 1998).

ASSESSMENT APPROACH

Traditional discipline-specific approaches to assessment often concentrate on evaluating distinct domains of function. This 'bottom-up' approach (Trombly 1993) focuses on the assessment of discrete component abilities that the therapist anticipates may be affected by the client's identified condition. The potential functional impact of these components may be inferred but is often not assessed directly. Therefore the 'link between deficits in basic abilities and the functional problems the client experiences in daily life may never become clear to him or her', which in turn may raise doubts about the meaningfulness of the intervention (Coster 1998).

The top-down assessment approach is an alternative to the traditional approach described above. This approach begins by gathering information about what the person needs or wants to do, the context in which he or she typically engages in these various occupations, and any current limitations. The critical roles the person wishes or needs to fulfil and the context that defines the expectations of these roles are identified using this approach. The assessment needs to identify the specific aspect of task performance that is most limiting the child's engagement in important occupations. For example, the reasons for limited participation in playground occupations may range from limited skills to initiate and sustain peer interactions, to an inability to remember and follow basic game rules, to physical difficulty such as running. Consideration of activities in which the child is performing well may highlight areas of strength that can be tapped to help facilitate the desired changes. Performance components or more discrete abilities are assessed when clarification of the source of the performance limitations is needed, and to help determine the most viable option for overcoming these occupational performance challenges (Coster 1998).

In a top-down assessment approach the extent to which a person is able to construct a pattern of occupation engagement that meets their individual needs and goals as well as societal expectations matters more than the individual's abilities and disabilities. This approach is consistent with the World Health Organization's framework, the International Classification of Functioning, Disability and Health (2001).

The assessment of a child with a traumatic brain injury is comprised of a review of occupational performance and the occupational performance components. The assessment of occupational performance includes information regarding the child and family's lifestyle and the specific activities performed by the individual in their daily routine at home and in their community prior to injury. The level of skill, methods of carrying out activities and strategies used to facilitate performance, as well as the nature of any assistance required before injury, must be identified. This information should be interpreted within the context of the roles and responsibilities of the child within the family.

Assessment of occupational performance components includes the sensory, motor, perceptual, cognitive and behavioural skills that are impacted by the impairment. Children are typically measured against age-based expectations and standards.

This developmental approach emphasizes the underlying performance components or abilities as the critical determinants of behaviour (Coster 1998) and does not always take into account the context or the environment in which the child performs the occupation. Studies have found that in addition to component abilities (e.g. strength), contextual features of the task (including emotional, social and physical context) and personal goals have been identified as potential critical determinants of successful performance (Bronfenbrenner 1992, Dunn et al. 1994).

For a child with traumatic brain injury, the top-down assessment process extends beyond the traditionally structured one-to-one test situation. This approach does not elicit problems with skills such as attention, organization, memory, information processing or the effects of fatigue and distractibility. Furthermore, impaired executive functions result in difficulty generalizing or adapting what is learned from one situation to another (Toglia 1991, Ponsford et al. 1995, Boman et al. 2004).

The assessment process in occupational therapy is ongoing and dynamic. It occurs in a variety of settings/environments and times in the context of the child's daily occupations. This includes one-on-one controlled environment and semi-structured group settings, as well as less traditional environments such as the hallways when moving between sessions, school classrooms, recreational activities and the community. This assessment approach provides information that will support and guide therapists, clients and families to develop meaningful interventions and recommendations to support the child's participation in daily occupations.

ASSESSMENT OF OCCUPATIONAL PERFORMANCE

The assessment of occupational performance can be achieved through direct observation of the individual performing the task, or through interviews or questionnaires. In pediatrics the interviewees are typically the family or caregivers. Direct observation is made while the person performs a task in a natural or simulated environment, assessing the individual's performance. Direct observation, although more time-consuming, yields more appropriate information and allows for a greater understanding of the client's difficulties than other assessment methods (Klein-Parris et al. 1986). Questionnaires and/or interviews are most useful after the patient has left the hospital or rehabilitation centre as they will yield information on how the patient really manages in a natural environment (Dutil et al. 1990).

Standardized ADL assessments usually focus on individual tasks performed in a hospital environment in isolation from normal routines and settings. The imposition of structure and simplification of demands also inherent in this assessment may render it insensitive to the executive dysfunction associated with TBI. Bottari et al. (2006) describe ADL assessment as having serious limitations as it typically requires the evaluator as opposed to the patient to complete many components of the chosen task or give detailed plans for the task, thus leading to an inaccurate estimation of the severity of the consequences of TBI for daily occupations. These factors are likely to elicit the individual's best performance and may not reflect their capacity to perform the same tasks in their own home and community. Fluctuations in initiative, mood, motivation, fatigue and concentration commonly associated with TBI may lead to variation in the level of assistance required in daily activities.

Numerous tools to evaluate occupational performance have been developed and their use is dependent upon the population and environment in which the clinician practises. Examples of assessment tools that are utilized to measure occupational performance in a top-down approach include the Canadian Occupational Performance Measure, the Community Mobility Assessment, the Pediatric Evaluation of Disability Inventory, the Sensory Profile, the School Function Assessment and the Functional Independence Measure for Children (WeeFIM).

The Canadian Occupational Performance Measure (Law et al. 1990) assesses a client's perception of his or her self-care, productivity and leisure abilities or skills. This tool provides the child and their family with a framework to identify and prioritize how they are performing in everyday occupations and environments and how satisfied they are with their performance. The child and/or their family identifies their most important concerns and rates their performance and satisfaction with these occupations.

The Community Mobility Assessment (CMA) (Brewer et al. 1998) is an assessment developed for adolescents with acquired brain injuries to assess their safety in the community. It involves a pre-outing questionnaire and 40 functional activity items, which assess the client's strengths and weaknesses in both the physical and cognitive domains.

The Pediatric Evaluation of Disability Inventory (PEDI) (Coster 1998) is a pediatric functional assessment which has been standardized for children between the ages of 6 months and 7.5 years, but can be used to assess the performance of older children. It includes 197 items evaluating three domains: self-care, mobility and social function. The PEDI was found to be responsive to self-care changes at discharge from hospital, and one and six months after discharge, in children with mild and moderate brain injuries (Coster et al. 1994).

The Sensory Profile (Dunn 1999) is used to determine how well children aged 3 to 10 years process sensory information in everyday situations, and to profile the sensory system's effect on functional performance. Caregivers complete a questionnaire comprised of 125 items, reporting the frequency with which the child responds to various sensory experiences. Infant and adolescent sensory profiles are also available.

The School Function Assessment (Coster 1998) examines students' abilities to perform important functional activities that support or enable participation in academic and related social aspects of an educational program. The School Function Assessment is comprised of three parts: Participation, Task Supports and Activity Performance. The Participation element examines the student's level of participation in six major school activity settings, i.e. regular or special education classroom, playground, etc. The Task Supports element examines the supports currently provided to the student when he or she performs school-related functional tasks. The supports are classified as assistance (adult help) and adaptations (modifications to the environment or program, such as specialized equipment or adapted materials). Activity Performance examines the student's performance of specific school-related functional activities, such as moving around the classroom and the school, using school materials, interacting with others, following school rules, and communicating needs.

The WeeFIM (2003) instrument is derived from the items of the Functional Independence Measure. It was developed and designed to measure changes in function in children aged 6 months to 7 years. It includes 18 items in six areas: self-care, bowel and bladder management, transfers and mobility, communication, and social cognition. Ottenbacher et al. (2000) found that WeeFIM instrument ratings were the best predictors of assistance ratings provided by parents and teachers.

ASSESSMENT OF OCCUPATIONAL PERFORMANCE COMPONENTS

The assessment of occupational performance components provides information that is used to help determine how to intervene, but not what the goals of the interventions will be. These evaluations can determine whether the suggested impairments are possible contributors to the limitations seen, and enable the therapist to devise a goal-oriented intervention program. Assessments of performance components can range from developmental assessments of motor skills such as the Peabody Developmental Motor Scale (Folio and Fewell 2000), to the Bruininks–Oseretsky Test of Motor Proficiency (Bruininks 1978, Bruininks and Bruininks 2005). Cognitive component assessments may include measures to evaluate orientation, attention and functional memory skills, such as the Children's Orientation and Amnesia Test (COAT) (Ewing-Cobbs et al. 1990), the Rivermead Behavioural Memory Test for Children (Wilson et al. 1991), and the Test of Everyday Attention for Children (Manly et al. 1998), or measures of executive function such as the

Behavioural Assessment of Dysexecutive Syndrome for Children (BADS-C) (Emslie et al. 2003).

The method of dynamic assessment used in the assessment of categorization skills (Josman et al. 2000) provides additional clinical information on factors that facilitate task performance. Information such as the client's response to cueing, prediction, and ability to self-evaluate provides valuable information in the design and development of intervention goals. A wide array of assessments to evaluate occupational performance components exists and their uses are dependent upon the population and environment in which the clinician practises.

INTERVENTIONS – DAILY ACTIVITIES
INTERVENTION PRINCIPLES

Banja and Johnston (1994) described a paradigm shift in the field of rehabilitation. The shift is from therapy to remediate impairments without reference to cost, to the promotion of participation. The new paradigm involves the process of attaining maximal improvement in the person's quality of daily life, within financial constraints. In this paradigm, therapy is goal-specific, aimed at achieving independence in activities and participation in roles of importance to the individual. The child with TBI and their family are therefore required to be involved with the planning and decision making of the rehabilitation process. The effectiveness of this family-centred process is therefore measured in terms of client-desired outcomes.

Cicerone et al. (2000) stated that the primary concern in the rehabilitation of persons with TBI should be to improve everyday functioning, in order to reduce levels of disability and participation restriction. Outcomes of rehabilitation should reflect meaningful improvements in everyday activities. Ylvisaker et al. (2005) described the last twenty years of pediatric brain injury rehabilitation as being dominated by increasing sensitivity to contextual factors and integration across many domains of functioning and across service providers. These themes are consistent with the WHO ICF model which includes contextual factors (environment) and barriers in relation to meaningful participation in everyday functional activities. The family and the child's support system are an integral part of the rehabilitation process and need to be involved in the design and implementation of interventions at all stages of the rehabilitation process. Ylvisaker and Feeney (1998) noted that when the routine performance of everyday tasks is supported by others, the individual is afforded rich opportunities to practise important tasks and at the same time 'exercise' cognitive, executive system, communication and behavioural self-regulation processes and systems. This approach holds the promise of reducing impairment while also reducing disability and improving participation.

Trombly et al. (2002) examined therapy in terms of the paradigm of participants actively setting goals. Improvements in occupational performance were found when adults with TBI participated in goal-specific therapy programs combined with training in compensatory strategies. The scores did not improve after discharge from therapy, therefore spontaneous recovery alone was not seen as a viable explanation for the improvement seen.

Goal Attainment Scaling (GAS) is a goal-oriented model of evaluation in which systematic procedures identify, document, measure and evaluate unique program goals for individuals or groups. GAS involves setting goals in collaboration with the client, implementing the program and taking measures to determine to what extent the goals have been met (Mitchell and Cusick 1998). It has low construct and concurrent validity and is not intended to have high correlation with other measures. It assists in the assessment of client change over time, towards established individual goals.

INTERVENTIONS

Therapeutic interventions are planned and based upon theoretical knowledge. Interventions are:

- Client/family-centred
- Dynamic in nature
- Developmentally appropriate
- Meaningful
- Goal-directed
- Measurable
- Stimulating
- Reciprocal

Rehabilitation efforts in the acute care phase are aimed at preparing the child for, and promoting participation in, daily occupations such as self-care and mobility. Early rehabilitation efforts may include: positioning, range of motion exercises, sensory stimulation, orientation training, promotion of communication and mobility. Caregiver education is an important component of early rehabilitation interventions and continues along the continuum.

Interventions broaden in the intermediate phase of rehabilitation along with the child's motor and cognitive recovery. Interventions include: improving motor control, training in daily occupations, cognitive-perceptual remediation, and community re-entry skills. In the community re-entry and integration stage of rehabilitation, interventions focus on participation in home, school and community occupations through the development and use of strategies and environmental supports. Community-based rehabilitation provides support to the child and their family to assist them in participating in their daily occupations. Key transition times within the child's development – e.g. entry into the school system or transition to secondary school – frequently necessitate closer monitoring, increased support and interventions by occupational therapists.

Self-care

Functional deficits in self-care are often evident following brain injury (Dumas et al. 2001). A primary goal of inpatient rehabilitation programming for children with TBI is to improve basic self-care skills. Self-care recovery is important for easing caregiving, increasing social acceptance by peers, and facilitating independent living. Cognitive skills such as new learning, memory, visual perception and attention are particularly vulnerable to childhood brain injury and self-care skills require many of these underlying competencies (Coster et al. 1994).

Jaffe et al. (1995) found that children with mild, moderate and severe brain injury showed no significant deficits in independent living skills three years post-injury. Self-care routines are typically well-learned and performed within familiar environments studded with contextual cues, and are maintained through prompts, cues and structure in specific environments, contributing to successful outcomes. Ponsford et al. (1995) reported that long-term difficulties with personal care occupations tend to occur in those who have significant physical impairment, suggesting that dependence is not primarily due to cognitive impairments. Philip et al. (1994) used the WeeFIM to assess functional changes in 30 children aged 3 to 20 years with brain tumours and found that 60% of these children were independent in self-care on discharge, compared to 23% on admission.

Coster et al. (1994) found that children with TBI assessed at one and six months following discharge from hospital had a decreased function in self-care skills on the Caregiver Assistance scale of the PEDI. The authors suggested that because caregiver assistance is an indirect measure of executive functions, cognitive functions were the reason for limitations in self-care skills.

Children who sustain a brain injury before the age of 3 years often present with good physical recovery and the functional problems associated with cognition are easily overlooked. Coster et al. (1994) reported that it is important for occupational therapists working in early interventions programs to assess the amount of caregiver support a child needs to perform age-appropriate activities. Children may pass the items on a developmental scale but function in a manner atypical for their developmental level in terms of the external support needed. As greater developmental demands are placed upon the child, they may have an increased need for caregiver assistance due to challenges in processing new information and acquiring new skills.

Chen et al. (2004) examined rehabilitation outcomes in relation to the quantity of treatment in pediatric rehabilitation settings and found that children with traumatic injuries who were older than 7 years and had low functional levels on admission improved the most. It was not clear how age interacted with functional gains; however it was postulated that the older children with traumatic injuries had already learned most functional skills, in contrast to their age peers with a developmental disability such as cerebral palsy.

Feeding

Feeding is an intricate task involving the physical ability to manipulate utensils and food, the cognitive ability to sequence, attend to and make judgements about the task, and the perceptual skills to permit correct identification of food and utensils (McNeny 1999). Feeding is also a sensory experience requiring the individual to initiate and interact with others. Many children with acquired brain injury experience an alteration in their sense of taste, smell and oral tactile sensory input, impacting on the occupation of feeding. Impairment of oropharyngeal swallowing after TBI is found in as many as 30% of patients who enter a rehabilitation setting (Rosenthal 1999). The assessment of swallowing for children with TBI needs to focus on their cognitive control, the loss of neuromuscular control of the swallow sequence, and iatrogenic causative factors such as intubation, tracheostomy and medication. Feeding is a social activity, which is embedded in culture and has unique meaning for each individual. Consideration of these socio-cultural factors is important when developing feeding interventions for children.

During the acute stage of rehabilitation, team members (occupational therapists and speech language pathologists) work together to assess the child's feeding skills. Management of swallowing disorders (dysphagia) requires a comprehensive assessment of the child's cognitive, physical and communication skills to determine the appropriate food consistencies the child can safely manage (Avery Smith and Dellarosa 1994). Optimal positioning for feeding safety and skill development is an integral component of this assessment. An oral stimulation program is provided when there are sensory and/or motor impairments that are influencing safe oral feeding. An oral feeding program is only initiated once safety has been established and a feeding protocol developed for trained staff and family to follow. A referral for a videofluoroscopy swallow study is initiated if the child is identified as being at risk of aspiration following a clinical assessment. A program to expand the quantity and range of textures the child can tolerate is developed and their progress monitored.

Environmental issues that can lead to increased distractibility and the child's level of impulsivity or reduced judgement are addressed when designing a feeding program. Goals to promote self-feeding skills, from both motor and cognitive perspectives, are established. Feeding interventions may include: the use of adaptive equipment, postural positioning, environmental modifications, retraining of motor and oral motor skills, sensory awareness, especially with respect to the face, and body awareness. A therapeutic feeding program needs to be scheduled at every meal and caregivers need to be trained in feeding techniques and modifications that will support the goals and progression of the program. If feeding challenges continue on a long-term basis, community-based rehabilitation interventions will need to address environmental modifications to support the child's participation in feeding in home and school environments. Interventions may include the provision of education for community nursing, school and support staff on feeding safety, appropriate textures, positioning for safety, promotion of independence, the use of adaptive equipment, and oral motor training.

Dressing/grooming/hygiene/toileting

During the early stages of rehabilitation, changes in the performance of the self-care occupations of dressing, grooming, toileting and hygiene occur with motor recovery and as the child becomes increasingly orientated. Interventions to promote and maximize participation in self-care skills at an age-appropriate level are undertaken. Examples of activities at this stage include: establishing structure and routine, chaining of the occupations to successfully re-learn the steps, the use of visual schedules (a pictorial sequencing chart), and the introduction of adaptive equipment. Fine motor challenges commonly present as difficulties in managing fastenings such as buttons, zippers and shoelaces. Programming to practise these skills and/or the modification of clothing is frequently undertaken. The structured daily routine of a rehabilitation setting facilitates these activities. Upon discharge or return home, the child's performance may decline when these cues are no longer available. It is therefore important that the family are involved in learning how to structure and support these activities. Home- and community-based rehabilitation upon discharge from hospital may be needed to support the generalization of these occupations to the home and community. Interventions also include the prescription of appropriate equipment that will allow for increased participation in self-care activities and reduce caregiver burden in both home and school environments.

Children who experience long-term difficulties with self-care activities due to cognitive-behavioural impairments commonly exhibit problems such as lack of initiative or poor attention to detail in personal care, resulting in failure to shower regularly, clean their teeth or brush their hair. These individuals may require verbal cues in order to satisfactorily complete self-care tasks (Ponsford et al. 1995). Also, changes in personality such as rigidity may lead to the individual spending an excessive amount of time over personal care. Poor self-regulation manifested as impulsivity may compromise safety in tasks such as regulating water temperature or unsafe transfer techniques. Difficulty making decisions may be apparent in clothing selections that fail to take into account weather or activities that need to be undertaken during the day.

Intervention approaches such as error-free learning (Wilson and Evans 1996), environmental modifications and cueing can assist the child and family in their performance of these routine occupations. Interventions need to be developed within the context of the environment in which the child/teenager performs these daily occupations.

Mobility/transfers

Physiotherapy and occupational therapy interventions in the early stage of recovery address positioning and mobility needs. The interventions include range of motion exercises and splinting or casting, to prevent contractures, positioning, and use of equipment such as wheelchairs and strollers to promote mobility and to accommodate changes in muscle control. With cognitive and motor recovery, the rehabilitation program progresses to focus on more independence in ambulation and mobility. Family involvement is a critical component of this programming and it has been shown that when parents are well trained and supported to provide physical exercises within the context of everyday activities, the child's long-term physical outcome is superior to that produced by intensive clinic-based treatment (Ylvisaker et al. 2005).

Recovery of motor skills and mobility functions has been documented to occur for up to several years post-injury (Vander Schaaf et al. 1997, Dumas and Carey 2002). Dumas and Carey (2002) reviewed reports of motor skill and recovery outcomes for children and adolescents with TBI. They found that motor skill and mobility recovery is often complicated by premorbid conditions, associated traumatic musculoskeletal injuries and cognitive and behavioural deficits due to injury. Outcomes range greatly from dependence to community ambulation with recovery of age-appropriate gross and fine motor skills.

The selection and prescription of appropriate mobility devices for home, school and community environments is undertaken with input from the client, family and professional. This may involve equipment trials and home assessments to ensure safety and independence.

Therapeutic interventions must be planned and structured to address mobility skills across a variety of environments and conditions. Training is graded according to physical, cognitive and environmental demands. Children are trained in skills of ambulation and mobility in a wide variety of environments, ranging from a quiet treatment room, to an open concept gym area, to crowded hallways, cluttered and visually stimulating classrooms and play areas. Once indoor safety has been determined, mobility skills are practised in outdoor environments. Depending upon their age and community environment, children and teens are supported to ambulate around the quieter streets and parks, then higher-volume throughways, and to access public transit. Mobility training involves both the physical and cognitive demands of this task.

Promotion of independence is achieved by gradually decreasing direct client support. For example, children are initially accompanied to their therapy sessions, and progress to travelling independently to sessions and then calling back to notify staff of their safe arrival in the next session. Further progression to independence within the facility is promoted. A similar style of grading independence is employed in the community, provided street safety has been established and the child is at the appropriate developmental age. Technology such as the use of cell phones may be required.

Community mobility and orientation

Independence in community mobility is essential for the adolescent to fully participate in educational, vocational, social and leisure occupations. The Community Mobility Assessment (Brewer et al. 1998) is an objective measure that was developed to evaluate the safety and functional abilities of an adolescent with an acquired brain injury within the community. Physical and cognitive skills are evaluated through participation in a community outing. Safety considerations such as visual scanning and impulsivity are integral aspects of the training. Family and caregivers are provided with recommendations and strategies to assist with the ongoing development of these skills.

Topographical orientation is ideally trained within the natural environments in which the child interacts. Developmental and familial considerations of both the child and their family need to be accounted for in developing these interventions. A structured approach is used to familiarize the child with street names, landmarks and consistent routes in order to reach a predetermined destination. Adolescents are also taught to have an established alternative plan of action in the event of an unforeseen obstacle. Strategies include carrying a cell phone, contact numbers, and money.

Social and emotional factors are also key considerations in developing interventions to promote independence in community mobility. A client may have sustained their injury as a result of a motor vehicle accident in which they were a pedestrian, and community ambulation may have become a stressful activity for both the child and their family. Intervention strategies such as relaxation techniques and systemic desensitization may be utilized to assist the young person in increasing safety, confidence and skills for community ambulation.

INSTRUMENTAL ACTIVITIES OF DAILY LIVING

A distinction is commonly drawn between performance of routine self-care activities such as bathing, dressing and eating, and those tasks that are more complex. The latter are referred to as instrumental activities of daily living (IADL) and include home management skills such as caring for clothing, cleaning, cooking, financial management and following safety procedures. Independence in IADL determines an individual's ability to live independently in the community (Law 1993).

Families vary in their ability and availability to assist and encourage the child to perform self-care tasks and IADL. During adolescence, increasing independence in self-care tasks and IADL often determines if a child will 'fit in' with peers or be successful in obtaining a job outside of the school environment (Shepherd 2001).

Jacobs (1987) found that only 63% of his sample of adults living with the effects of an acquired brain injury were independent in higher-order tasks such as shopping, caring for personal health and safety, and money management.

Household management
During childhood, children learn home management tasks that help them to contribute to family functioning and promote the development of skills for independent living and work. Toddlers as young as 18 months begin to understand what it means to 'help out' in performing household chores. Contextual considerations such as age, gender, socio-economic status, geographical location, customs and values about self-sufficiency may influence home-making expectations, how they are learned, and when a child learns home management tasks. Shepherd (2001) outlines a developmental sequence for learning to perform home management tasks, from imitative play at 13 months, to learning to put away toys with reminders at 3 years, to cooking simple recipes at 12 years. The transition timeline developed at Bloorview Kids Rehab (see Table 11.2, p. 212) provides a guideline for the development of independence skills for children with special needs.

Challenges in the performance of household tasks vary for children with TBI. Physical impairments can result in difficulty accessing, manipulating and using typical equipment or completing the entire task. Cognitive impairments may result in challenges related to initiating and terminating the task, remembering the sequence and generalizing skills to other environments. A child with reduced impulse control and low frustration tolerance may not be provided with experiential opportunities for learning due to concerns about their safety.

It is essential that interventions include the presentation of natural cues within the child's environment, such as organization of supplies and use of visual schedules: checklists and sequencing charts are commonly used strategies to teach skills to children and their families. Safety in the performance of household tasks is an important consideration in assessing IADL and designing intervention plans. Knowledge of emergency procedures and ability to respond and access emergency services need to be evaluated.

Cognitive rehabilitation programs aim to teach children to develop plans for problem solving: how to attack problems through a step-by-step approach to each problem or task, and how to use compensatory techniques for problems in planning and organization. These are taught to assist the child in accomplishing activities of daily living at home. An example of this approach is the planning program (Mitchell and Cusick 1998). This approach is not aimed to restore executive function but to replace poorly organized behaviours with guided routines and strategies that can be performed more independently and are successful. The model teaches children to create personal plans for learning and planning strategies (the process) at the same time as they are taught skills or actions (the content).

Environmental modifications, task modifications, and adaptive equipment are examples of intervention strategies that have successfully assisted children with TBI to develop IADL skills. During rehabilitation the children and adolescents take part in organized group activities to promote skill development through home and community participation. For the school-aged child, activities such as a baking group may be a component of their therapy program. The purpose of this group is to provide the child with opportunities to participate in typically developing occupations. This involves working collaboratively with peers to follow the written directions of a recipe, and making choices and negotiating with peers to identify the baking projects. Concepts of time management and measurement, as well as the incorporation of physical skills within a natural environment, are utilized. Opportunities to explore adaptive equipment as required are provided. Cognitive skills such as attention, memory, sequencing, planning, reasoning and problem solving are natural components of this activity. The ability to work in a safe manner using age-appropriate skills, i.e. judgement for their actions, is promoted using a variety of teaching techniques, e.g. modelling. Similar skills development is promoted for adolescents in groups, such as a group cooking program called the 'Lunch Club', with the expectations being graded to meet the developmental, skill and experience level of the participants. These programs also provide children and teens with leadership opportunities.

Programming is graded to reflect the abilities of the participants by introducing skill development in more demanding environments. For example, a cognitive communication group offered in an outpatient program includes menu planning and grocery shopping as part of its curriculum. Group shopping at a local grocery store facilitates time and money management, social interaction, problem solving and visual attention, in addition to the physical demands of the task.

A metacognitive approach is used to increase the child or adolescent's self-awareness of their abilities and needs. Clients are guided to learn new ways to advocate for their own needs within the protective rehabilitation environment, transitioning to their home and community. Increased awareness results in ability to use compensatory strategies effectively (Toglia 1991). Clients are encouraged to participate to their maximum ability, which may include directing a caregiver for appropriate positioning and set-up of a task. Tasks are modified to accommodate physical abilities and safety concerns (for example, use of a microwave versus a stove top to heat meals).

Time management
Performance components of time management include the ability to organize available time to meet educational, social, recreational, home and family needs (McNeny 1999). Impairments of memory and executive dysfunction impact upon the child or adolescent's ability to manage time. The establishment of a structured

therapy schedule during rehabilitation is the starting point for training or re-training of time management skills. Environmental modifications, such as the positioning of clocks and calendars, provide support for clients who are relearning skills of temporal orientation and time management.

Rehabilitation interventions are designed to teach the child procedural learning strategies to assist them in developing or re-training the use of more effective time management skills. These activities are designed to reflect the demands placed upon children and teens in a developmentally appropriate manner. A school-age child may require support to assist them in remembering their personal belongings, whereas an adolescent may need support to help them independently plan and organize their school assignments.

During the inpatient stage of rehabilitation the children are provided with a structured daily schedule and an agenda which they use to document their daily activities. This technique also serves as a compensatory strategy to aid with memory impairments and as a communication tool with families. The therapists provide graded cueing to support skill acquisition, including carrying a compensatory device such as a schedule and routinely using the device for planning and as a memory aid. Other compensatory strategies include the use of checklists for daily routines, low-tech devices such as watches with signals set to remind the child of a specific activity, or high-tech devices such as the use of personal digital assistants and computers. These types of devices can be used to assist an adolescent to complete tasks consistently and correctly at the appropriate time.

Money management

The challenges a child with a TBI experiences in acquiring the skills to safely and effectively manage money frequently occur as a result of cognitive impairments of attention, memory, judgement, executive dysfunction and impulse control. Functional limitations associated with these deficit areas include poor initiation of tasks, difficulty remembering purchases, decreased speed of processing, disorganization, and impulsivity in spending patterns. Frequently the child or adolescent's disability is 'hidden' or not easily seen, impacting on their performance of money management skills. They are expected to perform activities similar to their peers when they actually require more supervision or support to do so, and the need for this supervision may not be easily recognized.

Interventions to learn skills of money management can range from practising money identification and change-making skills with school-aged children in play, to teaching skills of planning for activities such as banking, shopping and budgeting with teens and young adults. The teenager with a TBI may need to learn to respond to cues to learn strategies to assist them in remembering their purchases, or in controlling impulsivity in spending patterns. These cues need to be graded across environments.

Interventions in money management skills are frequently addressed in preparation for community integration and supported during the child's transition to their community by families and community health professionals. Life skills groups to provide these individuals with opportunities to practise these types of skills in new environments and contexts are part of the outpatient program.

PRODUCTIVITY

Play

Play is a primary occupation of children with inherent purpose and meaning (Parham 1996, Bundy 1997). It is highly complex and it is vital to a child's development. Play provides the forum for childhood skill development to establish competencies required for adult life and work (Parham 1996). It is the interaction between the child and their environment. Play is intrinsically motivated and influenced by developmental skills and abilities. It is comprised of elements of physical, social and cognitive spontaneity, as well as the suspension of reality, which may manifest in a sense of enjoyment (Lieberman 1977).

Children with disabilities are at risk for play deprivation (Brown and Gordon 1987). Medical conditions that affect children can place them in a situation of participation restriction and hinder the development of their play skills and behaviours, and accordingly their discovery of the world (Ferland 2005). Children with restricted mobility were observed to seldom initiate play and were given 'lower status' play roles by their peers (Tamm and Skar 2000). In a study by Harkness and Bundy (2001) involving children aged 2–12 years with physical disabilities, with an age-matched control group, no difference in playfulness was found. Studies of children with cognitive disabilities, including developmental delays, attention deficit hyperactivity disorder (ADHD), and autism, found that children with disabilities had lower playfulness scores, compared to their age-related peers (Restall and Magill-Evans 1994, Leipold and Bundy 2000, Okimoto et al. 2000).

Mortenson and Harris (2006) questioned the extent to which deficits in cognitive, behavioural, social and motor function acquired following a pediatric TBI would impact the child's participation in play. They found that children with TBI demonstrated the behaviours of playfulness, but to a significantly lower extent than their age-related peers. Children with TBI had more difficulty approaching and engaging in play. A discrepancy was observed in the types of play activities and interests in which the pre-adolescent children with TBI and their age-matched peers were engaging (for example, play with Barbie dolls vs. peer sports). These findings suggest that playfulness is negatively impacted by TBI and that strategies to legitimize and optimize playfulness need to be incorporated into therapy practice.

The Test of Playfulness (Bundy et al. 2001) was developed to assess and promote playfulness in children. It is reflective of four elements of play: intrinsic motivation, suspension of reality, sense of control, and framing. Framing is the ability to give and read social cues within the context of the play activity. Through play the child attempts to assimilate information and to gain mastery.

Inpatient rehabilitation programming recognizes the importance of play for child development and provides a therapeutic playroom environment for children from infancy to 6 years of age and their families. Children participate in developmentally appropriate programming developed by early childhood educators, in which goals are developed in collaboration with the child, family and rehabilitation teams. The environment provides opportunities for nurturing and unstructured play where children are offered choices in levels of participation depending upon their daily schedule. Emphasis is placed on providing a 'home environment', free from the scheduled demands of the hospital environment.

Play interventions in both therapeutic play environments and in individual therapy sessions acknowledge the importance of play for child development. Therapeutic play interventions provide opportunities for the child to interact with others in a safe and consistent manner. During the early stages of rehabilitation, play may assume a multi-sensory-based focus, such as using a Snoezelen room to stimulate visual attention, tactile activities such as textured toys, hot/cold, and physical movement (rocking, rolling, swinging).

As the child progresses through rehabilitation, play becomes more complex and multi-dimensional. Play opportunities are based upon the child's developmental skill level. Children are provided with an environment and context for play, such as a doll's house, building blocks, or simple games. Play activities are graded to promote success, positive interaction, exploration and potential mastery of skills. The uses of play activities have been found to be important predictors for improvement in fine motor skills. The creation of a playful environment not only motivates children, but also generally provides the 'just-right' challenges through which children can succeed and master the environment (Case-Smith 2000).

Through engagement in cooperative play and the promotion of creative and imaginative play the child learns to work within rules and guidelines and to problem-solve. Guided problem solving through experiential learning, where the outcomes are not always what the child intended, provides opportunities for real world learning, i.e. successes and failures. This allows the child to develop skills to manage the range of outcomes inherent in play. Opportunities for social contacts with siblings, peers, parents and classmates are built into play interventions. Opportunities for scripting allow the child to explore roles and their environment – for example, play with puppets is encouraged.

Community-based rehabilitation programming encourages the child to participate in play activities within environments that will promote the development of physical, cognitive, social, play and self-help skills. This may include participation in an early intervention or nursery school type of program. Occupational therapists often provide information to community staff on the sequelae of a TBI and strategies that will support the child's participation in structured programming. Cronin (2001) found that although children with TBI may pass the items on a developmental scale, they function in a manner atypical for their developmental level in terms of external support needed. This may be reflective of problems in cognitive functioning that emerge as the developmental demands on the child increase, and the need for ongoing support and consultation to assist the child in participating in meaningful occupations.

School

Academic difficulties in children with TBI are extensively documented (Lazar and Menaldino 1995, Shurtleff et al. 1995, Marschark et al. 2000, Cronin 2001, Savage et al. 2005, Ylvisaker et al. 2005). The child with a TBI must be supported in their transition to school and provided with continuing support 'beyond the point of apparent cognitive recovery' (Lazar and Menaldino 1995, Cronin 2001). The needs of the students with TBI can be expected to change not only as a function of the interaction between recovery and maturational process, but also in relation to the school demands that are placed on the child at that particular time (Lazar and Menaldino 1995). D'Amato and Rothlisberg (1996) stated that 'any child having a history of a TBI should be considered at-risk for academic problems' and should receive classroom monitoring.

Research strongly favours a supportive transition to school with assistance remaining in place even when all appears to be going well. The transition to school is complex and requires families to navigate a complicated system involving an array of meetings and assessments. Families are required to assume the role of advocates for their children and often report that this process is overwhelming. The ability of health care professionals to guide families through transition to either regular education with special services or special education is increasingly limited by pressures to shorten lengths of stay and cost-containing measures (Savage et al. 2005).

Preparation for school re-entry begins during the acute rehabilitation phase, focusing on skill development and the introduction of compensatory strategies. Through participation in structured individual and group programming, functional recovery and skill development are addressed both as an inpatient and as a day-patient. Programming to support increased awareness of self and environment, improvement in general endurance, and increased performance of daily occupations is supported through a collaborative goal-setting approach. Compensatory strategies and environmental modifications continue to be refined within the community phase of rehabilitation.

Specific examples of interventions used to support readiness for the return to school include the establishment of a daily routine and schedule and the supported use of an agenda. Group activities provide opportunities to learn and practise skills within a safe environment. Clients practise executive functioning skills of planning and organizing group activities, learning to give feedback to each other, and evaluating personal goals. Intervention approaches are modified to accommodate the child's varying chronological and developmental level.

Intervention strategies which can be used to support the student's re-entry into school include: school visits prior to discharge accompanied by family and therapy staff, a graduated return-to-school program, the development of scripts to assist the child in responding to peer questions, and presentations to fellow students by clients, teachers and therapists to discuss TBI and their experiences. Interactive presentations that provide students with opportunities to understand and experience some of the challenges their peer who has a TBI may face, such as performing activities with their non-dominant hand, wearing an ankle foot orthosis, or listening to a list of disorganized instructions, are often used. These types of presentation are used to support the student's re-entry into the classroom. Visits by school staff to the rehabilitation centre during the child's rehabilitation program, to support initial understanding of the changes post-injury and their progress, are encouraged. Ongoing consultations by health care professionals and trained educators following discharge and at critical transition points throughout the child's educational program should be provided by outpatient programs.

School must not only meet academic needs but also provide opportunities for socialization and peer identification. Often rehabilitation interventions are educationally focused and may not fully consider all the occupations of childhood. Plans for school re-integration need to reflect all the occupations the child is involved in during the school day. This includes support during recess or lunchtime, and at transition times such as changing classrooms. It is often during the less structured periods that children with TBI encounter difficulties and require additional support.

The need to modify classroom approaches to address the specific capabilities and challenges of a child with a TBI requires the use of a variety of academic accommodations. Table 11.1 outlines accommodations that are often recommended to families and schools to support the child with TBI to fully participate in educational programming.

Written productivity

Learning to write is one of the major occupations of childhood (McHaleand Cermak 1992, Amundson and Weil 2001). Handwriting is an essential skill required to participate successfully in educational activities (Sudsawad et al. 2002). Sassoon (1990) found that handwriting is still an essential skill and, despite modern technology, parents eagerly await these first visible results of learning. Children who cannot write well soon realize their lack of success by comparing their own performance with that of other children.

Written productivity can pose a significant challenge for a student with an acquired brain injury, due to physical and cognitive impairment. Occupational

TABLE 11.1
Recommended accommodations to support school re-entry for children with TBI

Physical and environmental supports	Educational/teacher support system	Testing/assignments	Assistive devices and equipment
Preferential seating	Reduced course load and modified schedule	Additional time for note taking, tests	Use of agenda/ electronic organizer/watch
Locker location near home classroom	Resource room support for regular review	Opportunity to write tests/exams in a quiet environment	Use of computer-based templates
Supervision for movement in halls	Access to an educational assistant for note taking and information processing support	Modification of testing materials, e.g. open book tests, multiple choice vs. open-ended questions	Opportunity to work on a computer
Access to copies of teacher/peer notes	Regular identification and review process	Structured timelines	Access to adaptive software for physical and learning needs
Transportation support	Support for the development of self- advocacy skills	Opportunity for alternative means of testing, e.g. verbal answers	Support and supervision for adaptive equipment, e.g. mobility devices, computer
Review of timetable and location of classrooms	Support for social network building	Parental support and input for monitoring and task completion of homework and assignments	Use of visual schedules
Building modifications, e.g. washrooms	Review and reinforcement of an agenda	Break assignments into small steps and schedule check-ins/ reviews at midpoints	Assign designated place to store materials
Buddies for carrying books, ensuring materials not left behind	Learning strategies course	Test in student's strongest learning mode	Colour coding of materials
Additional copies of textbooks for home use	Linking of information with previously learned material	Assignments/ outlines available on computer	Access to tape-recorders, videotapes

TABLE 11.1 (continued)
Recommended accommodations to support school re-entry for children with TBI

Physical and environmental supports	Educational/teacher support system	Testing/assignments	Assistive devices and equipment
Modification of physical education program	Repetition of information/ instructions Use of multi-sensory approach	Note taking support/scribe for exams	Alternative types of locks on lockers
Adequate seating/ surface and table tops	Provision of extra time for task completion		Software to enhance written productivity
Quiet workspace, study carrel	Development and use of a tracking sheet		Access to cell phone for emergencies during travel to and from school

therapists working in classroom settings frequently report difficulties with hand-writing (Cronin 2001). These may include difficulty with generation of text, formation of letters, legibility, spacing and speed of output. Difficulties attending to task, writing in high stimuli environments and organizing thoughts are often seen following a TBI.

King et al. (1999a) found that school-based therapy for children with special needs which addresses goals of productivity with written communication – includ-ing copying from the board, correctly holding a pencil, typing, and classroom productivity, as well as cutting, colouring, clicking a computer mouse, organizing a desk, and focusing on a task – is educationally relevant and addresses skills underlying and supporting academic performance. Positive change in performance was seen using goal attainment scaling.

Written productivity is supported through interventions that address the development of handwriting skills, combined with compensatory approaches such as the use of assistive technology both for physical access and for educational needs of scanning and organization.

Children with TBI may participate in interventions to improve written productivity on both an individual and group level. Group programming, such as a 'Pencil Club', has been developed to support the acquisition of pre-printing skills for children with a TBI entering the school system. Preschool-aged children are provided with opportunities to support the development of pre-printing skills, including visual motor control and fine motor skill development. Printing groups are offered for school-aged children to assist them to develop skills such as pencil grip, posture, letter formation, spacing, and line orientation. These interventions are also offered on an individual basis and may involve dominance re-training for children with hemiparesis.

When remedial writing practices fail to produce a significant improvement in written productivity, the use of a computer is commonly recommended as an alternative means of text generation (Amundson and Weil 2001). Children are frequently supported to use technology as a means of enhancing their written output and to assist in transferring their thoughts to paper. This technology includes both access systems and software programs that support a child's written output. An example of a software program is 'Word Q' – a word cueing and auditory feed-back program that provides assistance with text composition for individuals with learning difficulties (Tam et al. 2005).

Leisure and socialization
The literature suggests that residual social and behavioural difficulties may represent a more significant long-term factor leading to participation restriction than persistent cognitive or motor impairments (Lehry 1990, Willer et al. 1993). Students with TBI exhibit maladaptive behaviours, including disinhibition, impulsiveness, decreased frustration tolerance, reduced anger control, poor judgement, decreased motivation, and insensitivity to others. Glang et al. (1997) found that the most difficult and long-lasting effects of a TBI are the loss of friends, decreased involvement in social activities and lack of social support. This is felt across all severities of injury and impacts the development of a sense of autonomy (Willer et al. 1993).

Individuals who have had a brain injury experience not only a traumatic event, but also a personal loss (Mateer et al. 2005). Rehabilitation programming consequently needs to be diverse and inclusive to address the needs of the child and their family at all levels. Individuals who participated in supportive group therapy and psycho-educational interventions reported reductions in the levels of their cognitive/psychological symptom distress and improvements in understanding difficulties, and achieving a higher sense of well being (Schmitter-Edgecombe et al. 1995, Mateer and Sohlberg 2001).

Interventions aimed at the development of social skills and the building of social networks are critical to support participation in all daily occupations. Glang et al. (1997) described school-based interventions to build social networks for children and adolescents with TBI. This involved the use of a facilitator to build friendships and assist in organizing opportunities for socialization, such as a pizza party or playing in the school gym. Education for the student's peers, to teach about the experiences of a student with a TBI, was built into this program.

Psychological support and socialization opportunities must be built into a program across the continuum of rehabilitation. Peer interactions and opportunities for play and socialization are important considerations when planning interventions. Structured group programming in the acute phase of rehabilitation is offered in therapy, school and recreational programming. Peer play is facilitated in the play-room. Social communication skills are taught and modelled in cognitive re-training groups. Opportunities for leisure skill development with a peer group are promoted in recreation and in programs such as Magic Hands (Kassam 2005), an occupational therapy program which introduces magic to children and youth with disabilities. The outpatient program can offer group programs for school-aged children and teens and young adults which facilitate social skill development and provide the participants with opportunities to build social networks. Parent support groups are often included in these programs to provide support to the entire family system and to support greater transfer of skills in home and community environments.

TRANSITIONS TO ADULT ROLES AND ADULT SERVICES

Transitions to adult roles are defined as the purposeful, planned movement of youth with physical disabilities from child-centred to adult-oriented services (White 1996). The experience of children, families and health care providers working in pediatric rehabilitation is that transitions are typically unstructured, short-term, fragmented and challenging. Research findings indicate that the transition experiences of students with special needs are bleak, particularly in preparation for community and social participation after high school, gainful employment, and independent living (Kardos and White 2005).

A framework is needed to implement a long-term developmental approach in training children to share in age-appropriate management of their special needs. This shared management approach (Kieckhefer and Trahms 2000) between families and health care providers is a planned, systematic approach. The approach involves a gradual shift in responsibilities, in which the leadership for care is transitioned from the health care provider to the parents and, as developmentally appropriate, to the young person. The goal is to allow the youth to gain the knowledge, skills and experience necessary for self-management in the adult world.

This approach aims to provide transition services in a coordinated, compre-hensive, function-based, diagnostic-specific, wellness- and prevention-focused and accessible format. The development of a consistent, self-directed pathway that is responsive to the needs of every child, young adult and their family is one compo-nent of this process. Tools such as a transition timeline (Table 11.2) are being introduced and used with children and their families throughout their rehabilitation process to ensure that the multiple transitions experienced during childhood development are supported and coordinated.

Youth with TBI face many challenges in managing the transition to adulthood. This involves the development and acquisition of adult roles and access to an adult model of service delivery. Skills of communication, self-advocacy, planning and

TABLE 11.2
Transition timeline

	Birth to 3	4 to 6	7 to 11	12 to 16	17 to 21
Parenting	• Let your child know the world is a good place. • Take short breaks from your child to renew your energy. • Apply for Special Services at Home.	• Give your child choices so they learn to make decisions. • Teach your child the consequences of their behaviours and choices.	• Let your child make mistakes. • Teach your child to speak up for themselves.	• Advocate for yourself. • Talk about sexuality. • Look for older role models. • Use your parents as a resource.	• If needed, contact the Office of the Public Guardian and Trustee to begin guardianship process before age 18. • Contact Ontario Disability Support Program(ODSP) for Income Support before age 18. • Become a mentor for younger children.
Social	• Get involved in community activities that include children with and without special needs. • Talk with parents of children with and without special needs. • Take your child to playgrounds and parks.	• Let your child learn what they like to do by exposing them to different leisure activities • Host birthday parties. • Invite families with children your child's age to your home to play.	• Encourage hobbies and leisure activities. • Help your child make friends. • Support your child's participation in community activities without parents where possible.	• Join teams and clubs at school. • Get involved in activities outside of school. • Hang out with friends.	• Find out about community programs for adults that match your leisure or athletic interests. • Keep in touch with friends from high school or camp by phone, e-mail and make plans.

TABLE 11.2 (continued)
Transition timeline

	Birth to 3	4 to 6	7 to 11	12 to 16	17 to 21
Self Care		• Teach your child everyday skills like brushing their teeth. • Teach your child self care skills related to their special needs. • Give your child chores that match their abilities.	• Take your child shopping. • Take your child on public transit. • Teach your child their personal information such as address, phone number, etc. • Let your child choose how to spend some or all of their allowance.	• Direct your own personal routines. • Cook together. • Start to find your way around the community. • Talk with your parents about where you will live as an adult.	• Learn independent living skills. • Plan and prepare meals. • Practice budgeting and banking skills. • Look at housing choices including attendant services and supported living options.
Education		• When registering your child for school, request a case conference to decide on the best educational placement. • Keep a record of your child's educational history.	• Let your child do homework independently as much as possible. • Support your child with homework by letting them tell you when help is needed. • Begin asking your child what they want to be when they grow up.	• Take part in meetings about your education and keep a record. • Talk about career interests. • Find volunteer work or a part-time job.	• Going to college or university? Contact the Office for Students with Disabilities on campus. • Looking for work? Contact ODSP Employment Supports for help with job search and training. • Contact local Community Living Association for resources and training opportunities.

(continued)

TABLE 11.2 (continued)
Transition timeline

	Birth to 3	4 to 6	7 to 11	12 to 16	17 to 21
Medical	• Develop good working relationships with doctors and other service providers. • Keep a record of your child's medical history.	• Teach your child what their disability is called. • Teach your child about their special needs.	• Ask your child what they know about their special needs and fill in the gaps in their understanding. • Help your child talk directly with doctors and other service providers.	• Begin to look for adult health care providers. • Attend part of your medical appointments alone. • Start to make your own medical appointments and keep a record of your medical history.	• Transfer to an adult health care provider. • Get a summary of your medical record.

Source: Gall K, Healy H (2005) A Timetable for growing up. Life Skills Institute, Bloorview Kids Rehab, Toronto, Ontario (used with permission).

organization are embedded in this process and pose challenges for youth living with the effects of TBI often due to cognitive impairments. Savage et al. (2005) describe the conflict between holding on and letting go that faces the parents of children with TBI. Significant concerns such as impairments in judgement, attention, memory, communication and behavioural issues pose special challenges and risks for independence and community participation. 'Most families never forget the early shock and fear experienced when their child was first injured. Having almost lost their child once, it may even be harder to let go as the future becomes present' (Savage et al. 2005).

At Bloorview Kids Rehab, group programming, combined with the approaches of cognitive rehabilitation and a life skills model, has been developed to provide services to youth living with the effects of TBI. A continuum of programs – ranging from individual topic-based life skills groups, to a community-based summer independence program, to a weekend retreat – has been developed to provide opportunities for skill development that will assist these individuals in their transition to the adult world. The Family Support Service at Bloorview Kids Rehab is a psychosocial model of service delivery which provides services for youth between the ages of 16 and 25 years, and their families, living with the effects of an acquired brain injury. This service supports the young person's involvement in adult occupations and roles through its linkages and partnerships with adult service delivery providers.

The transition to post-secondary education and work involves a multidimensional approach of physical, cognitive, social and emotional programming. Research findings indicate that social and emotional support is an important component of transition programming. Marschark et al. (2000) found that college students with a history of mild TBI in childhood or adolescence intellectually had similar scores to their peers but reported more severe distress in terms of their general personal and emotional functioning. Educational programming that includes career planning, leadership training and mentorship can support youth in learning about themselves and their world. Participation in co-operative education programming will provide a student with experiential opportunities to learn about the world of work and to develop job-specific skills. The use of a job-coach to support the student in learning the tasks of the job, in addition to employment accommodations such as environmental modification, can support the student's participation.

SUMMARY

The aim of occupational therapy assessment and interventions for children with acquired brain injuries is to promote their participation in everyday occupations. The effects of a brain injury on a child's occupational performance are impacted by sensory-motor, cognitive and social-behavioural impairments sustained as a result of the injury. The effects of a traumatic brain injury (TBI) grow more complex as a child matures and therefore rehabilitation efforts need to continue throughout the child's growth and development and continuum of recovery. Occupational therapists work in collaboration with the child/adolescent, their family and other health care professionals to promote participation in present and future occupations in the areas of self-care, productivity and leisure.

REFERENCES

Adams RA, Sherer M, Struchen MA, Nick TG (2004) Post-acute brain injury rehabilitation for patients with stroke. *Brain Inj* 18(8): 811–823.

Adolescent Health Transition Project (1995) Transition timeline: introduction and contents. Seattle, WA: Center on Human Development and Disability, University of Washington. (Report)

Amundson SJ, Weil M (2001) Prewriting and handwriting skills. In: Case-Smith J (ed) *Occupational Therapy for Children.* St Louis: Mosby, pp 545–570.

Anderson V, Catroppa C (2005) Recovery of executive skills following paediatric traumatic brain injury (TBI): a 2 year follow-up. *Brain Inj* 19(6): 459–470.

Avery-Smith W, Dellarosa DM (1994) Approaches to treating dysphagia in patients with brain injury. *Am J Occup Ther* 48(3): 235–239.

Banja J, Johnston MV (1994) Outcomes evaluation in TBI rehabilitation. Part III: Ethical perspectives and social policy. *Arch Phys Med Rehabil* 75(12 Suppl): S19–S26.

Blaskey J, Jennings MC (1999) Traumatic brain injury. In: Campbell SK (ed) *Decision Making in Pediatric Neurologic Physical Therapy.* New York: Churchill Livingstone, pp 81–140.

Blosser J, Pearson S (1997) Transition coordination for students with brain injury: a challenge schools can meet. *J Head Trauma Rehabil* 12(2): 21–31.

Boman IL, Lindstedt M, Hemmingsson H, Bartfai A (2004) Cognitive training in home environment. *Brain Inj* 18(10): 985–995.

Bottari C, Dutil E, Dassa C, Rainville C (2006) Choosing the most appropriate environment to evaluate independence in everyday activities: Home or clinic? *Aust Occup Ther J* 53: 98.

Brewer K, Geisler T, Moody K, Wright V (1998) A community mobility assessment for adolescents with an acquired brain injury. *Physiother Can* 50(2): 118–122.

Bronfenbrenner U (1992) Ecological systems theory. In: Vasta R (ed) Six theories of child development: revised formulations and current issues. Philadelphia, PA: J Kingsley, pp 187–249.

Brown M, Gordon WA (1987) Impact of impairment on activity patterns of children. *Arch Phys Med Rehabil* 68(12): 828–832.

Bruininks RH (1978) *Bruininks–Oseretsky Test of Motor Proficiency (BOTMP).* Circle Pines, MN: American Guidance Service Publishing.

Bruininks R, Bruininks B (2005) *Bruininks–Oseretsky Test of Motor Proficiency, 2nd edn.* Circle Pines, MN: American Guidance Service Publishing.

Bundy AC (1993) Assessment of play and leisure: delineation of the problem. *Am J Occup Ther* 47(3): 217–222.

Bundy AC (1997) Play and playfulness: what to look for. In: Parham LD, Fazio LS (eds) *Play in Occupational Therapy for Children.* St Louis: Mosby, pp 56–62.

Bundy AC, Nelson L, Metzger M, Bingaman K (2001) Validity and reliability of a test of playfulness. *Occup Ther J Res* 21(4): 276–292.

Carney J, Gerring J (1990) Return to school following severe closed head injury: a critical phase in pediatric rehabilitation. *Pediatrician* 17(4): 222–229.

Case-Smith J (2000) Effects of occupational therapy services on fine motor and functional performance in preschool children. *Am J Occup Ther* 54(4): 372–380.

Case-Smith J (2002) Effectiveness of school-based occupational therapy intervention on handwriting. *Am J Occup Ther* 56(1): 17–25.

Chapparo C, Ranka J (1997) *Occupational Performance Model (Australia)*. Monograph 1. Sydney: Total Print Control, pp 58–61.

Chen CC, Heinemann AW, Bode RK, Granger CV, Mallinson T (2004) Impact of pediatric rehabilitation services on children's functional outcomes. *Am J Occup Ther* 58(1): 44–53.

Cicerone KD, Dahlberg C, Kalmar K, Langenbahn DM, Malec JF, Bergquist TF et al. (2000) Evidence-based cognitive rehabilitation: recommendations for clinical practice. *Arch Phys Med Rehabil* 81(12): 1596–1615.

Coster W (1998) Occupation-centered assessment of children. *Am J Occup Ther* 52(5): 337–344.

Coster WJ, Haley S, Baryza MJ (1994) Functional performance of young children after traumatic brain injury: a 6-month follow-up study. *Am J Occup Ther* 48(3): 211–218.

COTO (College of Occupational Therapists of Ontario) (2005) Draft standard for occupational therapy assessment.

Cronin AF (2001) Traumatic brain injury in children: issues in community function. *Am J Occup Ther* 55(4): 377–384.

D'Amato RC, Rothlisberg BA (1996) How education should respond to students with traumatic brain injury. *J Learn Disabil* 29(6): 670–683.

Depompei R, Blosser JL (1991) Functional cognitive-communicative impairments in children and adolescents: assessment and intervention. In: Kreutzer JS, Wehman P (eds) *Cognitive Rehabilitation for Persons with Traumatic Brain Injury: A Functional Approach*. Baltimore: PH Brookes, pp 215–235.

Dumas HM, Carey T (2002) Motor skill and mobility recovery outcomes of children and youth with traumatic brain injury. *Phys Occup Ther Pediatr* 22(3–4): 73–99.

Dumas HM, Haley SM, Fragala MA, Steva BJ (2001) Self-care recovery of children with brain injury: descriptive analysis using the Pediatric Evaluation of Disability Inventory (PEDI) functional classification levels. *Phys Occup Ther Pediatr* 21(2–3): 7–27.

Dunn W (1999) *Sensory Profile*. St Louis, MO: Elsevier.

Dunn W, Brown C, McGuigan A (1994) The ecology of human performance: a framework for considering the effect of context. *Am J Occup Ther* 48(7): 595–607.

Dutil E, Forget A, Vanier M, Gaudreault C (1990) Development of the ADL profile: an evaluation for adults with severe head injury. In: Johnson JA (ed) *Occupational Therapy Approaches to Traumatic Brain Injury*. New York: Haworth Press, pp 7–22.

Ehrlich JS, Sipes AL (1985) Group treatment of communication skills for head trauma patients. *Cogn Rehabil* 3(1): 32–37.

Emslie H, Wilson C, Burden V, Smith I, Wilson B (2003) *Behavioural Assessment of Dysexecutive Syndrome for Children (BADS-C)*. Bury St Edmunds: Thames Valley Test Company.

Engberg AW, Teasdale TW (2004) Psychosocial outcome following traumatic brain injury in adults: a long-term population-based follow-up. *Brain Inj* 18(6): 533–545.

Ewing-Cobbs L, Levin HS, Fletcher JM, Miner ME, Eisenberg HM (1990) Children's Orientation and Amnesia Test: relationship to severity of acute head injury and to recovery of memory. *Neurosurgery* 27(50): 683-691.

Ferland F (2005) *The Ludic Model: Play, Children with Physical Disabilities and Occupational Therapy, 2nd edn*. Ottawa: Canadian Association of Occupational Therapists.

Fleming JM, Strong J, Ashton R (1996) Self-awareness of deficits in adults with traumatic brain injury: how best to measure? *Brain Inj* 10(1): 1–15.

Folio MR, Fewell RR (2000) *Peabody Developmental Motor Scales (PDMS-2), 2nd edn.* Austin, TX: PRO-ED.

Fraser R (1998) Career development and school-to-work transition for adolescents with traumatic brain injury. In: Ylvisaker M (ed) *Traumatic Brain Injury Rehabilitation: Children and Adolescents.* Boston: Butterworth-Heinemann, pp 417–427.

Glang A, Todis B, Cooley E, Wells J, Voss J (1997) Building social networks for children and adolescents with traumatic brain injury: a school-based intervention. *J Head Trauma Rehabil* 12(2): 32–47.

Harkness L, Bundy AC (2001) The Test of Playfulness and children with physical disabilities. *Occup Ther J Res* 21(2): 73–89.

Hart T, Giovannetti T, Montgomery MW, Schwartz MF (1998) Awareness of errors in naturalistic action after traumatic brain injury. *J Head Trauma Rehabil* 13(5): 16–28.

Hayden ME, Moreault AM, LeBlanc J, Plenger PM (2000) Reducing level of handicap in traumatic brain injury: an environmentally based model of treatment. *J Head Trauma Rehabil* 15(4): 1000–1021.

Jacobs HE (1987) The Los Angeles Head Injury Survey Project: rationale and design implications. *J Head Trauma Rehabil* 2(3): 37–49.

Jaffe KM, Polissar NL, Fay GC, Liao S (1995) Recovery trends over three years following pediatric traumatic brain injury. *Arch Phys Med Rehabil* 76(1): 17–26.

Josman N, Berney T, Jarus T (2000) Evaluating categorization skills in children following severe brain injury. *Occup Ther J Res* 20(4): 241–255.

Kardos M, White BP (2005) The role of the school-based occupational therapist in secondary education transition planning: a pilot survey study. *Am J Occup Ther* 59(2): 173–180.

Kassam S (2005) Magic Hands. (Presentation at OACR conference.)

Kieckhefer GM, Trahms CM (2000) Supporting development of children with chronic conditions: from compliance toward shared management. *Pediatr Nurs* 26(4): 354–363.

King GA, McDougall J, Tucker MA, Gritzan J, Malloy-Miller T, Alambets P et al. (1999a) An evaluation of functional, school-based therapy services for children with special needs. *Phys Occup Ther Pediatr* 19(2): 5–29.

King GA, McDougall J, Palisano RJ, Gritzan J, Tucker MA (1999b) Goal attainment scaling: its use in evaluating pediatric therapy programs. *Phys Occup Ther Pediatr* 19(2): 31–52.

Klein-Parris C, Clermont-Michel T, O'Neill J (1986) Effectiveness and efficiency of criterion testing versus interviewing for collecting functional assessment information. *Am J Occup Ther* 40(7): 486–491.

Law M (1993) Evaluating activities of daily living: directions for the future. *Am J Occup Ther* 47(3): 233–237.

Law M, Baptiste S, McColl M, Opzoomer A, Polatajko H, Pollock N (1990) The Canadian Occupational Performance Measure: an outcome measure for occupational therapy. *Can J Occup Ther* 57(2): 82–87.

Law M, King G, Russell D, MacKinnon E, Hurley P, Murphy C (1999) Measuring outcomes in children's rehabilitation: a decision protocol. *Arch Phys Med Rehabil* 80(6): 629–636.

Law M, Missiuna C, Pollock N, Stewart D (2001) Foundations for occupational therapy practice with children. In: Case-Smith J (ed) *Occupational Therapy for Children.* St Louis: Mosby, pp 39–70.

Law M, Baptiste S, Carswell A, McColl MA, Polatojko H, Pollock N (2005) *Canadian Occupational Performance Measure, 4th edn.* Ottawa: CAOT Publications ACE.

Lazar MF, Menaldino S (1995) Cognitive outcome and behavioral adjustment in children following traumatic brain injury: a developmental perspective. *J Head Trauma Rehabil* 10(5): 55–63.

Leipold EE, Bundy AC (2000) Playfulness in children with attention deficit hyperactivity disorder. *Occup Ther J Res* 20(1): 61–82.

Lieberman JN (1977) *Playfulness: Its Relationship to Imagination and Creativity.* New York: Academic Press.

McHale K, Cermak SA (1992) Fine motor activities in elementary school: preliminary findings and provisional implications for children with fine motor problems. *Am J Occup Ther* 46(10): 898–903.

McLaughlin AM (1992) Addressing the psychological needs of children with brain injured relatives: an activity group model. *J Cognit Rehabil* 10(2): 12–18.

McNeny R (1999) Occupations of daily living. In: Rosenthal M (ed) *Rehabilitation of the Adult and Child with Traumatic Brain Injury.* Philadelphia: FA Davis, pp 242–253.

Malec JF (2004) Comparability of Mayo-Portland Adaptability Inventory ratings by staff, significant others and people with acquired brain injury. *Brain Inj* 18(6): 563–575.

Manly T, Robertson H, Anderson V (1998) *The Test of Everyday Attention for Children.* Bury St Edmunds: Thames Valley Test Company.

Marschark M, Richtsmeier LM, Richardson JT, Crovitz HF, Henry J (2000) Intellectual and emotional functioning in college students following mild traumatic brain injury in childhood and adolescence. *J Head Trauma Rehabil* 15(6): 1227–1245.

Massagli TL, Jaffe KM, Fay GC, Polissar NL, Liao S, Rivara JB (1996) Neurobehavioral sequelae of severe pediatric traumatic brain injury: a cohort study. *Arch Phys Med Rehabil* 77(3): 223–231.

Mateer C, Sohlberg MM (2001) *Cognitive Rehabilitation: An Integrative Neuropsychological Approach.* New York: Guilford Press.

Mateer CA, Sira CS, O'Connell ME (2005) Putting Humpty Dumpty together again: the importance of integrating cognitive and emotional interventions. *J Head Trauma Rehabil* 20(1): 62–75.

Miller L (1991) Significant others: treating brain injury in the family context. *J Cognit Rehabil* 9(3): 16–25.

Mitchell T, Cusick A (1998) Evaluation of a client-centred paediatric rehabilitation programme using goal attainment scaling. *Aust Occup Ther J* 45(1): 7–17.

Mortenson P, Harris S (2006) Playfulness in children with traumatic brain injury: a preliminary study. *Phys Occup Ther Pediatr* 26(1–2): 181–198.

Nelson DL (1988) Occupation: form and performance. *Am J Occup Ther* 42(10): 633–641.

Okimoto AM, Bundy A, Hanzlik J (2000) Playfulness in children with and without disability: measurement and intervention. *Am J Occup Ther* 54(1): 73–82.

Ottenbacher KJ, Msall ME, Lyon N, Duffy LC, Ziviani J, Granger CV et al. (2000) Functional assessment and care of children with neurodevelopmental disabilities. *Am J Phys Med Rehabil* 79(2): 114–123.

Parham LD (1996) Perspectives on play. In: Clark F, Zemke R (eds) *Occupational Science: The Evolving Discipline.* Philadelphia: FA Davis, pp 71–80.

Philip PA, Ayyangar R, Vanderbilt J, Gaebler-Spira DJ (1994) Rehabilitation outcome in children after treatment of primary brain tumor. *Arch Phys Med Rehabil* 75(1): 36–39.

Ponsford J, Sloan S, Snow P (1995) *Traumatic Brain Injury: Rehabilitation for Everyday Adaptive Living.* Hove, East Sussex: Lawrence Erlbaum Associates.

Porr SM, Rainville EB (1999) *Pediatric Therapy: A Systems Approach.* Philadelphia: FA Davis.

Restall G, Magill-Evans J (1994) Play and preschool children with autism. *Am J Occup Ther* 48(2): 113–120.

Rosenthal M (1999) *Rehabilitation of the Adult and Child with Traumatic Brain Injury*, 3rd edn. Philadelphia: FA Davis.

Sakzewski L, Ziviani J (1996) Factors affecting length of hospital stay for children with acquired brain injuries: a review of the literature. *Aust Occup Ther J* 43(3/4): 113–124.

Sassoon R (1980) *Handwriting: A New Perspective*. Cheltenham: Stanley Thornes.

Sassoon R (1999) *Handwriting of the Twentieth Century*. London: Routledge.

Savage RC, Depompei R, Tyler J, Lash M (2005) Paediatric traumatic brain injury: a review of pertinent issues. *Pediatr Rehabil* 8(2): 92–103.

Schmitter-Edgecombe M, Fahy JF, Whelan JP, Long CJ (1995) Memory remediation after severe closed head injury: notebook training versus supportive therapy. *J Consult Clin Psychol* 63(3): 484–489.

Shepherd J (2001) Self-care and adaptations for independent living. In: Case-Smith J (ed) *Occupational Therapy for Children*. St Louis: Mosby, pp 489–527.

Shurtleff HA, Massagli TL, Hays RM, Ross B, Sprunk-Greenfield H (1995) Screening children and adolescents with mild or moderate traumatic brain injury to assist school reentry. *J Head Trauma Rehabil* 10(5): 64–79.

Stuss DT, Benson DF (1986) *The Frontal Lobes*. New York: Raven Press.

Sudsawad P, Trombly CA, Henderson A, Tickle-Degnen L (2002) Testing the effect of kinesthetic training on handwriting performance in first-grade students. *Am J Occup Ther* 56(1): 26–33.

Swaine BR, Pless IB, Friedman DS, Montes JL (2000) Effectiveness of a head injury program for children: a preliminary investigation. *Am J Phys Med Rehabil* 79(5): 412–420.

Tam C, Archer J, Mays J, Skidmore G (2005) Measuring the outcomes of word cueing technology. *Can J Occup Ther* 72(5): 301–308.

Tamm M, Skar L (2000) How I play: roles and relations in the play situations of children with restricted mobility. *Scand J Occup Ther* 7(4): 174–182.

Taub E, Ramey SL, DeLuca S, Echols K (2004) Efficacy of constraint-induced movement therapy for children with cerebral palsy with asymmetric motor impairment. *Pediatrics* 113(2): 305–312.

Toglia JP (1991) Generalization of treatment: a multicontext approach to cognitive perceptual impairment in adults with brain injury. *Am J Occup Ther* 45(6): 505–516.

Townsend E, Canadian Association of Occupational Therapists (1997) *Enabling Occupation: An Occupational Therapy Perspective*. Ottawa: Canadian Association of Occupational Therapists.

Trombly C (1993) Anticipating the future: assessment of occupational function. *Am J Occup Ther* 47(3): 253–257.

Trombly CA (1995) Occupation: purposefulness and meaningfulness as therapeutic mechanisms – 1995 Eleanor Clarke Slagle Lecture presented at the Annual Conference of the American Occupational Therapy Association, April 1995, Denver, Colorado. *Am J Occup Ther* 49(10): 960–972.

Trombly CA, Radomski MV, Trexel C, Burnet-Smith SE (2002) Occupational therapy and achievement of self-identified goals by adults with acquired brain injury: phase II. *Am J Occup Ther* 56(5): 489–498.

Van Benthem K (2004) Family-centred practice: am I giving what it takes? *Occup Ther Now* 6(1): 5–9.

Vander Schaaf PJ, Kriel RL, Krach LE, Luxenberg MG (1997) Late improvements in mobility after acquired brain injuries in children. *Pediatr Neurol* 16(4): 306–310.

Walleck C, Mooney K (1994) Neurotraumatic head injury. In: Barker EM (ed) *Neuroscience Nursing*. St Louis: Mosby, pp 324–351.

Warren M (1991) Strategies for sensory and neuromotor remediation. In: Christiansen C, Baum CM (eds) *Occupational Therapy: Overcoming Human Performance Deficits*. Thorofare, NJ: Slack Inc, pp 634–662.

WeeFIM 11 System Interim Clinical Guide (2003) Uniform Data System for Medical Rehabilitation, Amherst, NY.

White P (1996) Resilience in children with disabilities – transition to adulthood. *J Rheumatol* 23(6): 960–962.

Willer B, Rosenthal M, Kreutzer JS, Gordon WA, Rempel R (1993) Assessment of community integration following rehabilitation for traumatic brain injury. *J Head Trauma Rehabil* 8(2): 75–87.

Wilson BA (1999) Memory rehabilitation in brain-injured people. In: Stuss DT, Winocur G, Robertson IH (eds) *Cognitive Neurorehabilitation*. Cambridge: Cambridge University Press, pp 333–346.

Wilson BA, Evans JJ (1996) Error-free learning in the rehabilitation of people with memory impairments. *J Head Trauma Rehabil* 11(2): 54–64.

Wilson B, Ivani-Chalian R, Aldrich F (1991) *Rivermead Behavioural Memory Test for Children*. Bury St Edmunds: Thames Valley Test Company.

Winkler PA (1995) Head injury. In: Umphred DA (ed) *Neurological Rehabilitation*. St Louis: Mosby, pp 421–453.

World Health Organization (2001) International Classification of Functioning, Disability and Health (ICF). Geneva: WHO. (Report)

Ylvisaker M, Feeney TJ (1998) *Collaborative Brain Injury Intervention: Positive Everyday Routines*. San Diego: Singular Publishing Group.

Ylvisaker M, Todis B, Glang A, Urbanczyk B, Franklin C, DePompei R et al. (2001) Educating students with TBI: themes and recommendations. *J Head Trauma Rehabil* 16(1): 76–93.

Ylvisaker M, Adelson PD, Braga LW, Burnett SM, Glang A, Feeney T et al. (2005) Rehabilitation and ongoing support after pediatric TBI: twenty years of progress. *J Head Trauma Rehabil* 20(1): 95–109.

12
EDUCATIONAL OUTCOMES

Pamela Speed

Traumatic brain injury (TBI) is the leading cause of acquired learning impairment of school-aged children. The issues faced by children and youth present a new phenomenon in the field of education, due to the complexity and uniqueness of needs created by injury. Outcome is embedded in the neuropsychological sequelae of the injury, premorbid learning profile, age of onset, and the child's psychosocial response, as well as the family's response. All of these factors intertwine to make a unique learning and recovery profile mapped over a changed developmental profile.

Although children and adolescents tend to recover physical functioning more rapidly than adults, persistent long-term cognitive, communication and psychosocial sequelae have been well documented (Ewing-Cobbs et al. in Ylvisaker 1985, Donders and Strom 2000, Silver 2000). Problems in the area of attention, memory and efficiently processing information and cognitive communication deficits result in poor academic performance and social isolation, which are common observations from clinicians (Blosser and DePompei 1991, Lazar and Menaldino 1995, Brookshire et al. 2004). Even subtle deficits may have a substantial effect on the child's overall performance. Interruptions to the acquisition of skills have a disintegrating and cumulative effect on academic, social emotional and behavioural development over time.

The functional ability of an individual to cope with the demands of academic learning is dependent on the interrelationship and simultaneous integration of many cognitive and language-based skills. Efficient and speeded performance of these skills must take place within a dynamic environment with multi-modal and extraneous stimuli. These are the demands of the classroom environment, which is the performance arena for children and youth. Educators and community practitioners may not understand weakness in performance, as individuals with TBI may perform well on skills in isolation, or they may do well in specific environments which support the efficient integration or expression of information and skill demonstration. This makes the educational sequelae following TBI highly elusive to identify and to assess.

PREVALENCE

There are a number of factors which are important to address in understanding the outcome of children and youth with TBI; first and foremost is the identification of this population of students within school systems. Despite a significant incidence and prevalence of acquired brain injury in the population of pediatrics, there is relatively poor recognition by educational legislation and special education delivery systems and subsequently a poor understanding of the learning needs of students with TBI (Savage 1991). This is due, in part, to the fact that in many school jurisdictions the prevalence of TBI is not monitored or tracked.

Incidence figures in the United States estimate that approximately 20,000 children and adolescents per year acquire new persistent disabilities and re-enter school in need of enhanced educational planning (Ylvisaker et al. 2005). This number is consistent with the findings of Glang and colleagues, who estimated a total of 130,000 students in the United States with special education needs following TBI (Glang et al. in Ylvisaker et al. 2005). In Ontario, Canada the Ontario Trauma Registry figures indicate that the frequency of TBI is approximately 150 to 250 cases per 100,000 population. In Ontario, this is the equivalent of approximately 6,355 school-age children per year who are injured with potential to cause educational disability.

The prevalence of TBI should direct an approach by educational systems for specific TBI-focused services and teacher training programs. Despite the United States Federal Legislation – Individuals with Disabilities Education Act (PL 101-476 IDEA), which introduced traumatic brain injury as an exceptional category, the United States Department of Education reported that only 14, 844 students received special education services under the TBI label, indicating that children with TBI are greatly underserved by school systems (Ylvisaker et al. 2005). Despite the prevalence, complexity and diversity of the educational needs of students with TBI, these children tend not to be well recognized within school systems. This is due in most part to the lack of awareness of the magnitude of TBI within the school-aged population.

MILD BRAIN INJURY AND POST-CONCUSSIVE SYNDROME

Discussion of the mild and post-concussive population warrants attention in a review of pediatrics, as it adds to a better understanding of the hidden disability so often witnessed, but misunderstood, in educational settings. Children and youth who sustain mild TBI and concussive disorders are not well identified in the school system. Many of these children may have sustained a concussion with short or no loss of consciousness and may not have been seen by medical professionals (Segalowitz and Brown 1991).

The assumption that all individuals fully recover from mild injuries has been challenged in the literature (Gerber and Schraa 1995, Mittenberg and Strauman 2000, Ruff 2005). Post-concussive symptoms persisting beyond six months were found in 40 to 45% of patients in a study conducted by Alves et al. (1993). Williams et al. (1990) found that patients with mild brain injury and lesions on computed tomography had neuropsychological deficits and outcomes that more closely resembled those of patients with moderate TBI than those with uncomplicated mild TBI. In a study comparing mild TBI patients with orthopedic participants, Gerber and Schraa (1995) found that memory impairments differentiated the mild TBI group from the orthopedic group, at the six-month mark. In addition, more mild TBI patients had problems at work and had a specific perception of disability characterized by cognitive symptoms.

With respect to children, a number of studies have correlated the age of onset with recovery of skills under rapid development, specifically expressive language skills, making younger children more vulnerable than adolescents (Fletcher et al. 1987, Ewing-Cobbs et al. 1989). Segalowitz and Brown (1991) found that age at injury correlated with subject preferences. Overall research in mild TBI has documented persistent cognitive, memory and information processing complaints in a small but significant group. The challenge in identifying a post-concussive syndrome (Mittenberg and Strauman 2000, Ruff 2005) clinically underscores the challenge of recognizing cognitive and processing impairment within an educational setting.

A number of mild TBI patients have presented with complicated educational and emotional challenges in clinical follow-up. It is important to recognize children with mild head injury because persisting cognitive problems can have a significant impact on psychosocial/emotional outcome (Cicerone and Kalmar 1995). As these children may not be captured by traditional medical referral and follow-up, the Hospital for Sick Children in Toronto has a protocol for referring children with mild injuries to the Bloorview MacMillan Centre outpatient program, for physician and community school follow-up, when symptoms persist. In the case of mild injuries and post-concussive syndromes, neuropsychological consequences may be subtle, yet may have a substantive effect on recovery and outcome, particularly within school settings. This warrants monitoring of pediatric patients and education provided to parents and teachers as to the effects of mild injury.

BEHAVIOURAL, EMOTIONAL AND SOCIAL FUNCTIONING

When addressing issues of recovery and educational outcome, it is necessary to also address the impact of the child/youth's emotional response to injury. The individual's personality, their ability to cope, and whether the injury affected mental flexibility create an interplay that is hard to predict, but which ultimately determines the individual's pattern of recovery and rehabilitation. Often the most prevalent challenges evolve post-discharge from the rehabilitation centre. Brookshire et al. (2004) found that adaptive functioning problems occurred not immediately post-injury, but three years after injury, with the delayed effects of interaction with community and with the increase in expectations in the child's life (Curran et al. 2000). The emotional response of family, especially parents, is an additional factor in this scenario (Singer et al. 1994).

Insight, as all rehabilitation professionals know, is a key factor in determining psychosocial outcome. An increased rate of behavioural problems in a group of patients with mild TBI was noted in a study by Asarnow et al. (1991), which may indicate that better awareness of premorbid abilities may trigger a greater emotional response to loss.

Mateer et al. (2005) propose that combined psychoeducational psychosocial/ emotional interventions are associated with improved insight, improved rehabilitation gains and achieving a higher sense of well being. Improved awareness of cognitive difficulty and direct instruction in compensatory and coping strategies form the basis of the First Steps program designed to remediate cognitive difficulties in adult inpatients (Niemeier et al. 2005). These authors found that, even in an acute rehabilitation setting, learning compensatory strategies led to improvements in functional status, especially skills for psychosocial adjustment (Niemeier et al. 2005).

In pediatric rehabilitation settings integrated cognitive groups, which focus on education about TBI and functional strategy training, have been effective, especially with social skills training (Stewart and Wiseman-Hakes 1998). Rehabilitation gains have been noted with more integrated treatments that mesh cognitive, emotional and motivational interventions (Lewis et al. 2000), rather than treating cognitive functioning, personality and emotional reactions as separate entities (Mateer et al. 2005).

Contextual behavioural interventions, which support the student with respect to stressors and recognizing antecedents, particularly those created by specific educational demands, are necessary (Kendall et al. 1997, Curran et al. 2000, Lewis et al. 2000). This has implications for intervention strategies and school discipline, which need to be as individualized and specialized as the profile created by brain injury. Developing psychological and behavioural interventions through collaborative relationships with parents, school personnel and community professionals has value in improving outcome for community reintegration.

DEVELOPMENTAL PERSPECTIVE
The natural growth and development of a child or youth are disrupted by an injury to the brain. The dynamic process of recovery is mapped over maturational and developmental changes in neural structures, as well as developmental changes in cognitive, behavioural, emotional and social functioning. The impacts of these deficits on learning all contribute to the achievement and academic outcome of a child or youth.

In the initial year post-injury, the consequences of psychological sequelae cannot be completely predicted (Moore and Anderson 1995). Emergent challenges based on cognitive deficits in areas of the brain that have yet to develop may impact the learning profile of even children with mild to moderate injuries (Lazar and Menaldino 1995). Environmental factors must also be considered, including family functioning, as well as the changing demands that the educational system places on children as they progress to higher grades (Silver 2000, Taylor 2004).

The view that there is greater sparing of function in children has been challenged successfully as a result of continued research on outcome of TBI in children and adolescents. Although alternative pathways may assume the function of the damaged area, these pathways may accomplish the task less efficiently. From a developmental perspective, the inefficient or dysfunctional cognitive process may not be apparent until later development in the teenage years, when the skill or ability naturally emerges (Taylor and Alden 1997, Ewing-Cobbs et al. 2004, Taylor 2004). Young children are at greater risk for residual impairments and poorer recovery than older children or adolescents (Ewing-Cobbs et al. 1985, Lazar and Menaldino 1995, Rumney et al. 2002). Younger children may be more vulnerable because they are still in the process of acquiring skills rapidly; whereas older children or adolescents have a more fully developed skill base (Brookshire et al. 2004).

In a study of long-term sequelae, utilizing the Mayo-Portland Adaptability Inventory (MPAI), Rumney and colleagues (2002) found that children injured prior to the age of 5 years fared worse in terms of long-term cognitive and behavioural problems, as this is an age of rapid development of foundational cognitive, language, social and self-regulation skills. A longitudinal study of the relationship between age at injury and degree of impairment found that children less than 7 years of age showed more impairment than those 7 years or older (Moore and Anderson 1995). These authors also found that children with mild injuries acquired at an early age fared less well in later age.

MYTH OF RECOVERY – IDENTIFICATION OF UNIQUE LEARNING ISSUES

The myth of recovery, which states that children and youth recover fully from mild to moderate injury, may lead to inappropriate support, poor educational monitoring, and lack of identification and misidentification of difficulties at school. Learning problems and frustration are seldom attributed to a change in neurological function. When the child fails to follow expected developmental progressions because of impairments in learning, attention and reasoning, the child's difficulties are commonly attributed to motivational and emotional factors or viewed as behavioural problems. The myth of recovery may lead to assumptions within educational systems that children and youth require less support in the years following injury, whereas the reverse may be true. The need for educational support and modification may increase as the child progresses to higher grades and educational demands increase.

The remarkable feature of TBI in children and youth is the relative sparing of previously learned academic skills and knowledge and the potential for recovery or relearning of skills. This feature of TBI adds to the myth that children and youth recover well from moderate to mild trauma. Those with post-concussive syndrome may not be viewed as having any residual problems at all (Mittenberg and Strauman 2000).

The aspect of learning that is most changed by trauma is the ability to efficiently acquire new knowledge and skills and to apply these independently. This essentially speaks to the significant influence of the executive functions on the learning process. Learning requires the ability to process, integrate, formulate and express information in an efficient and speeded manner.

Cognition and the act of learning involve the simultaneous and integrated use of many thinking abilities. Also, the loss of potential for new learning is measured by situational demands. For example, in order to follow a lesson a student must make meaning from language and visual information, must reason with that information by applying it to other knowledge, and may be required to instantaneously formulate a response, all the while ignoring background noise. Students following acquired brain injury may retain previously learned skills or may be able to perform complex skills in specific and single-demand situations. It may be the act of listening and taking notes, while trying to recall information presented earlier in a lesson, that taxes the cognitive processes. A student may be able to perform well in a task which requires the application of specific skills in isolation, but may not do well with tasks of seemingly the same level of difficulty when the task and situation demand independent, and integrated, application of skills. This is a key aspect of how students learn post-TBI.

Even the expression of understanding is contingent on the demands of each situation. For example, a teacher requesting a prompt answer may challenge the student's ability to formulate a response on demand. Subtle deficits in initiation to prompt the word retrieval process may create a breakdown in the student's ability to answer a question, even though the answer is within the student's knowledge base. To the teacher who knows that the student has the knowledge and skill, these lapses in performance may not be clearly understood, but are nonetheless attributable to the injury.

It is the integrated performance of these cognitive and language abilities contingent on each situation that makes TBI and the learning process so unique. This myriad of interrelated abilities controlled by brain function can be impaired in an equally diverse and complex pattern, which impacts the learning profile of the child or youth. In the dynamic environment of the classroom where information is fast-paced and dialectic in nature, the ability to integrate new concepts may be impaired.

The other aspect of TBI that makes the learning needs of children and youth unique is that, compared to children with developmental learning issues, children with TBI may appear to be much less delayed. Educators may make the mistaken assumption that the student with TBI requires less intervention and special education support than other special needs students. In fact, what is lost in this scenario is the individual's potential to make further recovery gains and to actually perform at their potential, which may be much closer to the student's original trajectory and distinct from that of a child with an inborn delay.

Learning takes place within a dynamic continuum of development and growth. Thus, it is important to address learning issues within the context of the whole child. The interplay of emotion and self-concept in cognitive abilities cannot be overestimated. A young student who retains a clear image of his/her abilities prior to injury may find his/her learning problems incredibly frustrating. The emotional strain of attempting everyday activities that were easy prior to injury may be overwhelming. Increased frustration and behavioural and social adjustment problems may become more serious than the cognitive and physical impairments from the injury (Ewing-Cobbs et al. 1998, Gioia and Isquith 2004). Also, the loss of friends is often noted as a discouraging reality. Cognitive problems may not be understood by educators as the more obvious behavioural issues receive attention.

In clinical practice, it is commonly observed that many students with TBI are not identified by school personnel as having problems in school, until they actually fail or eventually succumb to emotional breakdown. This sets in motion a negative cycle of failure, anxiety and assumptions of incompetence which may long outlive the actual cognitive sequelae of the injury itself (Ylvisaker 1989).

Research and clinical findings indicate a high drop-out and failure rate for students returning to school following TBI (Ylvisaker 1989, Rumney et al. 2002). Essentially, the difficulty of effectively assessing and understanding the impact of cognitive impairment on learning underlies the high rates of school failure and social and emotional difficulties that may arise for an individual following TBI.

The terms 'myth of recovery' and 'silent disability' have dominated literature on TBI and children. The fact that children and youth with moderate and even severe TBI tend to recover physically has led to the inherent challenge of understanding the long-term effects of TBI within school settings and the community.

ASSESSMENT OF LEARNING POST-TBI

In order to tap this complex relationship of interrelated abilities tied to contextual demands, researchers have developed a strong focus on assessment which addresses the overlay of executive functions. The ability to control and execute knowledge and skills is affected by impairment of executive functions of the prefrontal cortex. These interface with language and communication abilities. Memory and information processing are also determinants in this mix of taking-in information, making meaning and applying and expressing concepts and ideas.

Gioia and Isquith (2004) define executive functions as an 'umbrella construct', as a 'collection of related yet distinct abilities that provide for intentional, goal-directed, problem-solving action, which provide for control, supervisory or self regulatory functions that organize and direct all cognitive activity, emotional response and overt behaviour'. Traditional assessments have proved poor predictors of key adaptive consequences of injury such as problems in behavioural self-regulation, school performance and interpersonal relations (Ewing-Cobbs et al. 1998, 2004, Gioia and Isquith 2004).

With respect to children and youth with TBI, impairment of executive function may not emerge as an outcome until the individual has returned to the community from hospital or rehabilitation centre. Problems may surface much later during adolescence, with the increase in environmental, academic, behavioural and social demands on the executive system. Ongoing developmental aspects of children introduce varying factors, which may dampen the predictive power of neuro-psychological tests (Taylor and Aiden 1997, Silver 2000, Taylor 2004). Adolescents are also still developing, and functions in executive thinking emerge into early adulthood. It may not be possible to evaluate functional difficulties until the child matures, or until these deficits interact with increased demands in school and social contexts. Performance on traditional psychological tests may not fully describe the functional implications of TBI, particularly the interaction of executive control over more complex and detailed information processing and learning demands within dynamic communicatively interactive environments (Madigan et al. 2000, Silver 2000, Ylvisaker et al. 2002, Brookshire et al. 2004, Taylor 2004).

An elusive aspect of understanding and assessing the effects of TBI in children is the disassociation between academic competence and academic performance. Despite the fact that most children who sustain severe to moderate TBI recover to the normal range on traditional measures of intellectual and language function, Brookshire et al. (2004) found that impairments persist on measures of problem solving, planning, response modulation and production of oral and written narratives. Focal frontal lesions in children can disproportionately impair executive cognitive functions and emotional regulation with relative preservation of declarative memory (Brookshire et al. 2004). (See Chapter 9 for further discussion of a complete neuropsychological protocol.)

Researchers and clinicians have addressed the complexity of the performance factor with ecologically valid assessment protocols. Ecologically valid assessment addresses the paradox in the assessment of the executive functions that Gioia and Isquith (2004) identify as such that 'some individuals with significant deficits in specific executive function sub-domains may have significant problems mak-ing simple real-life decisions'. An example of an ecologically based interrelated assessment is the Behaviour Rating Inventory of Executive Function (BRIEF), which was designed as a means of obtaining and standardizing information provided by parents and teachers to assess behavioural manifestations of executive functions in children aged 5 to 18 by addressing domains of everyday behaviour (Gioia and Isquith 2004).

The perspective of impairment of the executive functions addresses the difficulty that educators and families see with respect to planning for students who have apparently recovered, yet who fail with respect to keeping up with the demands of a functional day. The real test becomes the evaluation of the key challenges and strengths of the student post-TBI, as they come into play in the classroom and social milieu of school.

LANGUAGE AND DISCOURSE

The area of language most clearly demonstrates the impact of cognitive communication and executive function abilities as predictors of school success. In particular, verbal fluency and discourse ability are influential on the ability to meet the requirements of educational and social contexts, as these tap real world functioning (Silver 2000).

Studies of macro-level processing in children have emerged to examine the full scope of cognitive communication problems in children with TBI, which have 'gone unidentified with the use of standardized cognitive and linguistic tests' (Chapman et al. 2004). Recovery of lexical structures and grammar is often measured by traditional academic or language assessments, but it is beyond the sentence level that challenges occur with the synthesis, interpretation and expression of complex information within sophisticated language. Challenges in the organization and succinctness of verbal and written expression may have a direct impact on the student's academic achievement, when the student fails to convey a meaningful response (Dennis and Barnes 1990, Chapman et al. 1992). The ability to summarize and extract key information involves working memory for the salient aspects of a story, while inhibiting unimportant information (Brookshire et al. 2004). Children with severe TBI demonstrate difficulty recalling the gist of information and formulating a synthesized, interpretative statement (Chapman et al. 2004). This accounts for a discrepancy between understanding of small amounts of information presented in a lesson and the inability to integrate new concepts, as demonstrated by inadequate performance on academic tasks.

A study by Chapman and colleagues (2004) reported that children with TBI had special problems in transforming story content, defined as 'the combining of ideas into more concise and generalized statements'. Difficulties with discourse macro-level processing were greater for children injured prior to 8 years of age, than for children injured in later years. These authors found that discourse macro-level summarization ability was significantly related to problem solving, but not to lexical or sentence-level language skills or memory.

Children who sustain a severe TBI early in childhood are at an increased risk for persisting deficits in higher-level discourse abilities, which has implications for academic success. Discourse macro-level deficits may contribute to learning difficulties that persist at later stages post-brain injury. Deficits in verbal memory and verbal fluency were associated, one year post-injury, with a change of school placement from regular education to special education (Kinsella 1995, Silver 2000). Research has shown that direct instruction of summarization skills improved levels of comprehension and memory skills. Collaborative relationships between educators and clinicians are important to develop an understanding on the part of educators of the impact of higher-level language processing difficulties post-TBI and of strategies for remediation.

INFORMATION PROCESSING

A clear predictor of performance within school and social settings is the speed of information processing. Although processing speed might not be considered an executive function, it is often included in assessments, because of its interaction with abilities such as problem solving and working memory which are negatively impacted by slower processing speed (Brookshire et al. 2004). Processing demands are vulnerable to diffuse axonal injury and focal lesions of the prefrontal cortex. Academic performance and achievement may be highly dependent on the pace, length and complexity of information presented and the interrelationship of memory impairment. The student may be able to comprehend information when it is presented at a slower pace in smaller amounts and with fewer auditory distractions. Madigan et al. (2000) found that, by reducing the pace of information and customizing it for the individual through compensatory strategies and environmental modifications, performance of the individual with TBI can be enhanced significantly.

Clinically it has been observed that secondary students, following TBI, have difficulty keeping pace with and taking notes from an information video, and invariably students are only able to process up to one to three minutes of information presented. When this is compared to the cognitive load of listening to a 70-minute lecture in high school or a 20-minute lesson typical of elementary school, the student with TBI is likely to have lost crucial information. This is a critical feature underlying the challenge of acquiring new learning for students post-TBI. The interrelationship between language skills, cognitive deficits, memory and speed of information processing has a direct effect on the acquisition of new learning. This accounts for eventual educational delay, despite the retention of basic academic skills and knowledge.

Processing speed is a hidden marker, predictive of school success. It is also an area of deficit which, once properly identified as a need, is easily compensated with organizational strategies, direct instructional approaches and opportunities for structured review, enhancing educational outcome (Madigan et al. 2000).

ACADEMIC ACHIEVEMENT

The fact that many children following TBI may perform well on tests of academic achievement speaks to the fact that previously acquired and rote skills are rapidly relearned or preserved. Recovery of skills and knowledge is not necessarily predictive of the ability to independently perform in socially dialectic and academically dynamic situations.

The discrepancy between standardized academic test scores and academic outcome is most clearly illuminated in the Perrotta et al. study (1991), in which no differences were found between groups of children with TBI and sibling controls on tests of reading, spelling and arithmetic administered between one and five years after TBI. However, parents and teachers rated school performance of the injured child as lower than that of their siblings, and approximately 50% of the injured children had failed one grade. The authors suggest that poor application, rather than poor skill development, may explain the discrepancy and aspects of school behaviour. This fits with clinical experience that skills and knowledge are not necessarily lacking in students with TBI; rather it is the ability to independently demonstrate skills and apply these in a functional, dynamic context.

Ewing-Cobbs et al. (1998) found a discrepancy between achievement test scores and achievement placement, two years post-TBI in children and adolescents classified by age and duration of impaired consciousness. In a review of academic placement, 73% of severely injured children were found to be receiving either modification in the classroom or withdrawal instruction and programming. A greater proportion of severely injured children receive this assistance compared to the mild to moderate injury group. More than one-third of the severely injured group had failed a grade. Despite satisfactory achievement test scores, many children were not functioning independently with regard to the demands of the regular classroom (Kinsella 1995, Ewing-Cobbs et al. 1998).

Donders and Strom (2000) measured academic outcome in terms of the degree of academic support within the first year of recovery, rather than in terms of achievement test scores. They found that within the first year of recovery, achievement was influenced by over-learned verbal skills. Often, academic supports are removed or gradually withdrawn around one year post-injury, because the student appears to have recovered, based on retained previously acquired skills. Essentially these verbal skills mask deficits and often it is not until the second year that problems at school are identified. Even though recovery occurs, the rate of learning does not keep pace with developmental and academic expectations. Verbal fluency and speed of processing textual and auditory information are the skills that are not well measured by achievement tests, yet they are the skills which greatly impact the acquisition of new learning.

Ewing-Cobbs and colleagues (2004) conducted a study of change over time, with growth curve modelling, to examine the joint effects of TBI severity and age at injury on changes in academic achievement. They found that younger age at the time of injury predicted slower post-injury progress on tests of arithmetic computations and reading recognition, but that severe TBI was associated with more rapid progress in spelling than was mild to moderate TBI. These results confirm the need to separate recovery of previously developed skills from acquisition of new skills and they support the hypothesis that early brain insults have a time-lagged effect on development (Taylor and Alden 1997, Taylor 2004).

This research into educational outcome indicates the need for structured interventions which support the integration and application of new learning, and the development of teaching strategies which assist the student to compensate for attention and memory impairment (Taylor 2004). The research underscores the importance of effective assessment and the need to educate teachers and parents as to the implications of impairment for learning and achievement. Supporting students within the context of the classroom and assessment based on activities within the normal academic day provide real-world assessment, which leads to more effective strategies and to more effective long-term planning.

BEST PRACTICES FOR EDUCATIONAL PLANNING

Effective educational planning is contingent upon accurate assessment and identification of learning impairment created by TBI, and upon adequate program planning and monitoring. This entails that students with TBI have access to special education services and that school systems and educators have an understanding of the implications of TBI for learning. When the student with TBI returns to school with adequate funding, resource support and appropriate intervention programs and strategies, then academic success, continued rehabilitation – attenuated by lifelong gains – and improved self-esteem, leading to fewer personal and family stresses, can be achieved. Unfortunately, documented outcomes demonstrate that school failure, frequent school absenteeism even with young children, anxiety and sleep disorders, social isolation and high levels of emotional and behavioural adjustment problems are common scenarios evidenced in clinical practice.

Effective Educational Interventions – Program Development

School systems are moving from etiological disability categories to functional strengths and needs assessment for the development of system-wide Special Education Plans and the development of Individual Education Plans (Savage 1997, Ylvisaker et al. 2001, 2005). Many of the existing special education programs, services and strategies are appropriate for students with TBI, as the learning needs and strengths created by TBI are not very dissimilar to those of other exceptional learners, when a functional educational perspective is taken into account (Silver 2000). However, it is important that the learning needs are accurately identified and addressed, as assumptions of full recovery still prevail. Ylvisaker has stated in a number of articles that there should not be a specific TBI educational curriculum (Ylvisaker et al. 2001). The diversity within the population precludes this. The cognitive, physical and behavioural profile of TBI varies due to the mechanism of injury, age at injury, previous psychological and emotional profile and family coping, which all contribute to a highly unique and diverse profile for individual students (Lazar and Menaldino 1995).

Often the strategies to assist students with TBI are familiar to educators. What is unique is the identification of underlying cognitive problems and the design of effective Individual Education Plans, which address the real difficulties. Accurate identification of learning needs is necessary, as assumptions about learning that are inherent for other populations may impede the development of effective strategies for students with TBI. For example, the student with TBI may succeed in a structured learning environment, but it cannot be assumed that this student can apply the same academic skills when there is less external support. If the student is incapable of independently initiating and self-cueing, it is common to see difficulty with independent assignment or homework completion. Thus the interplay of executive functions must be understood by educators.

Difficulties in prospective memory, working memory and maintenance of academic performance levels over time indicate a need for frequent reminders, efforts to break down task requirements and pacing (Ylvisaker et al. 2001). Deficiencies in meta-cognitive knowledge imply that some children with TBI have poor insight about what they know and how quickly they can learn. Children with these sequelae may profit from structured study routines and monitoring to ensure that sufficient time is devoted to new learning (Glang et al. 1992). As Chapman and colleagues (2004) emphasized, strategy training in text summarization may benefit children with weaknesses in this skill, particularly in light of evidence that these difficulties lead to poor mastery and limited retention of content.

Dynamic assessment and observation of the ability to cope with curriculum expectations is an example of ecologically valid assessment (Ylvisaker et al. 2001). An effective methodology applied in clinical practice is a curriculum-based assessment to determine where, along the continuum of information processing and cognition, a breakdown of performance occurs. For example, if the student is unable to integrate information at the first stage of presentation, working memory and speed of information processing may be the issue. Weak integration and application of new learning may relate to problem solving and cognitive communication deficits. Accurate assessment leads to meaningful interventions specific to the contextual demands and to the individual learning profile.

Many of the strategies for students with learning disabilities work well for students with TBI. Visual organizers, external cueing, written information and particularly self-prompting strategies work well (Lenz et al. 1987). The pace, complexity and amount of information presented in a regular education curriculum can overtax memory and information processing. The most effective support for students at various stages of development, recovery and transition is often reducing the amount of information presented. This includes reducing the number of courses and the amount of work within the courses, and increasing the time frames for completion of assignments, as well as providing more structure, direct teaching and cueing for the completion of assignments. A successful strategy for working with many students with TBI is to directly teach the organizational structure in which information is presented and to highlight key points. This assists with the ability to integrate and make sense of the information (Harris and Pressley 1991, Glang et al. 1992). Technology is also a highly effective means of providing external structure for the learning process. Computer programs that provide visual organizers, word prediction, scan and read, and voice to text are highly useful compensatory aids.

Sometimes simple specific supports can make a significant difference in terms of enhancing the individual's performance. For example, a grade 9 student, two years post-moderate brain injury as a result of a boating collision, who had intact academic skills, was struggling with the transition to grade 9 at a new high school; he began skipping classes and was failing at the end of the first term. When his courses were reduced from four to three, with resource room support, he reported that he felt as though, now, he were 'not trying to catch up to a speeding train'. This slight modification to his programming made a significant difference to his ability to demonstrate his understanding and knowledge. Without the reduction in the number of courses, he would probably have had to repeat the year. Originally, the school responded to his 'adolescent lack of motivation'; but once they understood the underlying cognitive impairment, a more proactive relationship ensued on the part of the student and the teachers.

The concept of learned helplessness, which has been applied to students with learning disabilities who rely too heavily on their external supports, is a false one to apply to students with TBI. The academic supports are as critical for the acquisition of learning and the demonstration of learning as external aids such as a wheelchair or walker are for a student who has mobility challenges. As with all external strategies that are used within the rehabilitation phase – such as prosthetic memory devices, calendars, watches with timers – educational strategies can be taught for internalization. It is crucial with all strategies to make them explicit, to enable the student to develop insight as to the reasons for the strategies and to develop means of internalizing the external structures.

Savage writes about schools utilizing outcome measurement and functional assessment to determine needs of special education students. The School Function Assessment (SFA) is an instrument developed at Boston University with a rehabilitation focus to assess the student's ability to function and achieve success based on school-related skills. The SFA does not just measure academic success but also the student's ability to maintain safety, regulate behaviour, follow social conventions, use functional communication and understand instructions. This appears to be an

TABLE 12.1
Research-based, cross-population instructional strategies related to characteristics of many students with TBI

TBI characteristic	Strategy	Description
• Fluctuating attention • Decreased speed of processing		Acquisition of new material is increased by delivering material in small increments and requiring responses at a rate consistent with a student's processing speed; assuming familiarity with the teaching routine, pacing may need to be fast, even for a student with slowed processing
• Memory impairment (associated with need for errorless learning) • High rates of failure	High rates of success	Acquisition and retention of new information tend to increase with high rates of success, facilitated by errorless teaching procedures
• Organizational impairment • Inefficient learning	Task analysis and advance organizational support	Careful organization of learning tasks, including systematic sequencing of teaching targets and advance organizational support (including graphic organizers), increases success
• Inefficient learning • Inconsistency	Sufficient practice and review (including cumulative review)	Acquisition and retention of new information is increased with frequent review, as well as with both massed and distributed learning trials
• Inefficient feedback loops • Implicit learning of errors	Errorless learning combined with non-judgmental corrective feedback when errors occur	Students with severe memory and learning problems benefit from errorless learning. When errors occur, learning is enhanced when those errors are followed by nonjudgmental corrective feedback
• Possibility of gaps in the knowledge base	Teaching to mastery	Learning is enhanced with mastery at the acquisition phase
• Frequent failure of transfer • Concrete thinking and learning	Facilitation of transfer/generalization	Generalizable strategies, general case teaching (wide range of examples and settings), and content- and context-embeddedness increase generalization; cognitive processes should be targeted *within* curricular content
• Inconsistency • Unpredictable recovery	Ongoing assessment	Adjustment of teaching on the basis of ongoing assessment of students' progress facilitates learning
• Unusual profiles • Unpredictable recovery	Flexibility in curricular modification	Modifying the curriculum facilitates learning in special populations

Source: Ylvisaker et al. 2005: 104.

TABLE 12.2

Integrated approaches to educational, behavioural, and social intervention that have a research base and are applicable to many students with TBI

TBI characteristic	Approach	Description
• New learning needs • Impaired strategic behaviour • Impaired organizational functioning		Organized curricula designed to facilitate a strategic approach to difficult academic tasks, including organizational strategies; validated for adolescents with and without specific learning disabilities
• Decreased self-awareness • Denial of deficits	Self-awareness/attribution training	Facilitation of students' understanding of their role in learning; validated for students with learning difficulties
• Weak self-regulation related to frontal lobe injury • Disinhibited and potentially aggressive behaviour	Cognitive behaviour modification	Facilitation of self-control of behaviour; validated with adolescents with attention deficit hyperactive disorder and aggressive behaviour
• Impulsive behaviour • Inefficient learning from consequences • History of failure • Defiant behaviour • Initiation impairment • Working memory impairment	Positive, antecedent-focused behaviour supports	Approach to behaviour management that focuses primarily on the antecedents of behaviour (in a broad sense); validated in developmental disabilities and with some TBI subpopulations
• Frequent loss of friends • Social isolation • Weak social skills	Circle of friends	A set of procedures designed to support students' social life and ongoing social development; validated in developmental disabilities and TBI

Source: Ylvisaker et al. 2005: 105.

ecologically valid assessment that taps executive functions. It is also a means of developing Individual Education Plans that fit with rehabilitative goals to enhance meaningful participation in all aspects of school life (Savage 1997).

Appropriate programming, a quiet environment and one-to-one support for remediation and review will maximize learning potential and eventually move students to greater participation in regular programs. Intensive support and opportunities for one-to-one assistance are crucial in the early recovery stages to facilitate this potential. Reactivation of special education supports at transition times and when there is an increase in academic expectations is also necessary. Early intervention and rehabilitation enhance lifelong gains. Tables 12.1 and 12.2 indicate integrated approaches to intervention for students with TBI.

SCHOOL SYSTEMS PERSPECTIVE – AWARENESS AND ACCESS TO SPECIAL EDUCATION PROGRAMS

Awareness of TBI as an educational disability is crucial to school systems and school-based planning. However, the academic learning potential of students with TBI is often greatly over- or underestimated, as the spectrum of needs and strengths can be highly diverse (Lash and Scarpino 1993, Savage and Wolcott 1995, Savage 1997). As discussed previously in this chapter, the prevalence of students with learning disability as a result of trauma and acquired neurologic impairment is currently greatly underestimated within school systems (Ylvisaker et al. 2005). School systems respond to planning for this group as a low incidence population. Also, assumptions of full recovery still prevail, as students with TBI are often compared with other disability groups who may have more obvious stable profiles of impairment. School systems may not attribute emergent learning, social and behavioural challenges to the traumatic injury (Begali 1987, Tyler 1990, Blosser and DePompei 1991, Lazar and Menaldino 1995).

The criterion for access to special education services (in many school jurisdictions) has been based on profiles for students with inborn delays. The inappropriate comparison of students with TBI to students with relatively stable developmental profiles further precludes the student with TBI from attaining their recovery and academic potential. Students with TBI are often precluded from access to special education programs, based on a psychoeducational assessment which documents previously acquired and retained skills. Thus, the crucial aspect of recovery and preserved skills may not be effectively addressed for students with TBI when accessing services. This has led to the situation where many children at primary school age (kindergarten to grade 2) do not receive services as they are not (yet) 'delayed' relative to peers on assessments of academic skills. These children are greatly at risk of not developing foundational literacy and numeracy skills, and increased behavioural and social adjustment problems emerge.

School boards often do not have mechanisms in place to monitor students with TBI over the duration of their school years, particularly if the student is not currently accessing special education services (Lazar and Menaldino 1995, Ylvisaker et al. 2001). Children injured at a preliterate or preschool age who have emergent learning challenges in intermediate and senior grades may not be appropriately served with respect to the challenges created by cognitive and executive function impairment (Savage 1991, 1997, Ylvisaker et al. 2001, 2005).

The second common scenario is of the middle or high school student who returns to school with previously acquired skills and knowledge intact and who has impairment of memory, cognition and processing skills. These students may not qualify for special education support, based on assessment of previously acquired and retained skills. As a result of the lack of special education support, they have significant difficulty coping with a regular school program. These students would benefit from transition programs that recognize the educational impact of TBI and which meld a rehabilitation cognitive focus with an educational one (Milton et al. 1991).

Knowledgeable rehabilitation teams are effective in terms of follow-up and advocacy with school systems to ensure that long-term monitoring is in place. Students with TBI may need models of support for the transition period of the first two years post-injury, and may need reactivation of supports over the years.

Outcome studies have not measured the costs of the loss of employability potential and of attrition from high school when individuals with TBI do not reach their potential. As evidenced in the United States, a profile of exceptionality under special education legislation for TBI would provide the superstructure for programs, funding mechanisms, and knowledge forums for the development of an effective model of service delivery for school systems (Savage 1997, Ylvisaker et al. 2001).

TRANSITIONS – MODELS FOR TRANSITIONAL PLANNING AND INTEGRATING REHABILITATION AND EDUCATION SERVICES
PLANNING FOR TRANSITIONS – THE 'GOLDILOCKS PROBLEM'

Transition through the elementary school years to secondary school essentially poses the 'Goldilocks problem'. How much special education support is too much and how much is not enough? The answer lies in the functional assessment and continual monitoring of the demands of the learning situation and how these interact with the individual's pattern of impairment. In clinical experience, it is a common scenario to see schools remove support once the student is performing well, not realizing that the support is crucial to the integration and demonstration of learning. The difficulty with transitional planning again is underscored by assumptions of ability and the need to address the impact of neuropsychological impairment on performance. As the complexity of social and learning environments increases in the interface of injury and development, a whole new profile of learning challenges may evolve (Silver 2000, Taylor 2004, Niemeier et al. 2005). A clear understanding of this dynamic is needed on the part of families and educators in order to effectively support and address new educational and rehabilitation needs, as these evolve (DePompei and Blosser 1991, Savage and Carter 1991, Lazar and Menaldino 1995, Singer et al. 1996, Braga and Campos 2000).

Developing best practice in the field of education should focus on transitional planning, ongoing monitoring and frequent program review. A program delivery model based on a continuum of service, gradually moving from highly supportive special education placements to more integrated mainstream classrooms, has been deemed crucial to positive outcomes of school success and emotional and social coping (Savage 1997, Ylvisaker et al. 2001).

INTEGRATED PLANNING BETWEEN REHABILITATION SERVICES AND SCHOOLS

Effective school planning requires coordination between rehabilitation and education services. Savage describes the need to develop 'new models for innovative partnerships between schools (and rehabilitation) and community service providers in order to create better program models and services for children' (Savage 1997). Savage (1997) reviewed a number of international programs which plan with school systems for re-entry and for transitions. Effective communication between the rehabilitation team and the school team is critical to planning the school reentry (Begali 1987, Blosser and DePompei 1991, Savage and Wolcott 1995, Ylvisaker et al. 1995a, 1995b, 2005).

The Bloorview MacMillan neurorehabilitation team coordinates school planning through a multidisciplinary outpatient team and the educational expertise of liaison teachers. In addition to the medical follow-up clinics, the team and liaison teachers provide long-term follow-up of students through various transition phases in the school system and on to work or post-secondary options. The role of the rehabilitation/education expert has been effective in bridging the gap between rehabilitation and education services, assisting both parties to integrate program goals for students (Ylvisaker et al. 2001). The role of the liaison teacher is to provide professional development to school and board level staff in order to improve knowledge and expertise within the educational community. The role of the neuropsychologist in an outpatient team has been highly effective in assisting school personnel to understand the learning profile of students, particularly in terms of implications for the classroom. Families often have the additional burden of attempting to bridge this gap between school and rehabilitation (DePompei and Blosser 1991, Savage and Carter 1991, Lash and Scarpino 1993), and the liaison role in collaboration with the neuropsychologist has been crucial in educating parents as to the effects of TBI, including empowering parents with strategies for advocacy.

Rehabilitation case management services are also an essential means of ensuring long-term follow-up, evolving rehabilitation plans, and coordination with schools. This role has been effective in accessing the services of a speech language pathologist, occupational therapist or tutor at various stages of recovery and ensuring that schools are involved with long-term follow-up and transitional planning.

TEACHER KNOWLEDGE AND IN-SERVICE PROGRAMS

Understanding on the part of educators is deemed a critical feature of successful school re-entry following TBI. With the inclusion of TBI as an exceptionality category under the United States Federal Legislation – Individuals with Disabilities Education Act (IDEA), students with TBI have a recognized status in US departments of education, for funding, program development, formal access to programs and services and training for educational professionals. Since the implementation of this legislation, awareness in the field of education has greatly increased, along with teacher training programs, manuals and websites regarding the educational disability of TBI (Ylvisaker 1985, Rosen and Gerring 1986, Begali 1987, Savage and Wolcott 1995, Savage 1997). The *Journal of Head Trauma Rehabilitation* devoted a complete 1995 issue to outcome studies for pediatrics and educational issues.

The IDEA legislation heightened professional discussion regarding best practice and educational study. Research in the field has addressed medical and cognitive outcome studies, in-service programs for educators regarding the unique learning needs of these individuals, service delivery models for education, and the transitional planning process from hospital to school (Begali 1987, Tyler 1990, Blosser and DePompei 1991, Ylvisaker et al. 1991, Shurtleff et al. 1995, Ylvisaker et al. 1995a, 1995b, Blosser and Pearson 1997, Ylvisaker and Feeney 1998). Many teacher training programs and manuals for educators, as well as websites and web-based courses, have also been developed (see Appendix I). Recently, research has taken a more in-depth look at vocational and post-secondary education (Fraser and Baarslag-Benson 1994, Hayden et al. 2000).

In-service and pre-service programs for educators are critical to developing an understanding of the unique learning needs of children and adolescents. Understanding by educators, educational assistants and administrators of the impact on learning created by acquired neurological impairment has been deemed a crucial factor in outcome (Tyler 1990, Blosser and DePompei 1991, Becker et al. 1993, Savage and Wolcott 1995, Savage 1997, Ylvisaker et al. 2001).

SERVICE DELIVERY MODELS AND RECOMMENDATIONS FOR EDUCATION

Students with TBI require dynamic models of service delivery, with flexible options for access to special education services along the developmental and recovery continuum. This means that recognition within school systems of the need for long-term follow-up and monitoring for the duration of the student's school years is beneficial, even for students currently not accessing special education support services (Savage 1997, Ylvisaker et al. 2001). Ongoing support, education of staff and intervention planning are possible with long-term follow-up and established protocols for team planning and communication between the school-based team and the community rehabilitation team. Ongoing communication will improve teacher understanding regarding the educational issues faced by a student with TBI. Collaborative planning with families, community rehabilitation and school-based teams will improve the format for sharing of information, assessment findings and intervention recommendations and will ensure that prevention of educational difficulties and planning for transitions ensue. The Individual Education Plan needs to be flexible and in place, and close monitoring should be in place for students with mild injuries or those students who are currently not receiving special education services.

In addition to the extensive recommendations of Ylvisaker et al. (2001), Savage (1997) and Blosser and Pearson (1997) for school planning, it is recommended that school boards develop a database of all students with TBI and significant post-concussive disorder entering their systems, to ensure that the students are appropriately tracked if and when school-related difficulties arise. Developing an intake screen for kindergarten and high school is necessary.

School systems can become more proactive in their planning to meet the challenge of educating students with acquired neurological impairment if they themselves begin to study the implications and prevalence of this disability within the educational population. This knowledge is essential to advocacy efforts to improve legislation, funding, awareness and development of faculty of education programs regarding educational issues for children and youth with acquired neurological impairment.

FAMILIES

Input from families is highly important in the development of the student's Individual Education Plan and the Identification Placement Review process. However, in clinical experience, families' concerns are not well understood by school systems, because the underlying profile created by the TBI itself is not well understood. Performance indicators of school frustration often appear as laziness or lack of motivation. For example, many parents report that their child experiences high levels of fatigue at the end of the school day and frustration with the hours it takes to complete assignments that previously were done in a third of the time. Also, input from families of teenagers is not commonly requested, as school personnel assume that the student should be making independent decisions.

In a large Brazilian study, efforts to improve parents' knowledge and competence in working with their children elicited improved cognitive and physical outcomes compared with clinical interventions delivered directly to the child (Braga and Campos 2000). The conclusion could be drawn that training educators and parents to help children cope with academic demands would have favourable results. This fits with models of community support and contextually relevant interventions which have become a strong focus in the literature on pediatric TBI (Lazar and Menaldino 1995, Silver 2000, Feeney and Ylvisaker 2003, Mateer et al. 2005).

Integrated psychosocial teams, which provide family support, are an effective means of ensuring long-term follow-up by providing individual and family counselling, social work and support for habilitation issues at work, school and home (DePompei and Blosser 1991, Fraser and Baarslag-Benson 1994). Essentially the psychosocial support of the team has implications for improved outcomes in all aspects of living. The value of integrated interventions to support families is witnessed in improved psychosocial coping of children and youth (Singer et al. 1994, Hayden et al. 2000, Ylvisaker et al. 2002, Mateer et al. 2005).

PREVENTION

TBI is an educational disability which disproportionately affects children and youth. Yet, very little has been written about the responsibility of school systems to educate youth about prevention. Essentially, the educational curriculum teaches very little about the effects of the number one killer and disabler of our children and youth. Researchers and rehabilitation professionals know the value and the positive effects of prevention programs. In the United States rates of TBI-related hospitalization have declined nearly 50% since 1980, due in large part to prevention programs and mandatory seatbelt and helmet legislation. There are many available resources for schools and for prevention awareness programs, including prevention of sports injuries and concussion (Appendix II). There needs to be a greater voice in education literature, in the curriculum and in public forums for giving prevention education a higher profile in public awareness.

BEST FUNCTIONAL OUTCOME: REDUCING LEVEL OF PARTICIPATION RESTRICTION

Outcome is not just based on the level of impairment; it is based on reducing the level of participation restriction. Environmental supports and training family members and community practitioners, such as the scout leader, or classmates on how to assist the child/youth add to the rehabilitation gains. Addressing the functional demands of daily living can assist in the continuation of rehabilitation gains, improved socialization and gains in the quality of life participation. In rehabilitation terms, it means balancing supports and the right type of supports at different stages and transitions, both for the immediate recovery period and for many years along the developmental continuum (Mateer et al. 2005). Most importantly, it means developing means for the individual to value themselves through experiences of success and re-establishing identity (Prigatano 1995). It is the optimism of recovery, and the hope which recovery brings to opportunities for learning, that drives rehabilitation professionals to continue to advocate for their patients.

APPENDIX I: RESOURCES AND MANUALS FOR EDUCATORS

Begali V (1987) *Head Injury in Children and Adolescents: A Resource and Review for School and Allied Professionals.* Brandon, VT: Clinical Psychology Publishing.

British Columbia Ministry of Education Special Programs Branch (2001) *Teaching Students With Acquired Brain Injury: A Resource Guide for Schools.* Office Products Centre, 742 Vanalman Avenue, Victoria, BC V8W 9V7.

Educating Students with Brain Injury: A Web Site for Teachers: www.axion. net/gfstrongschool

Educators' Guide to Teaching Students with Acquired Brain Injury. Ontario Brain Injury Association and Brock University. www.obia.on.ca

Mira M, Tyler J, Tucker B (1988) *Traumatic Head Injury in Children: A Guide for Schools.* Kansas City, KN: University of Kansas Medical Center.

Neuroskills website, which has a number of links to resources for educators which cite online courses: www.neuroskills.com

Rosen CD, Gerring JP (1992) *Head Trauma: Educational Reintegration, 2nd edn.* San Diego, CA: Singular Press.

Savage RC, Wolcott GF (1995) *An Educator's Manual: What Educators Need to Know About Students with Traumatic Brain Injury.* Washington, DC: National Brain Injury Foundation.

Tyler J (1990) *Traumatic Head Injury in School-Aged Children: A Training Manual for Educational Personnel.* Kansas City, KN: University of Kansas Medical Center, Children's Rehabilitation Unit.

Wolcott GF, Lash M, Pearson S (1995) *Signs and Strategies for Educating Students with Brain Injuries.* Houston, TX: HDI Publishers.

APPENDIX II: PREVENTION WEBSITES AND PROGRAMS

Neuroskills: www.neuroskills.com

PARTY (Prevention of Alcohol Related Trauma in Youth), Sunnybrook Medical Centre, Toronto, Ontario.

Safe Kids Canada: www.safekidscanada.com

Smart Risk: www.smartrisk.com

REFERENCES

Alves W, Macciocchi SN, Barth JT (1993) Postconcussive symptoms after uncomplicated mild head injury. *J Head Trauma Rehabil* 8(3): 48–59.

Asarnow RF, Satz P, Light R, Lewis R, Neumann E (1991) Behaviour problems and adaptive functioning in children with mild and severe closed head injury. *J Pediatr Psychol* 16: 543–555.

Becker H, Harrell W, Keller L (1993) A survey of professional and paraprofessional training needs for traumatic brain injury rehabilitation. *J Head Trauma Rehabil* 8(1): 88–101.

Begali V (1987) *Head Injury in Children and Adolescents: A Resource and Review for School and Allied Professionals.* Brandon, VT: Clinical Psychology Publishing.

Blosser JL, DePompei R (1991) Preparing education professionals for meeting the needs of students with traumatic brain injury. *J Head Trauma Rehabil* 6: 73–82.

Blosser J, Pearson S (1997) Transition coordination for students with brain injury: a challenge schools can meet. *J Head Trauma Rehabil* 12(2): 21–31.

Braga LW, Campos da Paz A (2000) Neuropsychological pediatric rehabilitation. In: Christen AL, Uzzell B (eds) *International Handbook of Neuropsychological Rehabilitation.* New York: Kluwer Academic/Plenum.

Brookshire B, Levin HS, Song JX, Zhang L (2004) Components of executive function in typically developing and head-injured children. *Dev Neuropsychol* 25(1&2): 61–83.

Chapman S, Culhane K, Levin H, Harward H, Mendelsohn D, Ewing-Cobbs L, Fletcher J, Bruce D (1992) Narrative discourse after closed head injury in children and adolescents. *Brain Lang* 43: 42–65.

Chapman S, Levin H, Matejka J, Harward H, Kufera J (1995) Discourse ability in children with brain injury: correlations with psychosocial, linguistic and cognitive factors. *J Head Trauma Rehabil* 10(5): 36–54.

Chapman S, Sparks G, Levin H, Dennis M, Roncadin C, Zhang L, Song J (2004) Discourse macrolevel processing after severe pediatric traumatic brain injury. *Dev Neuropsychol* 25(1&2): 37–60.

Cicerone KD, Kalmar K (1995) Persistent post-concussion syndrome: the structure of subjective complaints after mild traumatic brain injury. *J Head Trauma Rehabil* 10(3): 1–17.

Curran C, Ponsford J, Crowe S (2000) Coping strategies and emotional outcome following traumatic brain injury: a comparison with orthopedic patients. *J Head Trauma Rehabil* 15(6): 1256–1274.

Dennis M, Barnes M (1990) Knowing the meaning, getting the point, bridging the gap and carrying the message: aspects of discourse following closed head injury in children and adolescence. *Brain Lang* 39: 428–446.

DePompei R, Blosser JL (1991) Families of children with traumatic brain injury as advocates in school reentry. *Neuro Rehabil* 1(2): 29–37.

Donders J, Strom D (2000) Neurobehavioural recovery after pediatric head trauma: injury, preinjury, and post-injury issues. *J Head Trauma Rehabil* 15(2): 792–803.

Ewing-Cobbs L, Fletcher JM, Levin HS (1985) Neuropsychological sequelae following pediatric brain injury. In: Ylvisaker M (ed) *Head Injury Rehabilitation: Children and Adolescents*. San Diego, CA: College-Hill Press.

Ewing-Cobbs L, Miner ME, Fletcher JM, Levin HS (1989) Intellectual, motor, and language sequelae following closed head injury in infants and preschoolers. *J Pediatr Psychol* 14: 531–547.

Ewing-Cobbs L, Fletcher JM, Levin HS, Iovino I, Miner ME (1998) Academic achievement and academic placement following TBI. *J Clin Exp Neuropsychol* 20: 769–781.

Ewing-Cobbs L, Barnes M, Fletcher JM, Levin HS, Swank PR, Song J (2004) Modeling of longitudinal academic achievement scores after pediatric traumatic brain injury. *Dev Neuropsychol* 225: 107–133.

Feeney T, Ylvisaker M (2003) Context-sensitive behavioral supports for young children with TBI: short-term effects and long-term outcome. *J Head Trauma Rehabil* 18(1): 33–51.

Fletcher JM, Miner ME, Ewing-Cobbs L (1987) Age and recovery from head injury in children: developmental issues. In: Levin HS, Grafman J, Eisenberg HM (eds) *Neurobehavioral Recovery from Head Injury*. New York: Oxford University Press.

Fraser R, Baarslag-Benson R (1994) Cross-disciplinary collaboration in the removal of work barriers after traumatic brain injury. *Lang Disord* 15(1): 55–67.

Gerber DJ, Schraa JC (1995) Mild traumatic brain injury: searching for the syndrome. *J Head Trauma Rehabil* 10(4): 28–40.

Gioia G, Isquith PK (2004) Ecological assessment of executive function in traumatic brain injury. *Dev Neuropsychol* 25(1&2): 135–158.

Glang A, Singer G, Cooley E, Tish N (1992) Tailoring direct instruction techniques for use with elementary students with brain injury. *J Head Trauma Rehabil* 7(4): 93–108.

Harris KR, Pressley M (1991) The nature of cognitive strategy instruction: interactive strategy construction. *Except Child* 57: 392–403.

Hayden ME, Moreault A-M, LeBlanc J, Plenger P (2000) Reducing the level of handicap: an environmentally based model of treatment. *J Head Trauma Rehabil* 15(4): 1000–1021.

Kendall E, Shum D, Halson D, Bunning S, Teh M (1997) The assessment of social problem solving ability following traumatic brain injury. *J Head Trauma Rehabil* 12(3): 68–78.

Kinsella G (1995) Neurological deficit and academic performance. *J Pediatr Psychol* 6: 753–767.

Lash M, Scarpino C (1993) School reintegration for children with traumatic brain injuries: conflicts between medical and educational systems. *NeuroRehabilitation* 3(3): 13–25.

Lazar MF, Menaldino S (1995) Cognitive outcome and behavioral adjustment in children following dramatic brain injury: a developmental perspective. *J Head Trauma Rehabil* 10(5): 55–63.

Lenz BK, Alley GR, Shumaker JB (1987) Activating the inactive learner. Advance organizer in the secondary content classroom. *Learn Disabil Q* 10(1): 53–67.

Lewis J, Morris M, Morris R, Krawiecki N, Foster M (2000) Social problem solving in children with acquired brain injuries. *J Head Trauma Rehabil* 15(3): 930–942.

Madigan NK, DeLuca J, Diamond BJ, Tramontano G, Averill A (2000) Speed of information processing in traumatic brain injury: modality-specific factors. *J Head Trauma Rehabil* 15(3): 943–956.

Mateer CA, Sira CS, O'Connell ME (2005) Putting Humpty Dumpty together again: the importance of integrating cognitive and emotional interventions. *J Head Trauma Rehabil* 20(1): 62–75.

Milton S, Flanagan C, Rudnick FD (1991) Functional evaluation of adolescent students with traumatic brain injury. *J Head Trauma Rehabil* 6(1): 35–46.

Mittenberg W, Strauman S (2000) Diagnosis of mild head injury and postconcussion syndrome. *J Head Trauma Rehabil* 15(2): 783–791.

Moore CM, Anderson VA (1995) Pediatric head injury: the relationship between age at injury and their psychological sequelae. Presented at the 22nd annual meeting of the International Neuropsychological Society meeting, 2–5 February 1994, Cincinnati, Ohio. In: Lazar M, Menaldino S (1995) Cognitive outcome and behavioral adjustment in children following traumatic brain injury: a developmental perspective; *J Head Trauma Rehabil* 10(5): 55–63.

Niemeier J, Kreutzer JS, Taylor L (2005) Acute cognitive and neurobehavioural intervention for individuals with acquired brain injury: preliminary outcome data. *Neuropsychol Rehabil* 15(2): 129–146.

Perrotta SB, Taylor GH, Montes JT (1991) Neuropsychological sequelae, familial stress and environmental adaptation following pediatric head injury. *Dev Neuropsychol* 7: 69–86.

Prigatano GP (1995) 1994 Sheldon Berrol, MD, Senior lectureship: The problem of lost normality after brain injury. *J Head Trauma Rehabil* 10(3): 87–95.

Rosen CD, Gerring JP (1986) *Head Trauma: Educational Reintegration*. San Diego, CA: College-Hill Press.

Ruff R (2005) Two decades of advances in understanding of mild traumatic brain injury. *J Head Trauma Rehabil* 20(1): 5–18.

Rumney P, Johnson P, Thomas-Stonell N (2002) The use of the Mayo-Portland Adaptive Inventory. Presentation to the Toronto ABI Network Conference, 2002.

Savage R (1991) Identification, classification, and placement issues for students with traumatic brain injuries. *J Head Trauma Rehabil* 6(1): 1–9.

Savage R (1997) Integrating rehabilitation and education services for school-aged children with brain injuries. *J Head Trauma Rehabil* 12(2): 11–20.

Savage RC, Carter RR (1991) Family and return to school. In: Williams JM, Kay T (eds) *Head Injury: A Family Matter*. Baltimore, MD: Paul H Brookes Publishing.

Savage RC, Wolcott GF (1995) *An Educator's Manual: What Educators Need to Know About Students with Traumatic Brain Injury*. Washington, DC: National Brain Injury Foundation.

Segalowitz SJ, Brown D (1991) Mild head injury as a source of developmental disabilities. *J Learn Disabil* 24(9): 551–559.

Sherk Consulting Group (1999) Provincial review of services for children and youth living with the effects of an acquired brain injury. November (unpublished).

Shurtleff HA, Massagli TL, Hays RM, Ross B, Sprunk-Greenfield H (1995) Screening children and adolescents with mild or moderate brain injury to assist school reentry. *J Head Trauma Rehabil* 10(5): 64–79.

Silver CH (2000) Ecological validity of neuropsychological assessment in childhood TBI. *J Head Trauma Rehabil* 15(4): 973–988.

Singer GH, Glang A, Nixon C, Cooley E, Kerns KA, Williams D, Powers LE (1994) A comparison of two psychosocial interventions for parents of children with acquired brain injury. An exploratory study. *J Head Trauma Rehabil* 9: 38–49.

Singer GHS, Glang A, Williams JM (eds) (1996) *Children with Acquired Brain Injury: Educating and Supporting Families.* Baltimore, MD: Paul Brookes Publishing.

Stewart M, Wiseman-Hakes C (1998) Peer group training of pragmatic skills in adolescents with acquired head injury. *J Head Trauma Rehabil* 13(6): 23-38.

Taylor GH (2004) Research on outcomes of pediatric traumatic brain injury: current advances and future directions. *Dev Neuropsychol* 25(1&2): 199–225.

Taylor GH, Alden J (1997) Age-related differences in outcome following childhood brain insults: an introduction and review. *J Int Neuropsychol Soc* 3: 555–567.

Tyler J (1990) *Traumatic Head Injury in School-Aged Children: A Training Manual for Educational Personnel.* Kansas City, KS: University of Kansas Medical Center, Children's Rehabilitation Unit.

Williams DH, Levin HS, Eisenberg HM (1990) Mild head injury classification. *Neurosurgery* 27: 422–428.

Ylvisaker M (ed) (1985) *Head Injury Rehabilitation: Children and Adolescents.* San Diego, CA: College-Hill Press.

Ylvisaker M (1989) Cognitive and psychosocial outcome following head injury in children. In: Hoff JT, Anderson TE, Cole TM (eds) *Mild to Moderate Head Injury.* London: Blackwell Scientific Publications.

Ylvisaker M, Feeney T (1998) School reentry after traumatic brain injury. In: Ylvisaker M (ed) *Traumatic Brain Injury Rehabilitation: Children and Adolescents, 2nd edn.* Boston, MA: Butterworth-Heinemann.

Ylvisaker M, Hartwick P, Stevens M (1991) School reentry following head injury: managing the transition from hospital to school. *J Head Trauma Rehabil* 6(1): 10–22.

Ylvisaker M, Feeney T, Mullins K (1995a) School reentry following mild traumatic brain injury: a proposed hospital-to-school protocol. *J Head Trauma Rehabil* 10(6): 42–49.

Ylvisaker M, Feeney T, Maher-Maxwell N, Meserve N, Geary P, DeLorenzo J (1995b) School reentry following severe traumatic brain injury: guidelines for educational planning. *J Head Trauma Rehabil* 10(6): 25–41.

Ylvisaker M, Todis B, Glang A, Urbanczyk C, DePompei R, Feeney T, Maher Maxwell N, Pearson S, Siantz Tyler J (2001) Educating students with TBI: themes and recommendations. *J Head Trauma Rehabil* 16(1): 76–93.

Ylvisaker M, Hanks R, Johnson-Greene D (2002) Perspectives on rehabilitation of individuals with cognitive impairment after brain injury: rationale for reconsideration of theoretical paradigms. *J Head Trauma Rehabil* 17(3): 191–209.

Ylvisaker M, Adelson D, Braga LW, Burnett SM, Glang A, Feeney T, Moore W, Rumney P (2005) Rehabilitation and ongoing support after pediatric TBI: twenty years of progress. *J Head Trauma Rehabil* 20(1): 95–109.

HEAD INJURY: LOOKING TOWARDS THE FUTURE

Peter B Dirks

Although traumatic brain injury remains a significant cause of childhood morbidity and mortality, there is cause for optimism in the future for a number of important reasons.

The incidence of severe head injury appears to be falling as is the mortality. Prevention is truly the only effective cure. Public awareness of head injury and increased education efforts toward injury prevention and childhood safety are being very effective in places where these strategies can be implemented. Better motor vehicle childhood restraints, window safety, use of bicycle helmets in manual wheel sports (bicycling, in-line skating), safer playgrounds, and increased concern for head injury in recreational and contact sports are resulting in a reduction in the incidence of both minor and severe head injuries. Severity reduction also goes along with these measures. Graded driver's licensing and better awareness and stiffer penalties for impaired driving in many Canadian provinces may reduce the incidence of motor vehicle accidents involving teenagers.

Despite these improvements, many childhood deaths from injury remain preventable. For example, Canada is thought to have twice the childhood injury rate of Sweden, which has the lowest in the world. Falls remain an important target for injury prevention in younger children. In many communities efforts are required to reduce youth violence. Although many injury prevention programs obviously are sensible, it should be acknowledged that the effectiveness of a number of large-scale injury prevention programs still needs to be demonstrated (see the Cochrane collaboration). For example, although bicycle helmets have been shown to reduce the risk of head injury by 60 to 90%, the effectiveness of graduated licensing for young drivers is uncertain.

Despite the numerous improved and effective prevention strategies, accidental traumatic brain injury remains common in children. Once an injury occurs, treatment must move quickly to minimize secondary injury. In this regard, improved emergency care in the field, triaging injured patients to designated trauma centres, and the development of medical standards for trauma assessment and resuscitation have definitely led to improved outcome of minor and severe traumatic brain injury. Recognition that attention to ABCs precedes neurosurgical intervention has been paramount in improving patient outcome. With timely expert care and improved imaging, injuries are being more rapidly diagnosed. Although there are no truly effective neuroprotective drugs to treat secondary brain injury, the fields of clinical epidemiology and evaluative medicine are leading toward design of better studies. Traumatic brain injuries remain extremely heterogeneous from patient to patient and trials of effective therapy remain very challenging to carry out.

Advances in treatment of traumatic brain injury will come after there is improved understanding of the molecular and cellular mechanisms of secondary brain injury. The relationship between traumatic brain injury and genetic background is now being considered, with the identification of patients at risk for more severe sequelae from mild head injury with the presence of the apolipoprotein E epsilon allele in their genotype. Improved functional and anatomic brain imaging and increasingly sophisticated neuropsychological evaluation will be important for evaluating all patients with brain injury, but particularly those with 'minor' injury who will be at greater risk of neurocognitive sequelae. Attempts at defining concussion severity and use of appropriate return-to-play guidelines are important for preventing further injury.

Once injury has occurred, contrary to a long-standing dogma, it is now known that the brain has a capability to generate new brain cells, based on neural stem cell activity in restricted regions of the brain. Perhaps this activity represents a form of endogenous yet incomplete neural repair. Stem cells are being studied intensively in many models of brain injury in terms of enhancing endogenous activity and for delivery of exogenous stem cells (with or without transduction of exogenous genes) into injured regions of the brain to effect repair.

Finally, the concept of brain plasticity is drawing renewed attention with the discovery of neural stem cells. How do new neural stem cells integrate into the existing neuronal circuitry? Stem cells aside, how do existing circuits reorganize in response to areas of neuronal loss? How can circuit reorganization be potentiated to improve function? How does patient training or rehabilitation factor into brain plasticity or reorganization?

The field of neurobiology is advancing extremely rapidly. These advances need to be kept on the radar screens of clinicians treating patients. Clinical observations can be made more meaningful in the context of a deeper fundamental knowledge of the basic pathophysiology of brain injury and repair. Brain injury remains unfortunately too common and devastating to patients, their families, and society. With continued application of a 'full court press' on prevention and with advances in understanding of neurobiology, particularly a knowledge that our brains are surprisingly more dynamic than had been imagined, we should see a brighter future for children with traumatic brain injury, with further reduction in incidence and improvements in outcome.

INDEX

Note: page numbers in *italics* refer to figures and tables